SAY "AAAH"

A Common Sense A to Z Guide
to those "Aaahsome" Years
Newborn to Age 5

Dr. Michael (Mickey) Lester
B.A., M.D., F.R.C.P.C.

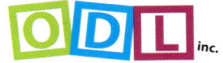

Copyright © 2011 by Dr. Michael (Mickey) Lester

All rights reserved. No part of this publication may be reproduced, stored in a retrieval system, or transmitted, in any form or by any means, electronic, mechanical, photocopying, recording, or otherwise, without the prior written permission of the author. Printed in Canada

For information about permission to reproduce sections of this book, write to Dr. Michael Lester, 71 King St. W. Suite 204 Mississauga, Ontario, Canada L5B 4A2

DISCLAIMER

The information in this book is true to the best of my knowledge and has been gained from more than 40 years as a practicing physician. The medical advice in this book is intended as an information guide only. It is not intended to replace or countermand the advice given by your child's doctor. I advise the reader to check with a qualified health-care professional before using any advice in the book where there is a question as to its appropriateness for your child. The author is not responsible for any adverse effects or consequences resulting from the use of any information in this book.

Library and Archives Canada Cataloguing in Publication

Lester, Michael, 1938-
Say aaah : an A to Z guide to those "aaahsome" years
newborn to age 5 / Michael Lester.

Includes index.
ISBN 978-0-9868837-0-5

1. Infants--Care. 2. Infants--Health and hygiene.
3. Child care. 4. Children--Health and hygiene. I. Title.

RJ61.L478 2011   649'.122   C2011-906391-3

Design: Angel Guerra/Archetype

This book is dedicated to my wife Karen
My children Danielle (Ruvan), Samantha (Mitchell), David (Vanessa) and Michael
My grandchildren Jamie, Lauren, Marley, Jacob, Sarah, Chloe and Sienna

Acknowledgments

It has taken me close to 25 years to complete this book. During this time I have updated the information numerous times as new information on children's healthcare has been brought forth. Even now, as my book is being edited, new information is being advanced.

There is, however, one constant – the art of medicine. The art of medicine is not taught during medical school or residency. It is learned by observation. This observation comes from my teachers, peers and the families I deal with on a daily basis.

I am extremely fortunate to have met three doctors who had a tremendous influence on my medical career. They taught me not only medicine and how to approach complex medical problems, but also and most importantly, how to practice the "art" of medicine. These doctors are Dr. Robert Farber, who in his mid-80s is still practicing, and Dr. Marvin Gerstein and Dr. Donald Hill, both of whom, unfortunately, left us too early in life.

I would like to also acknowledge the thousands of families who entrusted their children's healthcare to me. I now have in my practice children whose parents and grandparents I cared for as infants. I thank you for your trust. I thank you for helping to make me a better doctor. I thank you for constantly teaching me new things. I thank you for helping keep me grounded. I thank you for accepting and tolerating all my imperfections (I cannot think of any at present but I am sure my "parents" could write essays on them). I also thank you for questioning me. This has kept me on my toes and all of my neurons firing to capacity.

I would like to acknowledge my wife, Karen. There is hardly an evening that goes by when I do not discuss some medical issue that has concerned me that day. She sits patiently listening to me and always comes up with fresh ideas that help me problem-solve.

I would like to acknowledge my office staff, Darlene Hiscock, Judy Sharer and Maureen Payne. It would have been difficult for me to "survive" the past 20 years without their support. A special thanks to Maureen for helping me to organize my book with the use of her computer skills.

I would like to acknowledge all the help and support given to me by my consultant Arnold Gosewich.

I would like to thank all those parents who allowed me to take the photographs of their children for my book.

Lastly, I would like to acknowledge my editor Barbara Alter and her chief assistant Howie Alter. I now, after 50 years, know why I only received 51% in English during high school.

HOW TO USE THIS BOOK

I have tried to make it as easy as possible for readers to quickly obtain the information they seek. Unlike some traditional books dealing with healthcare, I have decided to arrange mine in alphabetical order. The format is similar to that of a dictionary or an encyclopedia.

Some topics may be quickly located in the table of contents, and the index has been cross-referenced to assist readers in locating exactly what they're searching for. You may, for example, look by common name under "F" for fever or "S" for sore throat, or for a particular illness by its medical name, such as Molluscum Contagiosum under the letter "M".

It is not possible to cover every illness an infant or child may develop. Accordingly, I have selected the most commonly occurring illnesses. The many photographs in the book will help you to identify the source of the particular problem, and the text will complete the picture. Happy reading, and I hope you find the book helpful and informative.

I have used the male pronoun throughout the book. This is for consistency only. I trust/hope my readers will not take offence as none was intended.

Dr. Mickey Lester

CONTENTS

Introduction   12

Abdominal Pain (Acute)   13
Abdominal Pain (Chronic Recurrent)   16
Allergic Reaction–Severe (Anaphylaxis)   18
    – Allergy (Dietary)   21
    – Allergy (Milk Protein)   22
    – Allergy (Seasonal)   24
Alternative Medicine   27
Antibiotics (Use and Misuse)   29
Anxiety   32
Anxiety-New Baby Blues   34
    –"Your Advisory Staff "   37
Asthma   38
Autism (Development)   52

Baby (Newborn Skin Care)   55
Bad Breath (Halitosis)   58
Bed Bugs   60
Bed Sharing (Co-Sleeping)   61
Bellybutton (see Hernias)
Birthmarks   62
Body Mass Index (BMI)   64
Breastfeeding – Getting Off to the Right Start (see also Feeding – Infant)   65
Breastfeeding – Weaning (from Breast and Bottle)   75
Breath-Holding Spells   78
Bronchiolitis   79
Bronchitis   81

Canker Sores (Mouth Ulcers)   82
Car (Motion) Sickness   83
Car Seats   84
Carotenemia (Yellow-Orange Skin Discoloration)   85
Celiac Disease (Gluten Intolerance)   85
Chicken Pox (Varicella)   86

Child Rearing (Discipline Tips)   89
    Child Rearing – (How-to's)   92
Circumcision (Advisability – Yes or No)   101
    – Circumcision (Procedure and Aftercare)   102
Cold sores (see Impetigo)
Colds   105
Colds and Flu   109
Colic   111
Constipation   113
Cord Blood (Storage)   117
Cough   118
Cradle Cap (Seborrhea) – Scalp   121
Croup (Tracheitis)   122
Crying Baby (What It Means and How to Deal with It)   125

Daycare (Choosing)   130
    – Daycare and Preschool-Entering Anxiety   131
    – Daycare syndrome   133
    – When to Exclude and When to Return the Sick Child   134
Developmental Milestones   137
Diarrhea (see Vomiting)

Ears – Middle-Ear Infection (Otitis Media)   140
    – Ears – Outer Ear Infection (Otitis Externa or Swimmer's Ear)   146
    – Ear Tubes (Myringotomy)   147
    – Ear Wax   149
Eczema (Atopic Dermatitis)   150
Epiglottitis   157
Eyes (Blocked Tear Ducts)   158
    – Eyes – Pink Eye (Conjunctivitis)   159
    – Eyes – Squint (Strabismus)   161
    – Eyes – Stye (Hordeolum), Chalazion (Lid Cyst), Dermoid Cyst   162

Feeding – Infant (Breast, Bottle, Solids)   163
    – Feeding (Overview)   176
    – Feeding – Vegetarian Diet   179
Fever (Overview)   181
    – Fever (Febrile Seizures)   187

– Fever – Fifth Disease ("Slapped Face Fever")   189
– Fever – Kawasaki Disease (Mucocutaneous Lymph Node Syndrome)   190
– Fever – Pain and Fever Control   191
Flat Head (Plageiocephaly)   193
Fragile X Syndrome   194

Giardiasis – bowel   194
Growing Pains (Legs – Night Pain)   195
Growth and Weight Gain   196

Hand, Foot, and Mouth Disease   197
Head Injury (Concussion)   198
Head Lice   200
Headaches   202
Hearing   204
Hepatitis A   207
Hepatitis B   207
Hernias (Hydroceles, Umbilical, Inguinal, and Granuloma)   209
Hives (Urticaria)   211
Holidays-Halloween   213
– Holidays – March Break   215
Hygiene (General)   216

Immunizations – Advisability (Yea or Nay?)   219
– Immunization (Pain Prevention)   222
– Immunization (Routine Vaccines)   224
– Side Effects of Vaccinations   226
Impetigo and Herpes Simplex (Cold Sores) Skin Infections   227

Jaundice (Newborn)   229

Labial Adhesions (Genital)   232
Lactose Intolerance   233
Lifestyle – Don't "Bug" Me!!   234
– Lifestyle – Keeping Fit   236
– Lifestyle – Obesity (Unhealthy Weight)   238
– Lifestyle – Shape Up   241
– Lifestyle – Sound Body, Sound Mind   243

Lymph Nodes (Glands)   245

Masturbation   246
Measles (German) Rubella   247
   – (Red) Rubeola   248
Medicine Administration – Method (By Mouth, Ear, Eye)   249
Meningococcal C Vaccine   251
Meningococcal Illness (A, B, C, Y, W135)   252
Molluscum Contagiosum   253
Mouth - white patches (See Thrush)
Mumps   254

Neck – (see Torticollis and Lymph Glands)
Neurodevelopment Assessment (18 Months of Age)   255
New Sibling Arrival (Management of the Older Sibling)   257
Newborn (Good News)   258
Night Sweating   267
Night Terrors   267
Nosebleeds (Epistaxis)   268

Orthopedic (Lower Limb(s) Problems)   269

Pacifier (See Thumb Sucking)
Penis – Foreskin   273
   – Penis (Structural Problems)   275
Picky Eater (Prevention and Treatment)   277
Pinworms (Bowel)   280
Pneumonia   281
Pyelectasis (Newborn Kidney Obstruction)   282

Rash (Diaper)   284
Ringworm Rash (Tinea Corpus)   287
Roseola (Fever and Rash)   288
Rotavirus (Gastroenteritis)   289

Safety (Home)   290
  –Safety – Summer Ouchies   291
  – Safety (Top-10 Summer Tips)   296

Sinusitis   297
Sleep   299
Snoring (Adenoids and Sleep Apnea)   305
Speech and Language Development   307
Spider Nevi – Veins (Telangiectasia)   316
Spitting up (Regurgitation)   316
Streetproofing   319
Stridor – Noisy-Breathing (Windpipe Narrowing)   320
Sudden Infant Death Syndrome (SIDS)   322
Sunscreen and Insect Repellent   324

Teeth Grinding and Clenching (Bruxism)   326
Teething and Dental Care   327
Temper Tantrums   330
Testicles (Undescended)   332
Throat Sore (Strep Carriers)   332
Throat, Sore – Tonsillitis, Viral or Strep   334
Thrush-mouth – Monilia (Yeast) Infection & Monilia Diaper Rash   338
Thumb Sucking and Pacifiers   340
Toilet (Potty) Training – Tricky, Very Tricky   342
Tongue Tie (Poor Latch and Speech)   345
Torticollis (Wry Neck)   345

Travel (Surf's Up) – Swimming   346
    – Travel Blues   348
    – Travel Tips   350

Urinary Tract Infections   353

Vaginal Irritation and Discharge   357
Visiting Your Doctor   358
Vitamin D   361
Vitamins and Supplements   362
Vomiting and/or Diarrhea (Gastroenteritis)   364

Warts   368
Index   370

INTRODUCTION

My book, *Say "Aaah"* is written for you, the parent. The advice is based on over 40 years of my experience in pediatric medical practice. Throughout the years I have prepared many handouts for my patients. Gradually, these pamphlets have expanded into volumes numerous enough to compile into a book. My philosophy has always been to keep things easy to understand and simple to apply. I endeavour to provide common sense solutions to the most frequent medical problems I have seen in infants, toddlers and young children. I have tried to give answers for every question a parent has asked me. Still, to this date, even at this writing, just when I think I've heard it all, a new concern will pop up which requires a new solution.

My book covers a large body of information. It is to be used for reference purposes as you need it. Consider it to be "the doctor who is in when the doctor is out" to be used as one of the first steps in problem solving, before you reach for the phone to call your pediatrician or before you visit your doctor, walk-in clinic or emergency department. At times, you may simply be reassured, and at other times you will be alerted to a potential problem which warrants medical attention.

Remember, although you are the caregiver and the onus is on you to make informed decisions concerning your child's well-being, during the first months, perhaps more than any other time in your baby's life, you should err on the side of caution. When in doubt, you should always seek medical advice.

As time has passed over the last 40-plus years, I find myself doing less "doctoring" in a traditional sense and instead providing more reassurance and counseling. I am now practicing a new subspecialty in medicine for the 21st century – the role of "Reassurance Agent". More often than not a hearty dose of reassurance works far better than a dose of medicine.

These days many parents prepare enthusiastically for the arrival of their new child by taking prenatal classes. Coached quite thoroughly, they are well informed to tackle labour and delivery. Too little time, however, is spent on preparing them for the period after the arrival of the baby. All too often they are less well-equipped to cope with the *aaahsome* responsibility of caring for their newborn, a being who is so completely dependent and vulnerable.

Sometimes, new parents become isolated from the potential resources offered by their own parents, grandparents, or siblings. On the other hand, they can also be provided with too much advice, given too freely, and this in turn, can fuel their anxiety. What is needed is a balance between these two extremes.

Parental stress and exhaustion can frequently lead to difficulties in parenting. Parents can lose confidence, good judgment and the ability to follow their gut feelings when it comes to understanding and interpreting their infant's symptoms; be it a startle, a change in cry, a digestive complaint or a breathing problem.

Common sense seemingly abandons new parents when a feeling of insecurity and doubt takes hold. This in turn complicates the issue of choosing appropriate healthcare options for their infant.

I hope my book (with a personal touch) will give the reader some degree of reassurance and confidence. In this way I can reach out and help the inquisitive, the perplexed, or the distraught caregiver.

Equally, I believe the book will educate and facilitate self-help. At the same time I stress again that when symptoms are of an urgent nature, immediately seek proper medical assistance!

We live in a fast and changing world in which medical knowledge is constantly advancing. New diagnostic tools and treatments are being brought forth on almost a daily basis. What is thought "true" today will be found "false" tomorrow. What is "in" today will be "obsolete" tomorrow.

No information book, including mine, is immutable or all-encompassing. As it is impossible to cover every variation of what I describe, it is not meant to be the final word. Always listen carefully to the advice of your child's physician. My book is never meant to contradict your doctor's advice. It may, however, provide a somewhat different perspective.

Abdominal Pain (Acute)

My definition of acute abdominal pain is the rather sudden onset of severe abdominal discomfort in a previously healthy child.

Appendicitis

The typical symptoms of acute appendicitis include the onset of a nonspecific abdominal pain around the belly-button area, which subsequently radiates to the right lower aspect of the abdomen. A low-grade fever as well as vomiting may or may not be present. The primary difficulty for making this diagnosis in children is the child's inability to communicate exactly where the pain is located in their abdomen. The discomfort is intensified with any movement. Often, their crying makes the physical examination difficult. Initially the symptoms are so nonspecific that the child is often sent home with the diagnosis of a "viral illness".

The delay in the actual diagnosis is the main reason that rupture of the appendix is much more common for young children than for older ones (who are able to communicate better and cooperate during physical examination). The initial diagnosis of appendicitis if missed will result in continuing inflammation and eventually the appendix will rupture. After this rupturing, the child will appear to be very ill and will act ill. The temperature is usually elevated, and there will be increasing resistance to any movement. The abdomen will become swollen and tender. The result: a very unhappy camper.

The white blood cell count is often elevated. Ultrasound of the abdomen frequently confirms this diagnosis.

The treatment is surgical removal of the appendix. If it is ruptured, intravenous antibiotics will be given, and if there is evidence of an abscess formation, drainage will be necessary.

Incarcerated Hernias

A twisting of bowel in an umbilical (belly-button) or inguinal (groin) hernia will result in the sudden onset of severe pain. The area will be tender and swelling from the bowel inflammation will not allow it to be reduced (pushed back in when pressure is applied). Vomiting may occur. Incarcerated hernias are a surgical emergency.

Stones

Although it is very uncommon, young children may get both gall bladder and kidney stones. With passage of the stones there is a sudden onset of excruciating pain. For the gall bladder the pain is in the right upper abdominal region. With kidney stones the pain is usually in the flank of the abdomen or the back. Blood may be present in the urine. Vomiting may occur with both.

With each condition the diagnosis again is suggestive by history. Children with any hemolytic diseases such as sickle cell anemia are more susceptible to gall bladder stones. The passage of kidney stones may have occurred in other members of the family. The physical examination usually reveals tenderness in the right upper abdomen for gall bladder stones or in the flank (side) or back for kidney stones.

Blood tests can help confirm a gall bladder problem. An ultrasound of the abdomen will reveal the presence of stones.

Blood present in the urine along with the above history and previously described physical examination indicators all point to a diagnosis of kidney stones. An ultrasound or flat plate x-ray of the abdomen may reveal the presence of the stone if it is radiopaque (composition which shows up on x-ray). An ultrasound and intravenous pyelogram (IVP) may be necessary to confirm the presence of and location of the obstruction. Treatment varies with each individual case.

Volvulus

This is a sudden twisting of the small bowel. The pain is severe and sudden at onset. It is often associated with repetitive vomiting which contains bile (dark green in colour).

Although volvulus may occur spontaneously, it is more common in children who have had previous abdominal surgery. Abdominal surgery may result in the formation of adhesions (fibrous bands). Loops of small bowel may become twisted around one of these adhesions. This results in impaired blood flow to the affected bowel. This in turn results in inflammation and varying degrees of tissue damage depending on how long the volvulus lasts.

This diagnosis is suspected with the above history, together with examination of an abdomen which is swollen, firm and tender when touched.

X-rays of the abdomen may show air/fluid levels in dilated loops of small bowel which suggest obstruction. An ultrasound and upper gastrointestinal (GI) series may be required.

The treatment is surgical correction.

Deceptively, the bowel may untwist on its own. When this occurs, all symptoms disappear. There will be no significant clinical findings. All x-ray and ultrasound examinations at this time may not show twisting.

The child, therefore, may have recurrent episodes of twisting and untwisting over a prolonged period of time. It is only with investigations during an acute episode that the diagnosis can be confirmed. If, however, the doctor is suspicious of recurrent volvulus, an upper GI series and follow-through may show an abnormality in the small bowel position, which may verify the suspected diagnosis of volvulus.

Surgical correction is required during an acute episode. If this procedure is carried out early, there will be no damage to the bowel. If untreated, the blood supply to the involved bowel will be diminished, leading to tissue damage and eventually tissue "death" to the involved section of bowel. The problem will require a more lengthy corrective surgical procedure along with a far longer period of recovery.

Intussusception

Intussusception is the most common cause of bowel obstruction in infants and toddlers.

It occurs when one part of the large bowel telescopes into another part. Imagine you have a large, long, sausage-like balloon. If you put your fist at the end and push in, the balloon will turn in within itself. This is what occurs in intussusception. The telescoping begins at the place where the small bowel meets the large bowel. The large bowel at this point herniates within itself. The distance of the herniation may be very short or long enough for the herniation to reach the rectal area. In this case it may even be observed protruding from the rectal opening.

The symptoms of intussusception are quite dramatic. The child suddenly screams in pain, as if his tummy had been hit with a cannonball. The child frequently doubles up in pain. There are often blood-streaked loose stools whose consistency appears to be like currant jelly. Vomiting may be present. Usually there is no fever.

If the child will cooperate long enough to allow the doctor to examine him, there will be tenderness, most commonly on the right side of the abdomen. Bloody stools may be present on rectal examination.

The diagnosis of intussusception may be suspected when an ultrasound of the abdomen is done. Confirmation is made by a barium enema. The barium will only go as far as the tip of the obstruction and no further.

Medical treatment is with the use of barium under pressure to push the obstructed bowel back to its normal position. This procedure is done under fluoroscopy. Complication may occur if too much pressure is applied (which can result in perforation of the bowel). If the obstruction has been present for more than several hours, or noninvasive medical treatment (barium enema) does not reduce the intussusception, then surgical reduction is required.

When there is spontaneous reduction of the obstruction a diagnosis of intussusception can be very difficult to make. During a spontaneous reduction all symptoms disappear. I have dealt with children who have had intussusception with "self-reduction" 2–3 times in a matter of several hours. Pain comes with the obstruction and resolves when it unobstructs. The diagnosis may be suspected but usually confirmed only during a painful episode. Occasionally it does not reoccur, but more frequently an "episode" which requires management will persist.

Constipation

I include constipation as a cause for acute abdominal pain because it is commonly implicated as its cause. In this paediatrician's eye however, constipation does not cause acute abdominal pain. Often a child with abdominal pain will have an x-ray of his abdomen which reveals a moderate amount of stool in the large bowel. The child is therefore diagnosed as being constipated, given a suppository or enema, and sent home with a laxative. However, when you review the child's history, there has been no change in the child's bowel habits and thus no clinical evidence of constipation. So my question is, "How can a child who shows no clinical symptoms of constipation be given that diagnosis to account for his severe abdominal pain?" He can't! All too often the diagnosis for the child's acute abdominal pain will be constipation, but in fact this diagnosis will be incorrect.

Constipation may lead to mild and very occasionally moderate abdominal discomfort, but not acute pain. If constipation were the cause, there would be a history of change in bowel movement habits to one of constipation, the physical examination would indicate the presence of stools when the abdomen is palpated in the left lower side, and lastly the rectal examination would usually reveal a very large amount of stool present. If these criteria are met, then constipation would be considered in the differential diagnosis of a child with abdominal discomfort.

Abdominal Pain (Chronic Recurrent)

Chronic recurring abdominal pain (C.R.A.P.) in a child under 4–5 years of age is always a concern. For older children and teenagers, it is frequently psychosomatic in origin – problems at home, problems at school or problems with peers, etc. For the child under 4–5 years of age psychosomatic abdominal pain is extremely uncommon.

When recurrent chronic abdominal pain occurs, there is most often no obvious trigger. Neither does it relate to mealtime, during eating of food or after. It may come on at any time of the day. It may last for variable lengths of time, from minutes on up to hours. The abdominal discomfort is most often located around the belly-button area. The quality of the pain is vague in nature, with the child saying "my tummy hurts" and nothing more. The pain seldom wakes the child up from sleep.

Anxiety experienced by young children may manifest with recurrent abdominal pain as one of its symptoms. However, other symptoms of anxiety are usually present as well and can be determined with a good record of the child's history. When the anxiety is dealt with, the abdominal pain will disappear.

The diagnosis of C.R.A.P. is usually made on the aggregate of history and seldom from the physical examination. The physical examination is usually normal.

The most frequent diagnosis for chronic abdominal pain is that there is no diagnosis found. Why the pain starts, and why it is lasts, is usually a mystery.

When a diagnosis can be made, the most common causes are chronic constipation, lactose intolerance, milk or dairy sensitivity, various food intolerances or a urinary tract problem. The uncommon causes would include celiac disease, irritable bowel syndrome, ulcer or inflammatory bowel disease.

The most common misdiagnosis is made by blaming constipation for the pain, even in the absence of a history of constipation. Remember, constipation is based on a history of constipation and not on a single x-ray of the abdomen which reveals stool in the colon.

Red flags

- the pain stops the child from participating in normal activities
- the pain wakes him at night
- it is associated with the time during or just after feeding
- loose diarrhea stools
- periodic fever
- blood in stools
- vomiting
- loss of appetite, energy and weight
- abdominal distention and the passing of a lot of gas
- a change in personality and behavioural pattern (child was happy and active and is now less so)
- a family history of hereditary bowel disorders

There are numerous investigations that may have to be done to rule out any underlying disorder. Blood tests, urine tests, stool tests, and abdominal ultrasound would be the first choices and the least invasive tests to try. Dietary manipulations may be attempted (such as a lactose-free diet). Depending on the results of these tests, further investigations would include an upper GI series, a barium enema, an endoscopic examination and, as well, a colonoscopy.

In the past 40 years I have seen a number of children with C.R.A.P. However, it has been awhile since I have had to carry out anything other than the least invasive of tests. If these tests do not point to the direction of the cause of the pain, then chances are slim that one can be found.

Bowel "sedatives" may help temporarily, but only by their placebo effect.

If food intolerances are suspected, an elimination diet is tried. Start by taking away lactose.

Allergy skin testing has been shown to be disappointing in determining the cause.

Seeing a naturopathic practitioner can lead to numerous tests which will result in a definite "diagnosis". Treatment will be instituted. Within a few weeks or more the child will get better. The bottom line, in this paediatrician's opinion, is that the child would have improved if left without any treatment. Having said this, if you wish to have your child seen by a practitioner of alternative medicine, I fully understand.

Chronic abdominal pain is frustrating for the child, the caregiver, and lastly, the doctor. No parent wants to see his child suffer. All parents want a definite diagnosis and a definite treatment plan to help the child. Unfortunately, in the real world more often than not there is no clear answer and essentially there is no specific treatment other than time. The longer the symptoms occur in a child who is also gaining weight and otherwise seems "well," the less the chance of finding the cause.

It is very important that you have good communication with your doctor. You both have to be in agreement with regard to the management of your child. Please do not go doctor hunting. One doctor should be at the centre of care for your child.

Remember, more often than not your "advisory" staff will only fuel your anxiety.

The bottom line is, if your concerns about your child's symptoms are escalating and you are increasingly frustrated and pressured by others, or the management suggested by your doctor is seemingly unsatisfactory, then by all means request a referral. I would truly understand this need and most doctor's feelings would not be hurt by your request.

Allergic Reaction – Severe (Anaphylaxis)

Picture the dot over the letter i in anaphylaxis. That dot is more than enough allergen to cause an anaphylactic reaction in a susceptible child.

Anaphylaxis is a serious allergic reaction that may affect many parts of the body and is potentially life-threatening. Symptoms may begin immediately, within a few minutes or even a few hours after contact with the allergen.

Symptoms involving the skin include hives, swelling of the face, and swelling of the hands and feet.

Symptoms in the mouth include itchiness of the tongue, swelling of the tongue, and difficulty swallowing.

Symptoms in the respiratory system include difficulty breathing, tightness in the chest, coughing, and wheezing.

Symptoms in the digestive system include nausea, vomiting, and diarrhea.

Generalized symptoms include a feeling of weakness, dizziness, faintness, loss of consciousness, collapse, shock, and death.

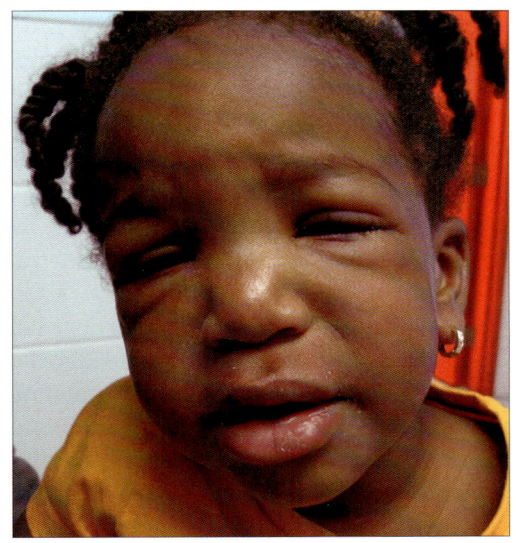

Swollen Face

All of this from one little dot. What allergens comprise potentially fatal triggers? They include peanuts, tree nuts, shellfish, stings from certain insects (hornets, wasps, yellowjackets, and bees, to name a few), certain drugs (especially members of the penicillin family), foods (soy, egg, milk and wheat are the most common, but almost any food can be implicated), latex, and even strenuous exercise. Peanut is by far the most common offender. Studies have found that up to 40% of individuals known to be allergic to peanuts will have an accidental peanut ingestion within four years of diagnosis – a very frightening statistic. Approximately 70% to 75% of food-allergic individuals have difficulty with only one or two foods. Up to 25% may react to three. The rest may react to four or more foods.

We do know that if there is a strong history of allergy in the family the potential for anaphylaxis is increased. Can anything be done to prevent this from happening?

Research has been undertaken to determine if anaphylaxis to any particular allergen can be prevented. Study results show that elimination of potential allergens from mother's diet during pregnancy, does not prevent potential anaphylaxis in the baby. Studies have been done on elimination diets during breastfeeding. The general consensus is that any elimination diet while breastfeeding will also be ineffective in preventing an anaphylactic reaction to any particular allergen. Some studies, however, have shown that elimination of a particular allergen, such as peanuts, during pregnancy and/or breastfeeding may delay the onset of a severe allergic reaction, but not prevent it. For those infants who have a very allergic background, delaying the introduction of solids until six months of age is recommended. But here again, anaphylaxis may only be minimally delayed, if at all. What about the formula-fed infant? Soy-based formulas have been ineffective. Special hydrolyzed formulas in which the protein has been broken down are also ineffective. There are no homeopathic or naturopathic remedies that are effective for either the prevention or treatment of anaphylaxis.

There is a growing body of evidence that there may be a narrow window of opportunity (between 7 and 9 months) when the introduction of foods we thought to be very allergy-promoting, such as peanuts, shellfish, and eggs, may not in fact result in food allergies, despite a strong family history. You may want to discuss this with your doctor.

Severe anaphylaxis only occurs when there is ingestion of the allergy-promoting food. If the contact is with the skin only, there may be a localized rash or hives, but not a full-blown anaphylactic reaction. Similarly, the inhalation of a small quantity of allergenic particles may result in a local reaction, such as nasal stuffiness and hives, but not a severe allergic reaction. Inhalation of a high amount of allergen, which may be present in certain atmospheric conditions, however, may cause anaphylaxis; for example, if a person is on a plane and everyone around him is eating peanuts at the same time, there may be a high concentration of peanut allergen in the air, resulting in anaphylaxis. In the school lunchroom, the gymnasium, the theatre, etc., it is highly unlikely that the air has a sufficient concentration of circulating allergen to cause anaphylaxis by nasal inhalation.

Deceptively, anaphylaxis may fail to occur until after numerous contacts with the offending allergen. Why this is so is not fully understood. Luckily, the offending allergen is usually easily identified; this is true, for example, after a wasp sting or after the ingestion of a particular food. The difficulty presents when the allergen is not known. Even the greatest detective cannot solve the crime when he does not have the clues. Allergy skin testing is most successful when a specific allergen is suspected.

What can be done? Remember the "three E's" – Education, Emergency and Epinephrine.

Education should be provided for your child, all caregivers, all relatives, all people whose home the child will visit, staff in daycare facilities, schools, and, in fact, whenever possible to every person who is going to be in contact with your child.

Your child should be wearing a MedicAlert bracelet.

Remember that the allergic reaction may start with minor symptoms. It should still be considered an **emergency**. Oral antihistamines have no place in the prevention or treatment of potential anaphylaxis.

Treatment is through the use of epinephrine by injection. There are two auto-injectable devices. One is the EpiPen, the other is Twinject. You and your child, as well as anyone caring for your child, should know the mechanics of how exactly to administer these treatments. A trainer unit (with no medication) should be provided for practice. Your doctor or pharmacist should assist you in learning how it is to be used. If possible, the child should be wearing or carrying the unit on his person. Extra units should be at home and also at any institution in which your child is spending time. Always check expiry dates (12–18months) to keep a current supply.

I would advise you to contact Anaphylaxis Canada for educational material. I would also highly recommend that you purchase *The Complete Kids Allergy and Asthma Guide* edited by Dr. Milton Gold, published by Robert Rose Inc.

I pray that, hopefully, you will never have to use your device!!!

Allergy (Dietary)

Any dietary restrictions, including milk, eggs and peanuts, during a mother's pregnancy will not prevent atopic disease (allergy) in her infant.

Avoidance of certain antigens, such as milk, egg and fish, in breastfeeding mothers may protect against eczema but not asthma or food allergy.

In high-risk infants, exclusive breastfeeding for 4 months reduces the risk of eczema and cow's-milk allergy during the first 2 years of life.

Extensively hydrolyzed formulas, such as Nutramigen, Pregestimil, and Alimentum, as well as partially hydrolyzed formulas, may delay or prevent the development of eczema in high-risk infants who are not exclusively breastfed during the first 4–6 months of life. With the use of these formulas in low-risk infants, prevention of the development of atopic disease is uncertain.

Soy-based formulas do not prevent atopic disease.

The delay of food introduction beyond 4–6 months of age does not prevent the development of atopic disease.

Recent evidence has shown that the early introduction of foods that were previously considered highly allergenic in nature (such as nuts, egg and seafood) may be helpful in preventing future allergies to these same potential allergens. They should be introduced between 7 and 9 months of age and continued. This holds true even when there is a family history of a particular food allergy. This premise of early introduction of these foods is well established in Europe and is just taking hold in North America.

New information concerning the prevention of allergies from occurring in children is rapidly becoming available. The above is only the "tip of the iceberg", and with ongoing research the management for the prevention of allergies will change.

Allergy (Milk Protein)

An allergy to cow's-milk protein occurs in approximately 2.5% of children.

Often there is a family history of a similar problem in other close members of the family (parent or sibling). There are 2 types of milk protein allergy. The first, which is immune mediated, is called IgE milk protein allergy. The second is called non-IgE milk protein allergy.

The symptoms of both begin in the first months of life.

Unfortunately, milk protein allergy, if it is to occur in an expected newborn, cannot be prevented. Restricting milk protein in the mother's diet during pregnancy will be ineffective.

IgE milk protein allergy – symptoms

The symptoms are rapid in onset. They include severe loose diarrhea, abdominal distention, irritability, crampy abdominal pain, and poor weight gain (or even weight loss). Blood streaks may be present in the stools. Non-intestinal symptoms include wheezing, hives, runny nose and eczema. Rarely, a severe anaphylactic (allergic) reaction may occur, which is a medical emergency (see Anaphylaxis).

Non-IgE milk protein allergy – symptoms

The symptoms are usually more gradual in onset. There are mucousy loose stools which may or may not contain blood. Fussiness and the excessive passage of gas is often present. Poor weight gain will be noted. Non-intestinal symptoms are usually confined to eczema only.

The diagnosis of a milk protein allergy is confirmed by history and response to dietary changes. A RAST blood test for the presence of IgE milk allergy or an allergy prick test will help differentiate between the 2 types of milk protein allergy. If the condition is unrecognized, after a period of a month or longer, varying degrees of anemia will be present due to blood loss.

Some infants may have a combination of IgE and non-IgeE milk protein allergy.

Treatment

The treatment for both is initially the same — the avoidance of cow's-milk and soy protein. Mothers who are breastfeeding should be encouraged to continue. All cow's milk and dairy products, as well as soy products, should be eliminated from mom's diet. Formula-fed infants should be placed on a formula which has all its milk protein completely hydrolyzed (broken down). Partially hydrolyzed formulas have no role in the treatment of milk protein allergy. Similarly, soy formulas do not play a role in the initial management.

The introduction of solid foods should, however, not be delayed. All solids should contain no cow's-milk or soy protein.

It should be noted that approximately 15% of those with IgE milk protein allergy are also sensitive to soy milk. This means, however, that approximately 85% may tolerate soy milk.

Approximately 65% of those with non-IgE milk protein allergy are also sensitive to soy milk. This means only 35% or less may tolerate soy.

Depending on the medical centre where the child is being treated, follow-up management once the infant is stabilized may differ.

Once on a completely hydrolyzed formula, symptoms should improve within a few days to 2 weeks with those infants who are formula fed. Initial improvement may take longer for those who are breastfeeding, because cow's-milk protein may continue to be excreted in breast milk for a few days after mother is placed on a restricted milk protein diet.

Infrequently, if there is no response to the above dietary changes, the infant should be placed on an amino acid formula.

All infants should remain on the restricted milk and soy diet and closely monitored until all symptoms have disappeared and the infant is demonstrating an adequate weight gain (i.e., stabilizes).

Once this is attained, those infants with IgE-mediated allergy should be continued on breast milk as long as mother is willing and able. During weaning, babies may be tried on a soy formula. If they do well, they should remain on the soy formula. If they are sensitive to soy protein (i.e., allergy symptoms return), then they should be placed on a completely hydrolyzed formula.

Infants who have an IgE mediated milk protein allergy should have skin testing every 6 months. Once the skin test becomes negative, the cow's milk protein allergy has, in most cases, resolved. At that time cow's milk may be introduced and the infant closely monitored by the doctor.

Those infants, who have non-IgE-mediated milk protein allergy may be tried on soy formula at 1 year of age. If they do well, the soy formula may be continued until 2 years of age, and at that time the infant may be challenged with cow's milk. Alternatively, at one year of age the infant may be challenged with cow's milk directly. If no symptoms occur, then the infant has outgrown his cow's-milk protein sensitivity. If symptoms occur after the introduction of soy or cow's-milk protein, then completely hydrolyzed formula should be continued and the infant rechallenged every 6 months. Again, all solids should be free of soy and cow's-milk protein until the child outgrows the sensitivity.

Approximately 50% of those with milk protein allergy will outgrow the problem by 1 year of age, 75% by 2 years of age and 85% by 3 years of age.

The occurrence of other food allergies is more prevalent in those who have IgE cow's-milk protein allergy as compared to those who do not. The diet should be discussed with your doctor or allergist. Food allergy skin testing to common food allergens is advisable.

Allergy (Seasonal)

Spring has sprouted. Streams are running. Ahh – warm weather at last. The snow has melted, layers of clothing are removed, convertible tops are down – what could be better? However, with spring comes an increase in air pollution (smog) as well a high pollen count in the air. This may be fine for you but not for millions of children and adults who suffer from seasonal allergies. For them, breathing has become "hazardous" to their health. What is running for them are their noses and eyes. Eyes are red and itchy and throats are scratchy. Heads are ready to explode. "Take time to smell the roses" is not for allergy sufferers.

From mid-April to the end of June grass and pollens are the main culprits that trigger allergic symptoms. During the hot, hazy summer days the pollen index often increases to a dangerously high level. From mid-August to the first frost (November), it is ragweed season.

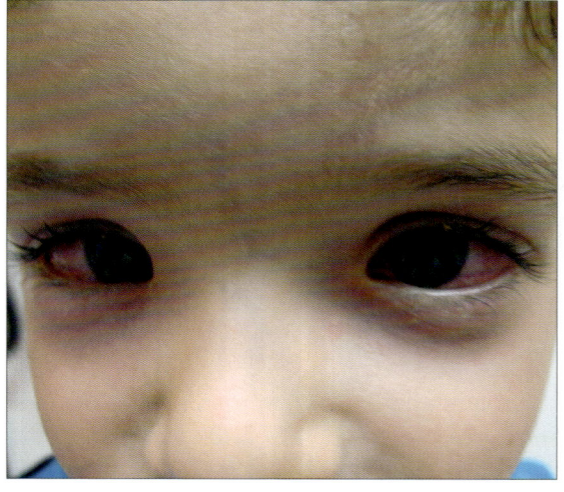
Allergic Conjunctivitis

Environmental allergies are a family affair. If one parent suffers from atopy (asthma, environmental allergies or eczema – in any combination) then there is up to a 40% chance that their child will suffer the same. If both parents are affected then the risk may rise to 60%. Children with eczema also have an increased risk of having both asthma and environmental allergies.

Although asthma and eczema may present within a few months after birth, environmental allergies normally do not present themselves in children until after a year and half to 2 years of age (more common after 3–4 years of age).

So what actually happens? A trigger, let's say pollen, is inhaled by a susceptible individual. The body recognizes this pollen as being foreign. It responds by initiating a cascade of immune events resulting in the release of histamines (and other substances). The areas targeted are the nose, eyes, throat and chest. The mucous membranes in the lining of these organs become swollen with the increased production and release of mucus and tears. The end result – allergy symptoms.

No one has successfully explained why a person may be free of symptoms only to develop allergic responsiveness sometime later in life when nothing in their environment has changed.

The nose symptoms include sneezing, nasal stuffiness, persistent clear nasal discharge, itchiness, and pain in the sinus areas. The typical child with nasal symptoms can be spotted from a distance by his "nasal salute" – a constant rubbing of his hand upwards over his nose to help alleviate symptoms.

The eye symptoms include redness, itchiness, and excessive tearing, puffiness of the eyelids and dark circles under the lower lids ("allergic shiners").

The throat symptoms include excessive mucus in the throat which constantly has to be cleared, a scratchy feeling, and a cough from irritation of the lining in the back of the nasopharynx.

Some individuals with environmental allergies only have a problem with pollens and grasses in the springtime. Others only have ragweed problems in the fall. Many have both.

Over the past 40 years, I have dealt with thousands of environmental allergy sufferers. Some cases, fortunately, are mild while others make people miserable. They become grumpy, do not function close to their potential and are not pleasant to be with (everyone around them seems to suffer in one way or another).

With young children, behaviour, performance and social activities all suffer.

Is there a cure? At best we can control the symptoms. Environmental allergies result from living in a large city in a northern climate with seasonal changes. Symptoms can be minimized only by moving to an "environmentally friendly" area such as Arizona.

So what is the solution? Well, you could keep the child in an air-conditioned room, with windows always closed, and have a HEPA air filter running at full blast. Meals and school work could be slid under the door. He would be allowed to leave to clean up and use the toilet. Finally, when the allergy season is over, he would emerge from his room. I do not feel that most parents would find this an acceptable solution.

Allergy skin testing and subsequent immunosuppressive desensitization may have to be considered. After skin testing, a solution containing the substances to which the child is allergic is compounded specifically for him. Starting with a very dilute concentration, weekly injections are administered. Slowly the amount and concentration of the solution is increased. After 1 to 2 years the frequency of injections is every 2 weeks. They are then spread out over longer periods of time – monthly. In 4 years therapy is complete. Hopefully, by then, the child's immune response to the allergens that he has been desensitized to will be diminished. The symptoms will have either disappeared completely or been greatly reduced. Although desensitization therapy done in this manner works extremely well, it is time consuming and drawn out over a long period of time. Most busy families will have a problem keeping to the prescribed schedule.

Personally, I do not usually recommend skin testing when all the allergic symptoms seem to strictly relate to a season of the year (spring or late summer). You can be fairly certain as to what the allergic triggers are. Secondly, I know of no child (or adult) who is happy about receiving weekly injections. Thirdly, there are now many safe medications available that specifically target some point in the immune cascade and prevent the release of histamine and other complexes which cause the allergic symptoms. Most of these medications have no side effects. Many can be used in children as young as 3 years of age.

So if your child has seasonal allergies I suggest the following:

- use a HEPA filter on the furnace or in the bedroom
- have air conditioning so that you can keep the windows closed
- maintain room humidity at 45%–50%

There are now many safe, effective medications available to control all the symptoms that the allergic sufferer has. These not only include oral medications (Singulair can be very effective in children as young as 3 or 4 years of age) but also nasal sprays and eye drops. They must be used on a daily basis throughout the entire allergy season. Discuss with your child's doctor the appropriate medications for your child's particular needs, how and when to use them, and how often and how long to use them, as well as their side effects and possible drug interactions. There are both over-the-counter and prescription allergy medications that are helpful. All medications should be explained to you so that you fully understand their use.

Therapy should be initiated based on the previous year's time of allergy symptoms onset and response to medication. Initiate therapy 2–3 weeks prior to the onset of symptoms based on previous experience. Continue daily throughout the entire allergy season. It is best not to stop and start intermittently unless directed by your physician.

The use of long-acting slow-release injectable steroids or rapid desensitization by an injectable concoction of environmental allergens should be considered only if previous therapy, as described above, has not been successful and symptoms are still very distressing to the child (not the caregiver).

Holistic medications and/or other naturopathic remedies, although not entirely proven scientifically to be effective, may be considered. As long as they do not adversely interact with other medications, they may be tried.

This spring do not allow your child to be a "big drip" and suffer needlessly. I wish for you a sneeze-free, scratchy-throat-free, cough-free and itchy-eyes-free allergy season.

Alternative Medicine

In my mind the word "alternative" is a misnomer. If it were as successful as reported it would no longer be alternative but mainstream.

I am a believer in holistic medicine – treating the entire body, mind and spirit as an interconnected whole. I also believe that any treatment that does no harm and has the potential to be of benefit is worth investigating.

In Canada, close to 4 billion dollars are spent annually on alternative medicine and natural health products. Studies worldwide have shown that up to 35% of children have visited a practitioner of alternative medicine. These visits are for the treatment of asthma, eczema, ear infections, digestive problems and a host of other ills. The highest utilization of naturopathic medicine is typically seen in Europe. However, more and more, North American parents are turning to alternative medicine for the management of behavioural problems, learning disabilities, attention deficit hyperactivity disorder (ADHD) and even autism spectrum disorders.

A "holy" battle is in progress – traditional Western medicine taking shots at alternative medicine and the reverse. Integrated care, with Western and complementary medicine working together, is still in its early infancy in North America.

But why are more and more people turning their backs entirely on traditional Western medicine and embracing alternative medicine?

It may be that doctors receive no formal training in communication with their patients. This could lead to a host of problems, including misunderstandings or patients being not completely satisfied with the explanations. Doctors who are heavily scheduled cannot spend enough time to listen to the patient. The patient feels rushed. Patients feel frustrated when a diagnosis is not given (even if one is not available). Lab tests seem to be ordered indiscriminately. Too often there is a very long wait time for test results, for investigations and for referrals to be obtained.

On the other hand, contrast this with practioners of alternative medicines, who do receive communication skill training. They spend much more time with the patient. They are better listeners. They are very convincing. They always (or nearly always) give a specific diagnosis. They present a plausible and understandable plan of treatment. They constantly reassure the patients that they will improve, and giving hope of improved health leads in turn to greater trust. Patients are convinced of the benefit, and many "will" themselves into improved well-being: the so-called "honeymoon phenomenon" is at work.

I realize that what doctors are not "up on" they tend to be "down on". Notwithstanding this fact, the following caveats should still be kept in mind.

The expertise of any health provider is determined in large part by the amount of experience he or she has with any given illness or age group. The number of children a naturopathic practitioner deals with is small compared to that of a family practitioner or pediatrician, so when it comes to dealing with childhood problems, most practitioners of alternative medicine have quantitatively less experience.

Many naturopathic therapies are based on one or more combinations of treating the immune system, which is over- or underactive. Allergy, often is the basis of the problem – usually foods such as milk, dairy, soy, wheat, sugar, caffeine, gluten, food additives, artificial flavourings, and colourings. There is an overabundance or deficiency of one or more substances in the body. The body contains too many toxins or is infested with *Candida* (monilia) or lacks probiotic flora. The bowel or genital micro-organism flora is out of whack, causing digestive or urogenital problems. There is a misalignment of the skeletal system, a disturbance in the magnetic aura or the electrical field in or around the body.

The same treatment is frequently prescribed to deal with vastly different conditions, many of which may have no relationship to each other. Nevertheless, the one remedy or minor variants thereof are touted as a "cure-all".

Unfortunately, there are many naturopathic studies which have not stood up to scientific scrutiny and are debatable as to their findings.

Many herbal remedies are not regulated by government health and welfare agencies – they may vary in quality and proportion of ingredients and may be contaminated. This is especially true of Chinese medicines (especially herbs in pill form). A harmful rather than beneficial effect may result. Cross-reaction with other medications may occur and could be contraindicated – always discuss combinations of alternative and traditional medicines with your doctor or pharmacist.

It is possible that substituting naturopathic medicine investigations for traditional Western investigations could delay a serious diagnosis with life-threatening consequences.

Naturopathic management is often quite expensive, and treatment can take a long period of time. I often consider this added time to be the benefit as much as the treatment itself.

Practitioners of alternative medicine are often known to discourage routine childhood immunizations. In my view, this is a most serious mistake.

Some day both alternative and Western medicine will more closely ally themselves for the improvement of patient well-being. Until then – it is your body, it is your child's body, your penny, and lastly, your choice. Please be informed – if a pot of gold is promised, avoid the temptation of going over the rainbow.

For now I think we can all agree as to the benefits of grandma's chicken soup!

Antibiotics (Use and Misuse)

The story goes: A couple was having dinner at a restaurant. The waiter approached and suggested, "For dessert, I would recommend gateau d'Amoxil on a bed of crushed Biaxin tablets covered with a drizzle of Zithromax". Sounds absurd, doesn't it? Nevertheless, with today's tremendous abuse and overuse of antibiotics, it is not so far-fetched.

There are a number of reasons why man may be becoming an endangered species. Among these is the abuse and overuse of antibiotics. Bacteria are able to genetically modify themselves and to adapt to become resistant to antibiotics. This is occurring at a far faster rate than man's ability to produce new, more effective antibiotics.

So what's the solution? Who's to blame? Why is this happening? The answer is not a simple one. We live in a world with a need for instant gratification – a desire for immediate results. We are no longer capable of taking the time just to sit back and smell the roses. Our need for quick fixes is too often a detriment to solving the problem.

Similarly, with many illnesses we do not have or wish to allot the time needed to let nature run its course. Carly Simon said it best: "I haven't got time for the pain". We have too much stress in our lives to allow an illness to stress us further. As users of the medical system, we mistakenly believe, that when a doctor tells us we do not require medication, he is withholding treatment. We tend to think, "After all, what is the harm in trying an antibiotic? Other doctors prescribe them for the exact symptoms I am having, so why doesn't my doctor give them to me?"

Patients who request or even demand a prescription for an antibiotic put the doctor in a very difficult position. Yet, it is ultimately still the doctor who is writing the prescription. It would be much easier for him to take less time and write out a prescription for an antibiotic than to explain why it is unnecessary and inappropriate. Still, there is no excuse for the doctor who writes such a prescription merely to satisfy the patient's demands. I feel strongly that the doctor is the gatekeeper for medical care, and must bear the burden of blame for the mess we now find ourselves in.

Frequently, patients will go "doctor hunting" until they finally find one who will give them what they want – an antibiotic. Within 2–3 days they feel much better and attribute this to the antibiotic which they vividly remember was withheld by their own doctor and others. They are very upset with the non-prescribers. No credit is given to the fact that the clinical improvement was due to time and time alone, and not the antibiotic.

It is only through education that we are going to curtail the overuse of antibiotics and to use them responsibly and only when necessary. Not only does the public have to be educated, I am sorry to say, so do many doctors.

Exactly when are antibiotics not needed?

• Colds which are viral, with a runny nose and cough, do not require antibiotics. The presence of a green nasal discharge does not mean there is a bacterial infection.

• Bronchitis in children is a viral infection – no antibiotics.

• Fever is a symptom, not a disease. No antibiotics are required unless there is a bacterial cause.

• Children with an asthma attack and fever do not require antibiotics unless there is the presence of pneumonia on a chest x-ray.

• A sore throat, along with the presence of a cold, is most likely viral. A sore throat with watery eyes is for certain viral – no antibiotics.

• If more than one member of the family is ill with similar symptoms, it is most likely viral – no antibiotics.

• A sore throat which is considered to be caused by strep bacteria, only after a throat swab which confirms the presence of strep, requires an antibiotic. It is next to impossible for a doctor to diagnose a strep throat infection upon examination alone. The exception may be if the child clinically has scarlet fever. Even in this case a throat swab must be done. Never accept an antibiotic for a sore throat unless first a throat swab confirms the need. This is imperative!

• A cough on its own, whether loose, dry, day and/or night, spasmodic, associated with vomiting or prolonged for weeks, does not require an antibiotic unless a chest x-ray shows definite pneumonia (rarely so).

When are antibiotics required in the office setting?

• A child with a sore throat and a positive throat culture for strep

• Pneumonia which has been confirmed with a chest x-ray

• Whooping cough, if diagnosed within the first 2–3 weeks of onset of symptoms

• An abscess – to be decided on an individual basis

• Cellulitis (superficial bacterial infection near the surface of the skin)

• Impetigo which is spreading despite the use of antibiotic creams.

• Sinusitis – This is a difficult diagnosis to make. The child who has had a green nasal discharge for more than 10 days to two weeks, is ill, may be febrile, and has pain over his sinuses or swelling around the eye probably has sinusitis.

• A urinary tract infection – This should be treated only if there is significant growth of a single bacterium on a urine culture. A bagged-urine culture, even if positive, should not be treated, because of possible contamination. A child who cannot voluntarily void should have an in/out catheter urine specimen taken to confirm the diagnosis of a urinary tract infection.

• Some bacterial causes of gastroenteritis require antibiotics. This depends on the stool culture results.

• Otitis media (middle ear infection) – children under 2 years of age with a diagnosis of otitis media probably should be treated with a course of antibiotics. For older children, unless they are very ill, it is best advised to wait a day or two before considering antibiotics. The vast majority of infections are viral in nature, and will resolve on their own. A middle ear infection with the presence of eye discharge is usually of a bacterial origin — antibiotic eye drops, as well as oral antibiotics, are indicated.

Remember, when your child first starts daycare or preschool, he will be exposed to many other children. For several months, while building up his immunity, he will experience numerous infections, most of which will be viral in origin.

In the end, trust your doctor. Let him (or her) do the doctoring. Without this trust, medical care cannot be properly and effectively delivered.

P.S. The doctor's office should be an antibiotic safety-zone!!!

Anxiety (What, me worry?)

Quid, me vexari? As Alfred E. Neuman of *Mad Magazine* would say "What, me worry?" Yes, Alfred: you and everyone else. We all have worries and fears. Anyone who saw the shower scene in Hitchcock's *Psycho* had to be frightened. I was afraid to shower for months. Others switched to bathing only – a little extreme but fully understandable. We can, however, overcome these phobias and function normally when given a little time.

Anxiety, on the other hand, is characterized by an unrealistic fear. That is, a fear that manifests in the absence of danger. Up until the past 20 years or so, anxiety disorders were identified mainly in adults. Recently, we have seen the same phenomenon in younger populations – beginning with teenagers and now down to young children – even preschoolers. In fact, it has been estimated that 2%–3% of the pediatric age group suffers from anxiety. The incidence increases if another family member suffers from an anxiety disorder.

Why? Professionals are still scratching their heads. Similar questions have been raised regarding the rise in ADHD and autism. Is it partly genetic? Perhaps. Is it partly environmental, both in the sense of the environment that surrounds us and the environment in which we are raised? Nature and nurture? Perhaps. Are these children just "wired" differently, due to some in utero event? Is it because of too many ultrasounds, which may, with the proper trigger, promote such disorders as anxiety? Who knows? I, for one, believe that anxiety has multifaceted causes.

How can a nonaffected person understand what a child with an anxiety problem really goes through? Perhaps, if we could understand, we would be much more compassionate when dealing with an anxious child. Think of this: I put a board on the floor measuring 4 cm thick and 20 cm wide and 5 m long. If asked, you would not hesitate to walk along it, even hop or skip or jump along that board. Now, if I were to take the same board and raise it up as high as the top of the CN Tower and ask you again to walk across, would you hesitate? It is the same board, same size, yet I think you would think twice. Why? Because falling from an overwhelming height adds the element of danger to the equation.

I dare say not one of us would take that challenge. We would become completely immobilized. Our hearts would race and almost jump out of our chests. Our minds would become numb. We would sweat profusely. Our legs would feel like putty, with heavy lead weights around them. "Go on, you can do it. There is nothing to be afraid of." Easy for you to say. Clearly you would not be considered to have an anxiety disorder, because there is real danger. But perhaps you now have a better idea of just how paralyzing a real anxiety disorder, in the absence of actual dangers.

Many experts in the field recognize various subtypes of anxiety disorders:

Separation Anxiety – Here the usual fear is one of separation from a caregiver, who is most often the mother.

Panic Disorder – sudden intense episodes of anxiety, sometimes without an obvious trigger.

Social Phobia – Here the child is extremely shy and social situations become fraught with fear and are avoided as much as possible. For this child, speaking up at daycare or preschool is next to impossible. An extreme example of this is a selective mutism, a syndrome in which the child will only speak to certain individuals and in certain situations.

Obsessive Compulsive Disorder – the need for ritualistic repetition or avoidance of normal everyday events. Examples would be the precision-like repetitive manner that his toys are placed in order, the placement of clothes according to colour, the inflexibility to alter daily routines. Numerous other examples exist.

Generalized Anxiety – frequent/constant worrying about many different things.

Simple Phobia – excessive fear of a single situation or thing; for example, dogs.

Post-traumatic Stress Syndrome – exposure to a traumatic experience while lacking the mechanisms to cope with it. Examples would be abuse, illness or death of some loved one (even a pet) or witnessing a horrific event.

So, what can be done to prevent or help the child to manage an anxiety disorder?

Prevention – Prevention is difficult to accomplish because we do not know exactly what we are preventing. Certainly if a caregiver is anxious, the child may pick up on this and become anxious too. If you as a caregiver suffer from anxiety, you must work on yourself first. Do not overprotect or overprogram your child. Every child needs space and time to explore, to use his imagination, to problem-solve and to make mistakes.

If you recognize that your child is behaving timidly and is overly attached to you I call this the "Blue Garter Syndrome" after the bruise around your thigh caused by your child's arms clenched around your leg), then slowly try to wean him away from you. Plan activities that involve other family members or close friends. Walk through the mall. Go to the playground or library storytime. Plan a play date with another child. You can think of many more. This will slowly encourage independence. This in turn will build self-esteem, an all-important component of your child's make-up which helps him to cope and minimize anxiety. Maintain routines with consistency – children thrive on this.

Validation – If anxiety is present, let your child know that you too are aware of it, that you understand, and will help. Give the anxiety a name such as "my worry bug" or "Mr. Scary" to help you communicate with your child about the anxiety.

Confront the anxiety – The only way to overcome the fear is by helping him to confront it gently and gradually. The sooner you do this the better. Daily exposure to his fear in small doses will slowly desensitize the child and thus lessen the anxiety load. The child must be taught skills to cope and deal with the problem. Take your time; your impatience may only fuel further anxiety. Plan ahead as to how to deal with "Mr. Scary" by including your child in the planning of the coping strategies. Remember, what works for one child may not work for another. Diminish his anxiety in a special way – with a favourite doll or fluffy animal allowed in bed to protect him from "Mr. Nightmare". Giving the fear a special name helps communication with the child and zeroes in on the problem. Carrying a magic wand to ward off "the bogeyman" or a lucky charm to handle works well. A goldfish, turtle or hamster named appropriately may act as a constant helper or guardian against "evil". Allowing the child to carry a picture of you or of a pet to look at for reassurance when needed may also help. Using a spray-mist bottle with "special powers" such as "magic water" over the bed at night, the bathtub, or anywhere else where there is an unrealistic fear, is helpful.

Positive reinforcement – Give positive reinforcement when small steps have been achieved. The use of a star or sticker reward system or a bracelet or necklace to which coloured beads can be added will give concrete proof of the child's successful progress.

Relaxation Exercises – For the older child, deep abdominal breathing, relaxing each part of the body part by part, and regular exercise can all help to relax and clear the mind.

Inform daycare or preschool staff. Teachers and administrators can be a great help.

Many books are available to help a caregiver cope with the anxious child.

Do not fail to seek professional help – Do not be embarrassed to request for help in the form of behavioural therapy. It works wonders. Medication may also be required on a short-term basis.

If your child's anxiety is appropriately addressed, then he can live a fuller, more satisfying life – capable of interacting in a healthy manner both in and outside the home.

Anxiety – New Baby Blues

Throughout your entire pregnancy, you have been waiting and preparing for your newborn's arrival. Hopefully your pregnancy has been rather smooth and uneventful except for some fatigue and the usual discomfort. You have attended all the prenatal classes, which have prepared you for labour and delivery but have barely touched on the area of care once he arrives. Likely you had a typical delivery and spent one to two days in hospital getting used to the baby. If you are breast-feeding, a nurse or lactation specialist will have helped you to get started.

You arrive home with your newborn baby. You are tired and probably sore, but extremely happy. You are determined to be the best mother possible. Once on your own, however, you realize that you have the awesome responsibility for another living being. You will have to determine whether the baby's behaviours, and whatever the baby is doing, are normal. No one has prepared you for decoding the meaning of his cry, his jittery movements, the colour of the skin, his cold hands and feet, or the rash on his body, spitting up, sneezing, hiccups, etc., etc., etc.

In a few days, you realize how unprepared you really are for caring for a newborn. Lack of sleep commences to take its toll and begins to diminish your coping skills. You may start to get conflicting advice from your "advisory staff". Day by day the situation seems to get worse. Nights and days begin to be mixed up; one feeding goes well, the next, not so well; sometimes the baby burps and others times he does not; he spits up, becomes fussy etc., etc., etc. Your husband, although he is trying to be supportive, really is unable to meet your needs.

With your first visit to the doctor, you tell him of all the things that concern you about the baby and he quickly reassures you that all is well. But your feeling is that all is not well. This easy reassurance does very little to relieve your anxiety.

You take the baby back home, closing the door behind you – just you and the baby – alone.

Within a few days, because of sleep deprivation and worry, you can become both physically and emotionally drained. You begin to have difficulty making decisions about your baby's health. Common sense flies out the window. Your advisory staff only further confuse you with their unsolicited conflicting advice. Parenting becomes a burden rather than a task of love. You feel completely overwhelmed.

You may have further feelings of guilt because it seems that you are losing your bearings. You believe that you are letting down those around you including your spouse and other children. This only increases your feeling of isolation.

This scenario will often begin to develop during the first week of the baby's life. In my 40 years of experience as a paediatrician I have witnessed it all too often. Sometimes "the blues" can surface and are suspected very early, even during the initial examination of the newborn in the hospital, or during the first visit at a few days of age in the doctor's office. Mom will usually appear to be more anxious than she was in the hospital. At her first doctor's visit she is not smiling. There is usually a long list of concerns. These may include excessive crying by the baby, poor feeding, sleep patterns and a host of other issues. A pattern is beginning to emerge, not only of the mother's inability to care for her newborn but, as well, her inability to meet her own needs. These mothers require a tremendous amount of support right from the beginning. This can take a large portion of the doctor's time; however, any doctor worth his salt should recognize these early symptoms and put into practice whatever intervention is required to prevent its escalation. Helping a mother during this most fragile and debilitating period of time is a reward in itself. It will lead to happier times, and that is the joy every parent should experience.

It is important that the signs of baby blues be distinguished from a full postpartum depression. The doctor should be able to distinguish between the two.

What can be done?

The good news is that if you can survive your baby's first month of life, everything will start improving. There definitely is a light at the end of the dark tunnel that seems to have engulfed you. You may require more visits to the doctor for examinations just to reassure yourself that the baby is gaining weight and that nothing physically is wrong with him/her. A gentle, calm, continuing reassurance that all is well is of great importance. The mother needs to have complete trust in her doctor for this to succeed. Skillful questioning by an astute doctor often will reveal those underlying concerns that must be completely dealt with to the mother's satisfaction. Fathers, too, must be involved with the baby's care. Despite their work outside the home during the day, it's probably true that moms would gladly change places with them. Fathers need to be sensitive and supportive. They must take the baby out of the mother's hands and take charge for at least a few hours each evening and longer during the weekends. This should give mothers some time for themselves – perhaps to take a long, warm bath, to read the newspaper or a book, or to just put their feet up and have a cup of tea. Support can also be provided by a relative or friend. Notice, I said, support, and not "advice"!

Again, free time should be made available to mom. If there is a breastfeeding problem, a lactation consultant should be consulted. A single visit or more, if required, by the public health nurse can best assess the home situation and provide professional advice as well as communication of other concerns to the doctor. It also gives mom an opportunity and some time to speak to another, understanding and knowledgeable "human being" and perhaps share a cup tea. I find that suggesting that mom join a group for new mothers and their babies is often helpful – the idea is new mothers helping new mothers so they do not feel so isolated. Moms should get out of the house as often as possible: taking the baby for a long walk or sitting in the park or going to their favourite hangout to sip a coffee. Having someone babysit for a few hours in the evening, so wives and their husbands can go out for quick bite to eat or catch a movie, does wonders to lift the morale and refresh the energy (leave the cell phone at home).

Babies have been born for thousands and thousands of years, some under the most adverse conditions. The vast majority of infants thrive. It's unfortunate that often it is the mother who is overlooked during this critical care period and may fall by the wayside.

The words are very easy for me to say – "Take your newborn home from the hospital with confidence, common sense, a sense of calmness and a positive mental attitude." It is up to you, however, to take this advice to heart and make it a reality. I wish you the very best.

Your "Advisory Staff"

It is too bad that when a baby is born he or she does not come with an accompanying instruction manual for parenting, for times when the baby is healthy, as well as times of illness. But do not fear. You will always have your "advisory staff" to guide you – rightly or wrongly (usually wrongly!).

The very first record of a caregiver's advisory staff dates back to the time of the pharaohs in Egypt. When Moses was saved by the Pharaoh's daughter, an "advisory staff" was appointed to help guide her with his upbringing. The very first self-help handbook of advice was written on papryus.

Now, just who forms your "advisory staff"? How did they become your advisory committee? Did you appoint them or was an election held (one that you were totally unaware of)?

No, this committee was not appointed. No, its members were not elected. They are, however, a group of very dedicated and concerned individuals who have taken it upon themselves to guide you in looking after the baby's welfare – a group who suspects that your parenting skills may not be up to par (at least, not up to their standards). They are there to fill in the so-called gaps that they perceive in your child-rearing knowledge (and they know there are quite a few).

Their numbers vary depending on their direct access to you. Unfortunately, in these modern times, access is easy to come by. With computer technology the whole world has access to you. You cannot hide.

Who actually are "they"? Well, they may include your mother, your mother-in-law, your sisters, their mothers-in-law, your aunts, and your friends (with or without children), just to mention a few. You'll notice that they are mostly female. The men around you seem to hold back their advice unless they are asked. However, the more "hands-on" they become in child-rearing, the more likely men are to throw in their two cents' worth.

Always remember that to your mother you were always perfect and could do little wrong. However, to your mother-in-law you were never good enough for her son and you will never be the mother she was (a joke).

You will constantly be under a microscope. Your every move for baby's care will be closely monitored and scrutinized. If deemed to be "wrong" you surely will be advised and strongly "encouraged" to rectify your mismanagement.

How does this constant barrage of advice affect you? Is it welcomed? Usually not. Is it helpful? Usually not. Is it calming and reassuring? Usually not. Is it confusing? Usually yes. Is it undermining – usually yes. Does it cast doubt on your parenting skills? Usually yes. Does it heighten your anxiety? You bet!

Unfortunately, many individuals on your "advisory staff" do not see it this way. They feel strongly that they are helping you to problem-solve (even if there is no perceived problem). They strongly feel that you should be thankful for their being around just in the nick of time to save you from making so many disastrous mistakes. The bottom line is they really do not have confidence in your ability to problem-solve or parent – after all, in their day, parenting was a skill that "young folk" nowadays just do not yet have. Even your friends and siblings are more than willing to throw in a word or two, or even more, of advice.

All too often your advisors supply the fuel to escalate some concern of yours even though it may initially be minimal. A little cold becomes pneumonia. A small amount of gas becomes a milk allergy. Lack of weight gain (in the advisor's eyes) is due to insufficient breast milk – "You are starving your baby," they say. I could fill a whole book with a host of further examples. Unfortunately, the advice of the "advisory staff" often comes when you are most stressed and when you are most vulnerable. You could cave in to it or, worse, say something that you will later regret.

So what can you do? Well, you do have options. You can either listen to them or ignore them. Most of all, however, you have to be diplomatic. After all, the people you are dealing with are not just passersby. They actually love and care for you as well as the baby. You have to remember that they will be in both your lives for a very long time. My advice to you is to listen with ears "half-open". That is, let what you want to listen to penetrate, and that which you do not want to listen to be filtered out.

Do not let anyone undermine what you feel to be the correct course of action. The final decision is yours and your spouse's. A simple "thank you" for so much unsolicited advice is all that is needed.

Keep the following maxim in mind: It is always much easier to give advice and to bring up someone else's child than to follow your inner voice and bring up your own.

Asthma

Asthma is defined as a chronic lung disorder in which the lining of the very small airways of the lungs become narrowed due to muscle spasm in these airways. In addition there is inflammation and swelling of the cell lining. The airways are further narrowed when secretions from the inflamed cells fill the already narrowed airways. Asthma symptoms are a result of this narrowing. They include coughing (mostly at night), wheezing (problem with getting air out), tightness of the chest and shortness of breath (in mild asthma shortness of breath occurs with exercise only or with mild exertion such as climbing stairs).

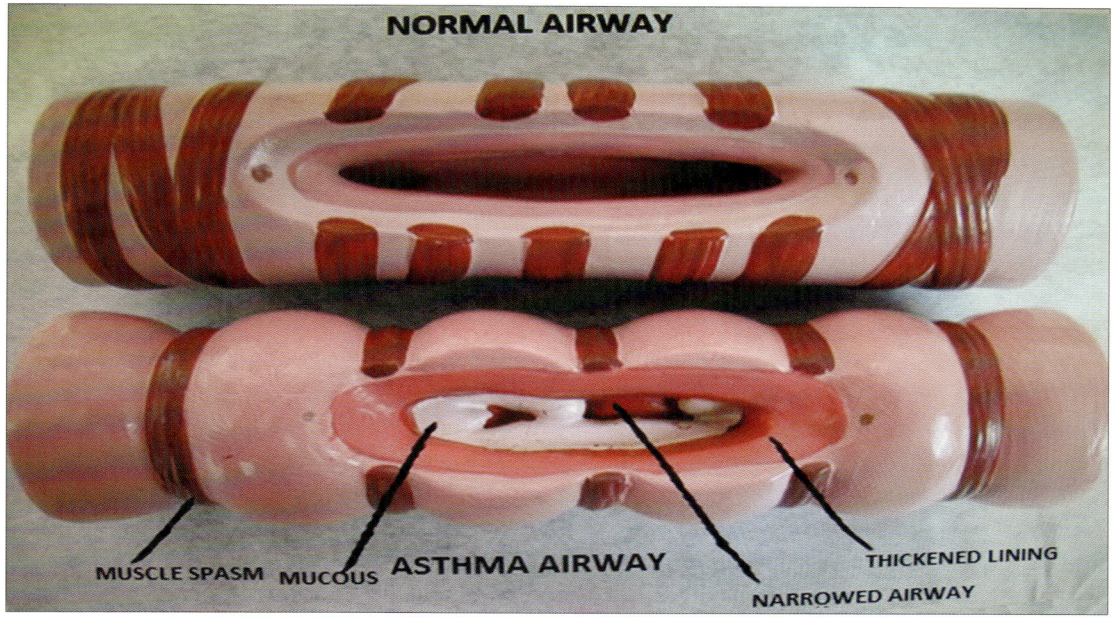

There are basically 2 types of asthma. The most common one is the one which is triggered by upper respiratory tract infections. These children usually outgrow their illness by 6–7 years of age. The second type is the one which is triggered by allergens. For this type, children, although they do improve with age, usually have the illness for life. Some children have a combination of both types.

Diagnosing asthma can be very challenging, particularly for children under 3 years of age. To confuse matters, most episodes with respiratory infections accompanied by cough and wheezing are common findings in children who do not have asthma. In fact, in the under-3-year- old age group, the younger the wheezing child, the less the likelihood of asthma. All that wheezes is not asthma!

Asthma is an extremely complex disease. Understanding its management may become overwhelming to a caregiver. There are many reasons for this. Although there are numerous causative factors in common amongst children with asthma, there are also many individual or nonspecific factors that may affect each patient in varying and different degrees. Each patient is an individual who has a common disease – asthma. Accordingly, each patient requires his own personalized plan for its management. Unfortunately, many of the drugs used (and, by the way, they are very effective in treating childhood asthma) are not labelled for use by children under certain ages. This is obviously a concern to the parents of an asthmatic child.

With the number of medications on the market (bronchodilators and anti-inflammatory), as well as different delivery systems, parents find it difficult to understand why one would be different from another or considered superior. More confusion results when different doctors prescribe different medications for the treatment of asthma in children who seem to have similar triggers. There are short-acting medications, long-acting medications and many possible combinations thereof. To further add to the confusion, new medications are constantly being approved for use. Advertisements in various media promote the superiority of their particular product. Parents think, "Why isn't my doctor using it?" Other parents of asthmatic children question their doctor's use of this or that medication. This uncertainty puts doubt in your mind as to your doctor's capability of caring for your child. You may wonder if other doctors are better equipped than yours to handle the problem of asthma.

How do I answer the above concerns? I do not specialize in the treatment of asthma. However, having been in practice for over 40 years and having managed numerous children of all ages with varying severity of asthma, I've found that the goal in treatment for asthma remains simple: It is to use the least number of medications, for as little time as possible, so that the child with asthma is mostly asymptomatic and without any limitations most of the time. This is the ultimate goal, but getting there may be a long and difficult process. On the parents' part it requires time, patience, and education. They should never be afraid to ask questions if concerns are not addressed. I cannot overemphasize that the most important aspect in managing a child's asthma is education of the parent. You owe it to the child to become as knowledgeable as possible in all aspects of his illness. This knowledge, in conjunction with your doctor's, is best found through your local asthma education centre. With time, your comfort level in dealing with your child's illness will increase. You will develop a "sense", or an ability to predict when an asthmatic exacerbation is about to occur. Remember, never hesitate to question as often as needed. Frequent refresher courses with updates in treatment are important to maintain. As stated, the goal of treatment is to lessen the severity and frequency of attacks so that your child is able to participate in all his routine activities. Plans for prevention should always be in place. An action plan should be at a state of readiness should an attack occur.

As previously stated, in young children, primarily those under 3 years of age, unless they have recurrent episodes of wheezing (in the absence of a respiratory tract infection or a cold), it may be difficult to diagnose the child's symptoms as those of asthma. There are no blood tests to confirm it. They are too young for pulmonary (lung) function tests. Allergy skin tests may be difficult to interpret as to allergy's role in your child's symptoms. A chest x-ray is usually inconclusive (findings of over-expanded lungs may be suggestive of but not conclusive for asthma). Other diseases may present with the same chest x-ray findings. Asthma is more likely in a young infant or toddler if he/she has eczema or food sensitivities or if he is known to have a family history of asthma or environmental allergies. Chronic persistent cough, especially at night, despite a clear chest when listened to, may be the only symptom of asthma. Equally, shortness of breath or coughing when exercising may be the only clue that the problem is asthma.

The bottom line: the diagnosis sometimes is only confirmed by the child's response to medication (inhalation of anti-inflammatory agent with a bronchodilator). In pediatric settings the only disease that responds to asthma medication is asthma! If there is an immediate response within a day or so, the diagnosis of asthma is most likely. If, however, after using the medications as directed with proper technique (that is, getting the medicine down deep into the lungs) for one month there is no significant improvement, then other diagnoses should be considered. Your child's symptoms may not be linked to asthma as the cause (see also the section below on why asthma medication does not work).

Can asthma be prevented? Maybe. Staying on a strict hypoallergenic diet during pregnancy will not help her to prevent the child from developing asthma. There is controversy as to whether breast-feeding helps to prevent the development of asthma. For formula-fed babies, hypoallergenic formulas (where the protein is completely broken down), as well as soy-based formulas, will not prevent or modify asthma. Neither does delaying the introduction of solids give protection against the development of asthma.

Recent research has shown that omega 3 (DHA) and 6 (ARA) may have an anti-inflammatory effect. Studies have shown that these 2 fatty acids may help reduce asthmatic attacks secondary to upper respiratory tract infections. Accordingly, I do recommend that all children over 1 year of age, with or without asthma receive a minimum daily dose of 200 mg of DHA along with ARA, either through the diet or by supplement. If less than 1 year of age, the infant with asthma should receive enough of these fatty acids from breast milk or by fortified formulas without the necessity of further supplementation.

There are many triggers of asthma. By far the most familiar trigger in childhood is the common cold virus. This is the reason asthma may not present itself or intensify until your child enters the "community" for the first time – for example, daycare, children's programs or school. This is also why there often seems to be an increased incidence of asthma attacks when children return to school – the so-called "September peak".

Other triggers may include: non-food allergens that are environmental in nature such as, pollens (grass, trees, weeds); animals (dogs and especially cats), saliva, urine, dander (skin scales); house dust mites, bed bug feces, drugs, and feathers (down). Animal allergy does not usually occur in children before 3 years of age.

Other environmental triggers for asthma include irritants such as smoke (tobacco or fireplace), cold air, weather changes, strong odours (perfume), harsh chemicals and pollution.

Other triggers include exercise, strong emotional outbursts, and elevated levels of stress.

Certain food allergens including nuts and peanuts, milk, soy, wheat, shellfish and eggs may produce wheezing as the only symptom of an allergic reaction. However, these foods may also produce a combination of symptoms including wheezing, swelling of the face and limbs, itchy throat, hives, difficulty swallowing, vomiting and diarrhea. Any combination of symptoms may indicate a severe allergic reaction known as **anaphylaxis** - a medical emergency.

Advances in our knowledge and management of asthma are being made as I write. A recent study indicated that children living in high-pollution areas, whose caregivers were stressed had an increased risk of developing asthma. However, there was no increase in the incidence of asthma caused by parental stress alone. In another study mothers who experienced stress during pregnancy and who also smoked cigarettes had babies who were 2-3 times more likely to develop asthma than babies exposed to cigarette smoke in utero whose mothers were not stressed – very interesting. We have a lot more to learn.

Asthma Management

Education

I must again emphasize the importance of caregivers receiving as much education about asthma as possible and especially how it relates to their child. An action plan should be in place if an asthmatic attack occurs. Early intervention will, in most cases, not only shorten the severity of the attack but its duration as well. Known triggers when possible should be avoided or eliminated. For recurrent bouts of asthma, a prophylactic (preventative) plan should be in place and continued as long as it is needed.

Remember, as a caregiver of a young child with asthma, you are the one who eventually teaches and hands over to him the responsibility of managing his illness. If the teacher does not know what to teach, the pupil can never learn the lesson.

Environmental Control

Aside from choosing where you live (pollution levels) you cannot control the outdoor air quality. However, you can and should try to, as much as possible, control the indoor air quality. There should be no smoking in the house or car (and I mean none anywhere – not even the furthest corner of the basement). Log-burning fireplaces should be replaced by gas or electric units. Carpets should be replaced by hardwood floors or linoleum tiles. Curtains should be replaced with blinds. Frequent dusting is mandatory. Indoor house plants provide a natural way to reduce indoor air pollution. Ceramic or clay pots reduce mould in the soil. A small plant can clean a room of excess carbon dioxide in about 8 hours. English ivy, bamboo plants and peace lilies are good choices. Choose green cleaning products which do not contain harsh chemicals. The filling for pillows, comforters and cushions should be composed of hypoallergenic synthetic materials. Mattresses should be covered with plastic hypoallergenic barrier covers. Maintain the humidity of the house at less than 50%. A central air purifier system is best – if you do not have one, put a HEPA filter unit in your child's bedroom. Keep stuffed toys to a minimum and wash them on a regular basis. Wash all bed sheets weekly at the highest temperature possible. In the summer, keep windows closed.

Pets can be a problem. If you intend to buy a dog or cat, let your child who has asthma come into contact with the breed several times before the actual purchase to ensure that there will be no asthma flare-ups. In the sales agreement insist on a statement specifying that you will be able to return the pet for refund if your child's asthma is aggravated once the animal is in your home. It is very difficult to decide what to do if you already have a pet (dog and or cat) that has been a family member for a long time. If the child's asthma is not worsened when he is with the pet – fine. If, however, asthma symptoms are occurring only in your house, especially when your child is in contact with the pet or pet's hair, you may have a problem. If in doubt, have your child allergy skin tested for animals. You must decide then as to what to do with Shep the sheep dog or Tigger the cat. If he has shown positive results on skin testing, immunotherapy (allergy needles) will take a long time to desensitize your child. When it comes to the intensity of animal allergies, cats are by far the worst of offenders.

All children over 6 months of age, especially those with asthma, should have a yearly flu vaccination.

Medical Management

There are basically 2 types of medications used in the treatment of asthma. The first are the bronchodilators, which help relieve the muscle spasm in the small airways. These are called your "rescue" or "reliever" medications. The second group are the anti-inflammatories (inhaled steroids), which reduce the swelling and secretions in the lining of the small airways. These are called your "controllers". Both can be given in 2 ways. First, there is dry inhalation with a metered-dose inhaler, disc or turbo inhaler. With the metered-dose inhalers a spacer is required to ensure their effectiveness. Second, there is wet inhalation, delivered by a machine which drives nebulized medicine through a tube into a mask which covers the child's face. Both are effective in the management of asthma, although dry inhalations are easier to administer and studies have shown that metered-dose inhalers with an AeroChamber are just as effective. Inhaled corticosteroids inhibit the production of cytokines. Cytokines are one of the mediators that cause inflammation of the airways.

Oral medications, if required, are also available. With severe asthmatic attacks during the acute phase, your child may be put on an oral steroid for a few days to gain control of the asthmatic process. Oral steroids may be required to be administered in small doses daily as part of maintenance therapy for those asthmatics who have frequent breakthroughs despite being on preventative maintenance therapy.

The production of leukotrienes (inflammation mediators) can be inhibited by medications such as Singulair. Singulair may be used in the prevention of exercise-induced asthma or in combination with other medications in a preventative maintenance program. These inhibitors have also been shown to help prevent upper respiratory tract infections (colds) from triggering asthma attacks. If, on returning to school each year, your child's asthma flares up due to respiratory tract infections (the September asthma peak), Singulair may help to prevent this from occurring. Starting Singulair 2 weeks before school and continuing it until mid-October may solve the problem. Singulair is useful for treating exercise-induced asthma, primarily, for example, during hockey or soccer season. Using Singulair on a daily basis during this period may help decrease exercise-induced asthma. Two preventative puffs of your bronchodilator (usually Salbutamol) may also be necessary prior to heavy exercise. An off-label side advantage of using Singulair is that it has been demonstrated to be of value for chronic recurrent hives. It is also a good alternative or additive when nonsedating allergy medications such as Reactine or Aerius, used to control environmental allergies, are not working alone or are found to be ineffective.

Side Effects (of inhaled bronchodilators)

Rescue medications usually have no side effects. Some children, however, may be very sensitive to these medications if mistakenly administered in more than the prescribed amount. Increased heart rate and heart palpitations are symptoms that indicate overdosage. Tremors of the hands may occur. Headaches or nausea and vomiting are very uncommon but may occur if the medication is abused. There are no long-term consequences to the proper use of these medications, but extreme overdosing can lead to cardiac arrest.

Steroids

Inhaled steroids may often take 48–72 hours before having a beneficial effect.

The word "steroid" strikes fear in every parent's mind. There are concerns about stunting a child's growth, damaging sexual development, adverse effects on the immune system and a host of other possible side effects. This results in reluctance by parents to accept the use of inhaled or oral steroids for their child.

There is still a dispute in the medical community as to the frequency and seriousness of side effects of inhaled steroids (especially long-term side effects). The only acknowledged short-term side effect is the development of oral thrush. This is very uncommon and if it occurs it is easily treated. It can be prevented by having your child rinse his mouth or have a drink after each inhalation. Currently, the consensus is that there is no suppression of the immune system. Suppression of the adrenal glands, which are important to produce increased "steroids" during sudden stress, such as a severe injury or during surgery, has been a concern. The amount of steroids absorbed into the blood system from the lungs after inhalation is minimal. However, it has been shown that the small amounts can suppress glucocortisol levels in the blood. Cortisol is required during stress and is produced by the adrenal glands. The assumption is that inhaled steroids may cause the adrenal glands to fail to react during a stressful situation. Without an increased production of glucocorticoids during stress, shock (low blood pressure and low glucose) may occur. In searching the literature this occurrence is very uncommon. It most likely would occur only if your child were to be on a very high dose of inhaled steroids or oral steroids for a prolonged period of time. Prolonged adrenal suppression may result in the production of non-specific symptoms such as nausea, fatigue, headache and poor weight gain. If the above symptoms are present, a cortisol blood level should be done along with any other investigations deemed to be required for that particular child. In my opinion, the beneficial effect of inhaled steroids far outweighs the risk of adrenal suppression. It has been shown that inhaled Fluticasone given in large doses (over 500 mcg per day) has more adrenal suppression then other inhaled steroids. There are also studies on inhaled steroids and their effect on growth which show that inhaled steroids taken frequently over a long period of time in high doses may curtail total growth potential, but only minimally.

Any child with a chronic illness (such as asthma) may not reach his growth potential because of the illness itself. It is difficult to sort out which factor in particular may affect growth the most – the illness or the inhaled steroids or both. Suppression of total growth potential by a combination of both factors would probably be by less than 2 cm. Yet, again, the beneficial effect of the inhaled steroids far outweighs the concerns for growth potential. There are also studies that have shown that the long-term use of inhaled steroids may result in demineralization (thinning) of bone, the result being that there may be an increased risk of fractures. Reported cases of fractures in such individuals are very rare and, again, do not outweigh the beneficial effects of inhaled steroids. Mineralocorticoids produced by the adrenal glands are not suppressed by long-term inhaled or oral steroids.

Other side effects have been attributed to steroids (especially oral ones), but the above-mentioned potential side effects are the main concerns. Some others could include an increase in blood pressure, the development of type 2 diabetes, breakdown of one or both hip joints, eye problems such as glaucoma, or psychosis. I should emphasize again that these occurrences are extremely rare and would occur only with long-term use of oral steroids at high dosage.

The bottom line – the beneficial effects of inhaled steroids and the occasional use of oral steroids far outweigh any adverse effect. If any of my own children or grandchildren were to have asthma, I would not hesitate to prescribe inhaled steroids and, if required, oral prednisone (also a steroid).

Every asthmatic should be treated on an individual basis. The treatment protocol depends on many factors – age, triggers, frequency and severity of attacks, response to treatment and compliance. Your doctor, asthma educator, allergist and asthma specialist may, in any combination, play a role in your child's therapy.

Immunotherapy

A small percentage of asthmatics may benefit from allergy skin testing and a subsequent immunotherapy program. This would include any patient for whom it is difficult to determine the triggers as well as those for whom it is extremely difficult to change the day-to-day environment in which they live. An immunotherapy program starts with weekly injections of a solution containing the allergens which were positive on the skin test. Initially, a weak solution is used and then gradually increased in strength. Desensitization may require 2–3 years of therapy. It is not 100% guaranteed that this will eliminate the trigger completely, but it may make the allergy more tolerable.

Holistic Therapy

If you wish to try alternative medicine either as a substitution for or as adjuvant to traditional therapy, discuss this with your doctor. My basic philosophy is that if something does no harm and seems to help, then it is worth trying. It is your child, it is your penny. However, if anyone promises you a quick cure, run the other way. I would not like to see you waste your money and/or time on any therapy that has absolutely no shred of scientific evidence to validate its efficacy. Because some naturopathic medications may interfere with previously prescribed medications, causing unwanted side effects, always check with your doctor.

Mental Health

Caring for an asthmatic child can become overwhelming for a caregiver. Caregivers may become so overprotective of the child that they deny themselves and their child a normal lifestyle. Asthmatic children add one more stress to the parent who may already be stressed. If this is the case for your family, you may require counselling.

Why Asthma Treatment May Not Work

For any asthmatic who is not responding to treatment, the following areas of management should be reviewed. In most cases the solution can be found.

The Child Does Not Have Asthma

Every medical student is taught "all that wheezes is not asthma". All too often this is forgotten, especially for young infants and toddlers for whom it may be difficult to distinguish a wheeze from a non-wheeze respiratory problem. When the caregiver says that his child is wheezing, asthma leaps into the doctor's mind right away. Wheezing refers to difficulty getting air out (expiration). A simple question to the caregiver is whether the child is having trouble getting air in, out or both, or if they really do not know at all. These descriptions will often determine if it is or is not truly a medical wheezing. The caregiver can be asked to reproduce the sound, if possible. The doctor may reproduce the sound. If uncertainty remains, the best way to correctly identify wheezing is to digitally record the sound.

In an infant between a few weeks and 8–10 months of age, air movement through a small amount of mucus at the back of the upper airway can be transmitted throughout the whole chest cavity. The sound is loud and wet and can be felt with the hand on the child's chest. If his chest is listened to with your ear, it sounds as if it is filled with seawater. Yet the child is happy, has no disturbance in feeding pattern, has good colour and has no interference with sleep pattern. The diagnosis in this case will be that he is a "happy wheezer" or mucousy infant. If he could clear his throat that would solve the problem – however at his age he can't. He therefore will clear the airway with an occasional big cough or just by swallowing the mucus. These symptoms are of great concern to the caregiver but of little or none to the child. This pattern may persist until 8–10 months of age. It will not respond to asthma medication. Nor will it respond to a change to a different formula. No treatment is required except patience and time. Do not listen to your "advisory staff", as this will only make you doubt yourself further. If you have concerns, speak to your doctor. If the noisy respirations are not bothering your child but are more bothersome to you or your advisory staff then leave the child alone.

Infrequently, wheezing can be heard even without a stethoscope from the other side of the room. Most times, however, it cannot. It essentially requires the chest to be examined by the doctor. A careful examination will reveal if bronchospasm (wheezing) is present or not. If the child is crying or upset, it will make it almost impossible to get an accurate account of air movement in the chest. It is mandatory to wait for as long as it takes until the child settles down and allows his/her chest to be examined.

A postviral cough can last for many weeks. This usually occurs in the healthy child who has developed a viral illness with a cough. All the symptoms except for the cough may disappear. It is usually worse at night, often repetitive in nature and not infrequently associated with vomiting. The cough during the day is much less noticeable. When the symptoms for this kind of cough occur, it becomes most difficult for a doctor to convince caregivers that time alone is the best treatment.

There are numerous other causes for a persistent cough with or without wheezing: a congenital abnormality blocking the airway structure, a foreign body doing the same, cystic fibrosis, whooping cough, the 100-day cough, a postnasal drip, immune problems, congenital heart disease, gastroesophageal reflux (small amounts of food are refluxed up the esophagus and spill over into the windpipe), on entering daycare or school for the first time – here the child may contract numerous respiratory infections due to contact with other children. This may last up to 8–10 months. With frequent coughs, asthma may be considered, but it is not the problem. "Whooping cough–like virus" or "100-day cough" is very common, especially during the winter season. It is caused by a virus. It usually starts with a mild upper respiratory tract infection. The child soon begins to have loose, congested coughing spasms, mainly at night (*cough-cough- cough-cough-cough cough-cough*) until the child loses his breath and also vomits thick mucus. The only difference between the 100-day cough and whooping cough is that with whooping cough, during coughing spasms there are periodic loud, harsh, inspiratory sounds as if the child were trying to catch his breath – the typical "whoop". The cough may be so severe that a hemorrhage may appear in the white of the eye. Small hemorrhages into the skin called petechiae may also occur. Both of these will resolve. The above described cough is not asthma and is to be considered a postviral cough. Treatment with asthma medication most often does not alter the symptoms or the duration of the symptoms. They may be tried, but if there is no significant improvement in 2–3 weeks then they are not going to help.

Finally, if the diagnosis of asthma is contemplated after reviewing the history and family history, but cannot be confirmed by examination, then a one-month trial of asthma medication may be required. This should be monitored closely by the treating doctor.

To my mind, every newly diagnosed asthmatic should have at least one chest x-ray. This should be done to rule out a host of other medical conditions.

Problems with Medication

In the treatment of asthma there is no indication for the use of cough medication or oral decongestants. Both of these suppress the cough and dry up the secretions. The medications for asthma do the opposite – they loosen the secretions so that they may be coughed up and expelled. Using asthma medication with cough suppressants and decongestants is like trying to move a stalled car – with you at the front pushing backwards and someone at the back pushing forwards. Guess what? The car doesn't move.

Proper dosage of both bronchodilators and anti-inflammatory medications must be used. Often an insufficient amount of anti-inflammatory is used in the dosage. During an acute attack, oral steroids should not be withheld if the child is having difficulty breathing and is not responding to inhalation therapy. Oral steroids can be safely used for a few days and then stopped. Oral steroids will lessen the severity of the attack as well as its duration. The philosophy is to "hit the disease hard" to get its attention and to control it and then taper the oral medication to a lesser dose, or discontinue it completely after a few days.

Note: It is important to start medications as early as possible rather than to wait until the airways become further narrowed.

Once the symptoms have been relieved, the bronchodilator may be discontinued. However, the anti-inflammatory (controller) alone, at a reduced dosage, should be given for a further 10 to 14 days to ensure that the "twitchy" airways are completely put to rest. If you stop the anti-inflammatory inhalation too early without allowing the airways to return to normal, there is a risk of a rebound asthmatic episode.

One of 2 common reasons why asthma medication fails to work is improper technique. Unless the medications are delivered to the small airways they will not work. Each time a patient comes to the office because of his asthma he should bring in with him his medications for reassessment and review. Technique for their use should also be reviewed. When delivering medication, if the child is crying, insufficient amounts will reach the small important airways – the medication may therefore be ineffective.

The second reason why asthma medication does not work is because of poor compliance; that is, the patient is not using the medications as prescribed. It goes without saying that if the medication stays in its canister it will not help with an asthmatic attack. Both the acute and preventative plans that have been put in place must be carried out as directed. There is no point in increasing the dosages or changing the medications if the usage technique and/or the patient's compliance are a problem.

Patient compliance when on long-term prophylactic medication can become a problem. With diabetes, for example, if you forget to take your insulin you quickly become ill. However, with asthma, if you forget to take your medication, at first occasionally and then more often, for a short period of time this will frequently create no problem. The reason the child was put on prophylaxis in the first place was to prevent recurrent asthmatic attacks. If the medication is discontinued too soon, one runs the risk of his asthma returning as before. If you feel your child no longer requires prophylaxis, discuss this with your doctor before discontinuing the medication on your own.

Problems Concerning Environmental Control

Caregivers who are resistant to becoming educated about the importance of creating as "friendly" an environment as possible are a real problem. They are doing their child a great disservice.

Problems with Triggers

Too often, an asthmatic will repeatedly encounter the same hostile environment only to have his airways triggered into hyper-reactivity each time. Often it is next to impossible to get someone else to alter the hostile environment to accommodate the asthmatic child. Prime examples of these situations are:

- visiting grandparents whose house may be dusty and where grandpa may be smoking a pipe.

- spending the weekend at dad's apartment with dust, smoke and Shep the shedding sheepdog.

- playing a vigorous sport, such as baseball, hockey or soccer.

In each of the above examples, it is very difficult to avoid the hostile environment. However, the triggers may be prevented from firing. Remember, no good gunfighter enters a shootout without his guns blazing. I, therefore, suggest that when anticipating entering a hostile environment, initiate anti-inflammatory medication for the child 2–3 days beforehand and have him continue taking it until he leaves that environment. There are some studies that have shown that with viral-induced asthma, the use of inhaled steroids at the first signs of a cold, in an effort to prevent the cold from triggering asthma has not been effective. Other studies have shown the reverse. Therefore it is worth trying in order to see if your child is one of the candidates for whom inhaled steroids work to prevent an asthmatic attack.

Peak-flow meter monitoring in children over 7 years of age is an excellent way to predict and thus prevent airway hyper-reactivity. It is a simple device that the child breathes forcibly out into. It measures his ability to exhale air on a scale. Comparing this result against his best result (done when well), one may predict the presence of reactive airways even before symptoms appear. The measurement may also predict the severity of reactivity. It is an excellent tool to monitor the child's airways on a daily basis. Each asthmatic should have his peak-flow zones established for reference.

The truth is that a lot can be done to lessen both the severity and duration of an asthmatic attack. Education, proper medication and dosage, proper usage technique and compliance are the basic cornerstones for controlling asthma. Each asthmatic should have an acute attack routine, a preventative routine, and also a long-term prophylactic routine if necessary – all are based on individual patient needs.

Tips

A spacer device should be used with any child who is on a metered-dose propellant inhaler. Ensure that it is the correct size. Do not share spacers. All new spacers should be washed before use. This will eliminate any electromagnetic charge on its inner surface which may impede the delivery of the medication mist. Wash the spacer in soap and water frequently (depending on how often it is used, at least every 1–2 weeks).

Studies have shown that, unfortunately, when a child is crying during an inhalation, very little medication is deposited in his lungs. This is one of the main reasons why the medication will not work. I suggest that you practice with him as often and as long as it takes, using the mask if you're giving wet inhalations or the spacer for dry, until the child becomes accustomed to the treatment and does not resist by crying.

How do you know when the metered-dose inhaler is empty? One way is to shake it to hear the movement of fluid inside. The other indication is if the medication fails to deliver any relief; then the canister may be empty.

Asthma Prophylaxis – for chronic reactive airways

If any of the following are true, your child's asthma is **not** under optimal control:

- He requires reliever medication 4 times a week
- He has a persistent night cough, tightness of the chest or congestion 4 times a week
- He has shortness of breath or coughing during exercise
- He is missing a lot of school or activities because of asthma

Prophylaxis medication given on a daily basis to prevent an exacerbation of symptoms may be required. Medications prescribed are either an inhaled steroid and/or a montelukast inhibitor(Singulair). With inhaled steroids a low dose is tried first. If there is poor response a double low dose is tried.

If either medication on its own is beneficial, prophylaxis should be carried out for 3–4 months or longer depending on the individual case. Your doctor will advise you.

If neither of the above medications is helping on its own they should then be tried in combination. Failing this, inhalers that contain a combination of both inhaled steroid and salbutamol should be tried. The Singulair should also be continued. Long-acting beta antagonists (LABAs) may be needed if the child still does not respond to the above treatments (for children over 8 years of age).

In children with cold (viral) induced asthma, using high dose inhaled steroids at the first symptoms of a cold may be all that is required to prevent an asthmatic attack. Daily prophylaxis in such cases would be unnecessary.

A newer medication omalizumab is administered every 2 weeks by subcutaneous injection. Omalizumab has been shown to be very effective in helping to reduce the need for continuous steroid therapy in children. Omalizumab acts on the immune system to help prevent release of mediators which cause airways to become reactive.

The bottom line is that if prophylaxis is required, the most conservative protocol should be utilized– the one in which the least amount of medication keeps the child as free as possible from asthma symptoms. Many do well on less while others need more. Remember, every child with asthma is different. Do not compare one child with another or one doctor's regime with another's. All questions should be answered by your doctor until you are satisfied.

For exercise-induced asthma Singulair may be tried during the season of activity (for example, – hockey season). It may also be tried 1 to 2 hours before high-exercise activity. A dose of salbutamol (Ventolin) may also be used alone a half-hour prior to physical activity or in combination with Singulair. A child should not be kept out of sports or gym classes at school because of asthma.

All possible attempts should be made to discover the trigger or triggers which cause the airways to be continually reactive. Once identified, these triggers are to be avoided. A referral to an allergist or childhood asthma respirologist may be the optimal next step.

The ultimate goal is to reach a level at which your child can live as asthma-free as possible with the least amount of medication.

Essentially, there are many ways to travel from A to B. Getting to that destination is what counts. There are so many different ways of handling the management of asthma for a child. If there were only one way, life would be a lot simpler for the patient, caregiver and doctor. Keep in mind that standards of care from doctor to doctor, as well as within different communities, may vary.

To conclude, we have covered a lot. Reading the above 2 or 3 times or more may be necessary to help absorb all the information you require. You can use it as a handy reference when needed.

The above is the way I see the management of asthma at this time.

Autism (Development)

Autism is a neuro-developmental disorder.

In some surveys over the past 2–3 decades the incidence of "classic" autism has been estimated to have dramatically increased to approximately 1 per 150 children, while other surveys have put the incidence as 1 per 1000 children. Autism is approximately 4 times more prevalent in boys than girls. The million-dollar question is why?

One reason for the rise in the incidence of autism is known. It is due to the expansion of the diagnostic criteria which now makes possible the inclusion of a broader demographic than has been previously found to fulfill these criteria.

What is the cause?

Unfortunately, we do not know the cause. We do know that autism does have a genetic component. In fact, if one child in the family has autism, the risk of the second child's having this condition is 20–50 times higher than for the general population.

Using MRI, as well as other neuroimaging techniques, researchers have found structural differences in areas of the brain in many autistic children. Most experts in the field agree that something "triggers" the illness in susceptible individuals. What makes an individual susceptible is not clearly understood. Genetics certainly plays a role. At this time at least 15% of children with autism have been found to have an underlying genetic cause. This number will certainly rise. At present it seems to be that the gene defect is a sporadic change in gene composition that occurs soon after the sperm has entered the ovum at the time of conception. Genetically, the parents do not show this defect. A gene defect on the X chromosome resulting in autism could explain the higher incidence in boys. Males have only one X chromosome. Females have 2 X chromosomes. In girls, the normal chromosome seems to protect against autism developing, even if the other X chromosome has the gene defect. Does having the gene defect automatically result in autism or are there external factors that trigger the gene to express the disorder? What those exact triggers are still remains unknown. Yet, why has there been such an increase in its incidence in the past 30 years? Environmental triggers present in our outside environment, as well as those inside our bodies, are a strong possibility.

Here are some "far-out" speculations as to why. Is there a link between autism and paper diapers? Coincidentally it was about 30 years ago that we began to switch from cloth to disposable paper diapers. Could there be some neurotoxin that is absorbed through the skin, especially if the latter is irritated? Is autism the result of the increased use of prenatal ultrasounds and ultrasound stethoscopes that may trigger some change in brain development? There are many more speculations, however none has been subjected to the rigors of research and shown to be the cause. Why is autism more common in boys? Why are there pockets in North America where the incidence of autism is much higher than for the general population? These questions and a thousand more concerning autism are yet to be answered. As more and more research in this area is done, I feel the answers will soon be uncovered. When this happens, prevention may become the reality and treatment greatly improved. Pre- or postnatal screening may become available to enable early diagnosis. Drugs may be available to treat the neuro-biochemical imbalance and thus modify the symptoms.

The MMR vaccine, (as well as other vaccines) has not been implicated as the trigger or cause of autism, despite previous claims that were based on flawed data. There have been many well-controlled scientific studies that have confirmed the finding that there is no relation between the

MMR vaccine and autism.

The symptoms

Autism is characterized by the impairment of communication (speech and language) skills, by the impairment of social skills and by the presence of repetitive behaviour patterns.

The following is a list of symptoms, which may not all be present:

- failure to develop social gestures such as smiling
- failure to babble or show interest in sounds around him
- disinterest in surroundings
- dislike of being held or cuddled
- poor eye contact
- child fails to respond to his name
- delayed speech/language development (no understandable words by 15 months of age)
- child does not use gestures to show or point
- repetitive movements of whole body or parts of body such as:
    – constantly moving fingers
    – excessive hand or arm flapping or body rocking
    – excessive spinning or running in circles
- plays with toys inappropriately – i.e. would rather throw the toy than play with it or prefers to spin the wheels of a toy car rather than play with it appropriately
- fascination with parts of objects
- would rather play by himself; relates poorly to others – shows a lack of interest in socially interactive play with other children
- echolalia – repeating what is said to him as if an echo
- increased sensitivity to or interest in tactile sensations, for example:
    – child is difficult to dress and undress
    – likes to continually feel certain materials or stroke mother's hair
- excessive temper tantrums (often without obvious provocation)
- hyperactivity – always "on the go"

If autism is suspected, the child should have a neuro-development assessment to confirm the diagnosis. A hearing test may be indicated. A speech-language assessment is necessary. Chromosomal analysis should be considered if conditions such as fragile X syndrome are suspected to be a possibility.

Treatment

The earlier the diagnosis is made and the earlier treatment begins, the better is the prognosis. Children with autism fall into a continuum of severity, but no matter how severe, the child's "upper potential limit" can be reached (not surpassed), but only with early intervention. At present, for many reasons the diagnosis and treatment may be delayed by 2–3 years. The fault sometimes lies in a lack of parental awareness, the doctor's own failure to consider the diagnosis, the lack of diagnostic facilities, or the scarcity of knowledgeable, trained therapists for the management of autism. In this pediatrician's eyes, treatment should be available a maximum of a few months after the diagnosis is confirmed.

Treatment includes behavioural modification programs, intensive socialization-based programs, speech and occupational therapy or a combination of some or all. In all cases, the earlier treatment is begun and the more frequent and intensive the therapy, the better the outcome. Unfortunately, many of these programs, most often offered privately, are prohibitively expensive for most families.

A Few Words of Caution

There is no magic cure for autism such as specialized diets, consuming supplements, any kind of manipulation, whether chiropractic or the laying on of hands to change the body's aura or magnetic field, removal of excessive toxins or heavy metals, treatment of any pathogen such as yeast (monilia) or manipulating the intestinal flora. Many other so-called cures have been suggested. Simply put, there is absolutely no scientific evidence to support the above listed "cures".

Recently, hyperbaric oxygen has been used for the treatment of autistic children. There are anecdotal comments and 1 or 2 small studies that show that hyperbaric oxygen may have the potential to improve some symptoms of autism. At present there has been no definitive statement supporting its use. Larger, well-controlled studies are now under way to confirm the long-term beneficial effects of the hyperbaric option. The results of these studies are not yet available.

I do realize how devastating the impact of the diagnosis of autism is on parents. Most parents would do anything, go anywhere, and sacrifice all in order to help his or her child. A parent placed in such a vulnerable state can easily be taken advantage of by those who give false hope, professing to hold the "cure" for their child.

More hopefully, there have been cases where children who receive intensive, early intervention using recognized therapy methods, in time no longer meet the criteria for a diagnosis of autism.

Baby (Newborn Skin Care)

Your infant has arrived – so have flowers, presents, good wishes and more than enough advice on parenting.

The worst is over – or is it? Your baby has jumped from his protective internal environment to a new and ever changing one. Furthermore, he has all of the built-in natural equipment to make such an adaptation. Remember, babies have been born for thousands of years under incredibly adverse conditions – through blizzards, in deserts and even in the back seats of dirty taxicabs. They all thrive.

The first days and weeks are the most difficult and are going to test you to the maximum. Some parents seem to pass through this adjustment period with ease. Others become overwhelmed and depleted both mentally and physically. Be assured that this trying time is temporary and soon you will be able to return to a more normal routine.

Fathers – this is your baby too. More and more fathers are taking an active role in raising even the youngest and smallest of infants. Of course, no one expects you to breastfeed, but you should be more than just a bystander. You are not a mere spectator watching a sporting event. You are part of the team. Your wife needs your help, support, caring and understanding. Newborn baby care outside of breastfeeding should be shared between both parents. Your baby needs your attention. Luckily, you are able to retreat back to your work. Your wife does not have this luxury. She may be physically and mentally stressed, with no place to retreat – left at home to care for and make decisions about a new life. I cannot emphasize how much she needs your support at this time, even though she may look fine and say everything is okay – for mom, the outside world's expectations of motherhood must feel overwhelming.

Skin Care

General

Some babies have beautiful skin and never get a rash. Others have very sensitive skin and as soon as one rash comes and goes another one arrives. Most newborn rashes require very little care. As a general rule if the rash appears moist then dry it (powder) and if it appears dry then moisturize it.

During the first 2 weeks after birth, the baby's skin may appear to be very dry and flaky. This is normal and moisturization is not necessary. All products used for bathing and washing the baby should be ones specifically designed and manufactured for baby's use. Do not use adult products, which may contain chemical additives that can irritate a baby's sensitive skin.

Bathing

Remember to wash hands before and after you change the baby's diaper or bathe the baby.

Sponge the baby (face, neck, hands, and diaper area) with lukewarm water until the umbilical stump has fallen off and the belly button has healed and dried. This process will take approximately 2–3 weeks. During this time, use a cotton ball or cotton-tipped stick dipped in alcohol to dab the belly button stump and the skin around it twice daily. Once the stump has fallen off, clean the area twice daily with soap and water. Dry thoroughly with cotton balls.

Once the navel has dried you may bathe the baby daily, or every two days or whatever suits your schedule. The room should be warm. All your "equipment" should be within arm's reach —tissues, baby wipes, cotton balls, washcloth or natural sponge, soap, shampoo, moisturizer, powder, hair brush, small comb with rounded edges, cotton-tipped sticks, and a large fluffy towel. When you begin to bathe your baby, you may find the sink (at a good height) or a baby bathtub easier and more comfortable to use than an adult bathtub for up to 6 months of age. Keep the water depth no more than 10 cm (4 in.) and again lukewarm. When using an adult bathtub a suction-cupped rubber bath mat will prevent the baby from slipping. Remember to support his head with one hand while bathing him with the other. The baby's hair may be washed daily or 2–3 times weekly in warm water. Rinse well with a washcloth from the forehead back. Clean the diaper area last. After bathing, wrap and dry the baby off in a soft towel. Don't forget to towel baby in all the creases and folds, especially under the chin and between the fingers and toes – keep them dry. Style the hair as you wish. When finished, give your baby a good cuddle and take a great big sniff – nothing smells sweeter.

Remember, babies can squirm like a freshly caught bass. Be gentle but hold them firmly. Never run the water while your baby is in the bath. Always check the temperature of the water before putting the baby into it. Never, ever leave the baby unattended in the bath. When moving the baby in or out for bathing, place one of your hands on the baby's upper back for support, with his head resting on your wrist. Place your other hand between his legs to support the lower back.

No special care is required for a boy's foreskin. You do not have to retract it. For infant females, clean the vulva region by gently opening the labia and then wiping from front to back (to prevent germs from spreading into the vagina, which may cause an infection) with a cotton ball soaked in baby oil – one swipe only for each cotton ball. Do not become a "hyper wiper". Excessive wiping will result in irritation of the area, with a subsequent rash. It is unnecessary to clean the vaginal opening of mucus. Mucus flow from the vagina is normal and helps clear out bacteria.

If the baby's skin after drying appears rash free, you do not need to apply any product to the skin before diapering (see also Rash – Diaper Rash).

Remember, safety first. Accidents happen in a fraction of a second. Most are avoidable. Ensure that wherever you are bathing, drying, dressing or just changing a diaper is secure – the closer to the ground the better. A baby, before developing head control, may drown if face down in as little as a saucer of water.

Ears

Clean the outer ear with a moist warm washcloth. Never insert cotton-tipped sticks into the ear canal to remove wax that you can visualize. If this is repeated on a regular basis, wax will be gradually pushed deeper into the canal, causing impaction. This could result in a mild hearing loss and continuing discomfort. Removal of impacted wax can be very difficult for the doctor. It may be required in order to visualize the eardrum if there is a suspicion of a middle-ear infection. Removal of impacted wax is usually very discomforting for the child (as well as distressing for the parent). A general rule – nothing smaller than your elbow should ever enter your child's ear.

Eyes and Nose

You may notice some discharge in the corner of the child's eyes. Using a cotton ball moistened with warm water, wipe the eye from the inner corner outwards. Use a clean cotton ball with each wipe and when finished, dry with a cotton ball. Removing mucus from the baby's nose is unnecessary. It is most often bothering you and not the baby. If you really cannot stand it then gently remove the mucus with your fingertips – nothing else.

Nails

The baby's nails are quite soft and grow quickly. They may be bitten off or cut with infant nail clippers or infant nail scissors when you feel it is required (frequently if he continually scratches his face). It is much easier to cut the nails while the child is sleeping. I will never forget when my own daughter asked me to cut my granddaughter's nails for the first time. "No problem," said I. Once the bleeding had stopped she said thank–you and never asked again!

A word about cotton-tipped sticks: never insert them in any opening (eyes, nose, ears, genitalia or rectum).

Caring for your baby should be a pleasure and not a chore. Talking or singing to the baby during sponging, diaper changing or bathing will help to calm an apprehensive infant. A mother's voice is one of the best "pacifiers" a baby can have!

Bad Breath (Halitosis)

Halitosis, or "jungle breath", as it is commonly called, surprisingly can occur from early infancy. More often than not there is no cause to be found for it and it usually disappears with time.

In infants, milk residue on the baby's tongue can cause an odor. Clean the tongue with a washcloth or toothbrush.

In an older infant or child, the following are possible explanations for bad breath:

• Morning breath

- Mouth breathing – due to enlarged tonsils and adenoids
- Dental decay
- Gum and gingival disease
- Chronic sinusitis
- Chronic inflammation of the tonsils and/or adenoids
- Food that becomes lodged in the crypts of the tonsils or between the teeth
- A foreign body in the nose
- Diet
- Postnasal drip
- Recurrent esophageal reflux (spitting up) – usually not an obvious cause because the child swallows the vomitus and it goes undetected
- A retropharyngeal pouch – this is an out-pouching of the upper swallowing tube. Food may become trapped in the pouch and decay there. This results in bad breath. This condition is rare and can only be diagnosed by scoping (looking at) the esophagus. In small children this would require a light general anesthetic.

Morning breath, which occurs after prolonged sleeping or napping, is caused by the lack of saliva flow while sleeping. The saliva in the mouth remains stagnant, along with any debris found there. In this low-oxygen environment anaerobic (not requiring oxygen to thrive) bacteria produce sulfurous compounds. It is the production of sulfur that causes bad breath. This condition most often clears up within an hour or two after the child wakes, when the flow of saliva (which contains oxygen) resumes.

Continuous mouth breathing due to an obstruction (enlarged tonsils and adenoids) can cause drying of the mouth, also resulting in a sulfurous odor. Removing the tonsils and adenoids would be considered only if the halitosis is affecting the child in social settings and if other methods to increase saliva flow, such as chewing on sugarless gum or sucking on sugarless lozenges do not correct the problem.

The diet is reviewed. Symptoms of gastroesophageal reflux (spitting up) are investigated. Often the child is too young to communicate the markers for this. A persistent cough, especially when he lies down, which is relieved only when he sits up or stands, may be the only symptomatic clue.

The management of this condition depends on the cause. Sometimes it is the caregiver himself who has an over-sensitive sense of smell. Frequently when I examine the child, I can detect nothing abnormal, yet the parent insists that a foul odor is present.

Certain ethnic diets may result in a breath odor which is foreign to others. This should not be considered halitosis.

Brushing the teeth twice a day with toothpaste (no fluoride until 4-1/2 to 5 years of age) is most often all that is necessary. If a fluoride-containing toothpaste is used, the amount should be no more than the top of a matchstick. If the child can gargle, any mouthwash may be used. Breath freshener mints are fine. Sugarless gum for the older child will help keep the saliva flowing and thereby diminish bad breath. Any of grandma's "home-brewed" remedies may be tried, including chewing on mint or parsley. A trip to the dentist should definitely be considered.

Chronic sinusitis (a persistent green nasal discharge) is a very uncommon cause of bad breath. It really can only be confirmed with a CAT scan of the sinuses. A postnasal drip which causes mouth odor is also frequently present with chronic sinusitis.

A foul-smelling discharge from one side of the nose may be caused by a foreign body and be mistaken for halitosis. Once it is removed the odor quickly disappears.

The bottom line is as follows: seldom is the cause for bad breath determined. It is usually self-limiting. More often than not it bothers the caregiver and not the child. If others do not notice or comment on your child's breath, then it is likely that you are over-sensitive and concerned over very little.

Bed Bugs

Do not read the following article if you are at all squeamish or have just finished eating.

All you need to know about bed bugs that you wish you never had to know: Bed bugs are really nasty little critters – the vampires of the insect world.

Bed bugs are pale, oval, and flat in appearance and measure approximately 4–9 mm in length. After feeding on human blood they become bloated and turn dark red. They are found widely distributed around the world.

The lifespan of these bugs is approximately one year. Females during this time can lay up to 400 eggs. They are laid in clusters of 10–50 eggs. Eggs hatch in about 10 days.

These bugs can be found anywhere where there is a crease, crevice or small crack in bedding, furniture, floorboards and walls. Cribs and children's mattresses are not excluded from these bugs' hunting ground. They can be transported on clothing, in suitcases and by many other modes of transportation.

The bugs live on human blood. They can survive up to 6 months after a single feed.

They hide during the day and feed at night. The most common bite sites on humans are on exposed areas (the face, neck, arms, hands and legs). Often the bites appear in a straight line in a group of 3. These have been nicknamed "breakfast", "lunch" and "supper". Oftentimes, the presence of blood smears (crushed bugs) on the bed linen or dark spots of dried bed bug excrement along mattress seams are signs suggestive of an infestation of bed bugs. Similarly, fecal brown spots, shed skins and egg casings can be found near their hiding places.

The lesions of a bed bug's bite appear as small red or white firm swellings. They are very itchy. Bed bug phobia may affect individuals, resulting in stress, insomnia and anxiety.

Treatment consists of preventing scratching by keeping the fingernails short and by using an oral antihistamine. Continued scratching may cause infections that require either topical or oral antibiotics. The bites are not contagious.

Getting rid of bed bugs is a difficult task. They are considered by many experts to be the most difficult pests to exterminate. Treatment of the infested area requires the elimination of all bugs and eggs. This can be extremely difficult to do without professional help. With the ban on many types of insecticides (such as DDT), bed bugs have become resistant to many of the pesticides now being used. Many extermination companies are using trained dogs to sniff out bed bug hiding places.

Most professional companies use a combination of pesticides, vacuuming and steam cleaning. More expensive yet more environmentally friendly methods of ridding bed bugs include using either extreme heat or freezing techniques (must be frozen for at least 2 weeks).

Prevention is difficult. In hotels, apartments and motels avoidance can be very challenging. Be wary when purchasing secondhand furniture or beds. Examine them closely before they are purchased and brought into your home. When travelling, it is prudent to examine the bed and furniture before unpacking. Keep luggage off the floor on luggage racks.

Be cautious of any unproven advertised treatments that promise complete eradication. The majority of them do not work and are a waste of your time, effort and money.

My advice is: if you have a problem with bed bugs, call in the professionals. Review their credentials and ask for 2 or 3 names and phone numbers of satisfied customers to check the company's references.

The good news is bed bugs do not carry any disease. The bad news is that until they are removed they are a troubling disruption to your daily routine and cause a great deal of emotional stress.

Bed Sharing (Co-sleeping)

Newborns, infants and toddlers have been sharing beds with their parents since the beginning of time. The chief reason was necessity – there was only one place to sleep. Two more reasons are given for bed sharing. The first is that it is extremely convenient for the mother to breastfeed her child. The second explanation is based on the hypothesis that bed sharing gives the infant more security. It was thought to promote better bonding with parents than sleeping separately in a crib.

No studies have ever shown an increase in bonding or the feeling of security in children who have co-shared a bed with their parents for any length of time, as compared to those who have not.

On the other hand, there are hazards involved that parents must be made aware of, should they decide to co-sleep with their infant. There is a 40-fold increased incidence of suffocation in infants who bed share. Some of these deaths are related to SIDS. Most, however, are related to an obstruction to breathing. There are many situations that are causes for obstruction; a parent who rolls over onto the infant during sleep; an infant smothered under the breast of the mother; an infant's face gets covered by a pillow, or blanket, or the infant ends up faced down on a loose blanket; the infant becomes lodged between the bed and the headboard, bedside table or wall. These are only a few situations that could result in infant suffocation during bed sharing.

If you have still decided to bed share, I suggest the following:

- If you are a heavy sleeper, don't bed share at all!
- Never smoke, drink alcohol or take medication that may cause increased drowsiness while in bed.
- A firm mattress (no waterbed) with a well-fitted, tight bottom sheet is required.
- Pillows, comforters or heavy blankets should be avoided.
- The mattress must be tight up against the headboard, the footboard, the wall and the side tables.
- No cords should be hanging within reach of the infant.

In this pediatrician's view, bed sharing should not mean sharing the bed but sharing the room. If you wish the baby to be near you, then place his crib next to your bed. This is the best and safest place for him to sleep. It also provides you with a convenient place which gives easy access to your baby in order to meet his needs.

Also keep in mind that with bed sharing, you may have a titanic struggle later on when you eventually decide to switch the baby to sleeping in his own crib, own bed or own bedroom.

PS: Intimacy between caregivers is much improved if there is no baby sharing your bed. Where is dad sleeping? In the basement?

Birthmarks

Mongolian Spots

Mongolian spots are bluish discolorations that lie flat on the skin. They look like bruises. They may occur anywhere on the body but most often are found on the lower back and buttocks. There is a well-defined edge between them and the surrounding normal skin. They are non-tender. Over a period of a few years they will slowly fade and disappear completely.

Port Wine Stain

A port wine stain is a reddish-blue discolouration in the skin. It is flat and non-tender. Its margin is quite distinct from the normal skin.

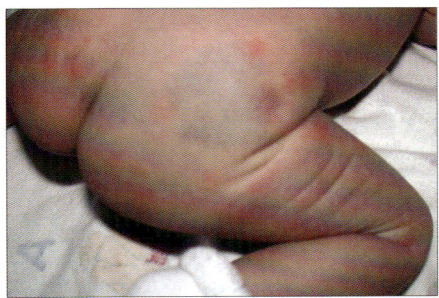
Mongolian Spots

Port wine stains remain for life and will increase in size as the child grows.

Port wine stains on the face may be associated with small areas of calcification in the brain. Together they are called Sturge-Weber syndrome. Depending on the degree of brain involvement there may be developmental delay and seizures. Intracranial lesions are diagnosed by skull x-rays, CAT scan or MRI. Laser surgery, if it is desired for cosmetic reasons, will greatly diminish the intense colour.

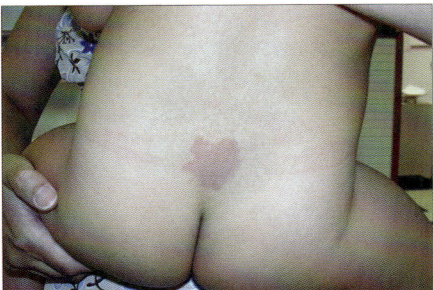
Port Wine Stain

Capillary Hemangioma

Capillary hemangiomas may be present at birth or appear at any time during the first year of life. They are usually raised, blood-red and have a "bumpy" feel. They are composed of tiny capillary blood vessels. They turn white when pressed with the finger.

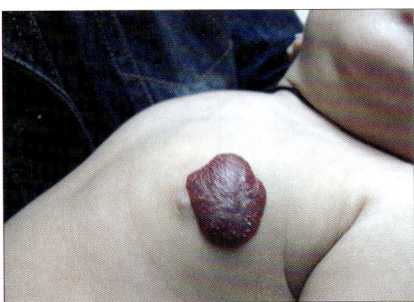
Strawberry Hemangioma

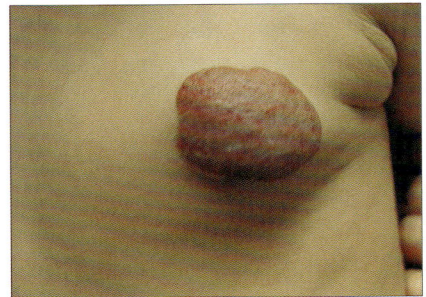
Pale Areas of Hemangioma – signs of blood vessel regression

During the first year of life they may increase in size. Thereafter, they may spontaneously regress and completely disappear by 5–6 years of age or earlier. Little further regression will occur after 6 years of age. With regression of the blood vessels the surface of the hemangioma will start to have a whitish appearance. With increased regression the whitish area of skin will increase in size. With complete regression the overlying skin may have a completely normal appearance. There may, however, be a small degree of depigmentation and a "weathered" look and roughened feel to the overlying skin.

Laser surgery after 6–7 years of age, if cosmetically desired, will aid in its resolution.

Café au Lait Spots

These are light to dark brown pigmented flat areas of skin of varying sizes and shape. They may have excessive hair growth (hairy nevus). They are painless. They do not disappear and they increase in size as the child grows.

They are of no concern unless they are many in number. A condition called Von Recklinghausen's disease or neurofibromatosis has as one of its characteristic findings numerous café au lait spots (more than 8–10 with at least one spot over 2 cm in diameter).

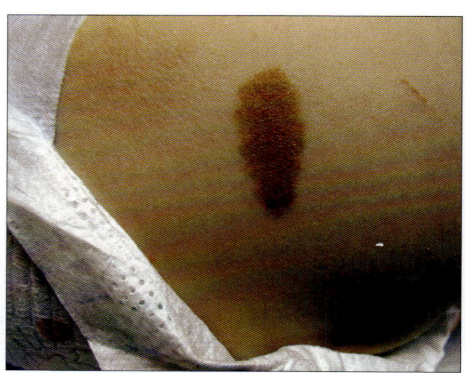
Café au Lait Spot

Body Mass Index (BMI)

The BMI is an excellent indicator to determine if your child's weight is appropriate for his height. It enables the doctor to measure the child's body fat in order to determine if there are risks for his being underweight or overweight.

The doctor will use a body mass index for the age percentile chart, along with the BMI, to plot the percentage of body fat your child has as compared to standards for children of the same age and sex.

If your child's BMI is above the 95th percentile he is considered to be overweight. Those who are in the 85th to 95th percentile range are considered to be at risk of becoming overweight.

If the BMI is less than the 5th percentile the child is considered to be underweight. If the BMI is below the 15th percentile, there is a risk of becoming underweight.

For both boys and girls between 2 and 3 years of age, a BMI of over 18.5 is considered to be an indicator for being overweight (above the 95th percentile).

For boys between 3 and 6 years of age a BMI over 18 is considered overweight (above the 95th percentile).

With girls between 3 and 5 years of age a BMI over 18 (or a BMI over 19 between 5-6 years years of age) is considered an indicator for overweight (above the 95th percentile).

To calculate your child's BMI use one of the following formulas.

For pounds and inches (imperial):

Multiply the child's height x height. Divide this number into the child's weight. Multiply that number by 703. The resulting number will be the child's BMI.

For centimetres and kilograms (metric):

Multiply the child's height x height. Divide this number into the child's weight. The resulting number will be the child's BMI.

The BMI can be calculated and then plotted on a percentile chart on an annual basis, or even more frequently when there is concern about your child's progress or lack thereof. There are 2 variables to watch out for concerning weight: the pattern of acceleration, or too rapid an increase, which indicates an overweight child; or a pattern of slowed weight gain or deceleration, which is an indicator for an underweight child.

If the child is either overweight or underweight, appropriate investigations on an individual basis will be done to rule out any medical cause or if found, correct it. Overeating or undereating, as well as any social issues present, will be addressed.

Breastfeeding (Getting Off to the Right Start)

The Art and Skill

When I first started in practice some 40 years ago, it was customary for hospitals to allow a seven-day stay for mothers and infants who had been delivered vaginally. Those infants born by Caesarean section and their moms were given 10 days to recoup. Now, with the early discharge program, infants and moms are sent home 48 hours (some as soon as 24 hours) after the postpartum birth or 72 hours if the birth was by Caesarean section

These days during childbirth education classes, the majority of time is spent preparing mothers for labour and delivery. It is lamentable that not enough time is spent on follow-up postnatal care. Most notably, this includes learning the art and skill of breastfeeding.

At present in Canada 80% to 90% of mothers initiate breastfeeding. After 4 months approximately 40% were still exclusively breastfeeding. By the time the baby is 6 months of age, less than 10% are still exclusively breastfeeding (50% are giving some breast milk along with formula). Anecdotally, in my own practice (composed of a highly diverse ethnic mix) I would estimate that at least 40% of mothers who initiate breastfeeding have already supplemented their baby with formula by bottle on a regular basis by 3 days of age. The incidence today, as compared to 20 years ago, of mothers who initiate breastfeeding has improved only marginally. However, I strongly suspect that the number of mothers reportedly still breastfeeding their infants exclusively at 4 and 6 months has greatly diminished. I would not be surprised if newer statistics were to show a significant decrease in mothers who initiate breastfeeding and no longer exclusively nurse their infants by the one-month birthday. This does not bode well for something that is natural and beneficial and so important for both mother and her baby.

So, the question is, "Why are more mothers choosing not to breastfeed, and why are so many stopping breastfeeding before baby reaches 6 months of age?" There are numerous reasons and circumstances for this, many of which can be avoided. Unfortunately, many are not. This is distressing.

During the prenatal period so many mothers are not properly educated and prepared for both the emotional and physical strains that they will experience after the process of labour and delivery. Mothers are sent home, perhaps too early, from hospital before there is adequate supervision and education as to how to get the baby to latch and suckle. Added to this, mothers at this time are very uncomfortable from the delivery, very tired, and mentally drained. A crying baby is hard to tolerate. Mom's advisory staff (the unelected – mother, mother-in-law, etc.) will all too often advise her to supplement. Many hospitals are still sending a breastfeeding mother home with a formula supplement "just in case"!! There it is, sitting in the cupboard, very handy to use. The end result is that within one day of discharge (or earlier), the baby who is "on the breast" is also being supplemented with a bottle of formula. The baby seems to be more content with this arrangement. A bottle will drip just from holding it upside down, and because of this it seems so much easier for him to get milk from the bottle than the breast. Within a short period of time more formula and less and less breast milk is given. Without proper technique and frequent breastfeeding, the mother's breast milk will soon "dry up". Breastfeeding is doomed from the beginning.

I have mentioned some of the deterrents to successful breastfeeding, so now let's go over some of the positives and the advantages.

In this day and age there are very few products that you can get that are free of charge, already prepared and ready to use, packaged in very nice containers, fully natural (having no additives) and laying claim to be the finest "health product" on the market. Breast milk is one such product (probably the only one).

We all know the many beneficial health reasons to breastfeed. Recently, it has been shown that infants who are exclusively breastfed, as compared to those who are bottle-fed and introduced to solids at less than 4 months of age, are 6 times less likely to become obese as adults. Now, that is a real bonus and a further incentive to breastfeed your infant for at least 6 months or longer. By the way, delaying the introduction of solids until at least 4 months of age and preferably closer to 6 months of age reduces the risk of obesity in formula-fed infants.

To successfully nurse you require the following – mammary glands, a commitment to breastfeed (not just saying "I can try"), and a positive mental attitude which says that you can and will successfully breastfeed your baby ("I will do it"). Add to this your willing customer (the baby), and success will be yours and his. For this to work you must try your utmost to relax. The more stressed you are, the more difficult it is to be able to produce breast milk. Despite all the advances in supplemented formula composition, no substitute comes close to the excellence of breast milk. Breast milk provides the baby with better immunity, the best building blocks for both his short and long term health, and breastfeeding is the best way in which mom and baby can bond. Remarkably, recent studies have shown too that breast-feeding significantly reduces the incidence of breast cancer in mothers who nurse who also have a strong family history of this disease (by as much as 50%).

Get as much rest as you possibly can. You should try to sleep when your baby sleeps. Have your husband do as many of the daily household routines as he can tolerate so that you can concentrate on your strength in order to meet the baby's needs.

During pregnancy the breasts are being prepared to breastfeed. They become larger and are already producing milk. A little milk may leak from the nipples. When breastfeeding is initiated, a hormone called prolactin is produced. This hormone stimulates the milk glands in the breasts to produce milk. The first milk the baby receives is called colostrum. As soon as baby enters the world the milk "factories" are primed and ready to go. As soon as the baby is placed on mom's tummy, after birth, he should be put to the breast. Most babies will show a desire to latch and suckle within 30-40 minutes of being born. You have the milk and he has the equipment to get it. As the baby suckles there is the release of another hormone in mother called oxytocin. This hormone signals the breasts to let the milk flow. It also helps mother's uterus to contract.

There is no set feeding schedule. Feed the baby on demand. Remember, every baby is different, so do not compare one with another. Demand-feeding essentially means that you feed the baby whenever he is hungry. How do you know he is hungry? Frequent wakening, crying, rooting (sucking motion of lips) and sucking on fists are the most common symptoms that your baby is hungry. Whether you feed the baby every 2 hours or 4 hours is established between you and the baby. Six to 12 feedings over a 24-hour period is the norm. At night if the baby seems satisfied and is sleeping, you may let him go for 4–5 hours before feeding him again.

Unfortunately for mom, the baby may not recognize the difference between night and day. For him a day is a day – 24 hours. Keep it bright and noisy during the day and the reverse at night. Eventually he will catch on.

In the early days babies may breastfeed very frequently – called cluster feeding. This is normal and occurs during growth spurts. It does not mean that you do not have enough milk.

This first "milk" that baby gets is called colostrum. This "pre-milk" is rich in antibodies, which helps give the baby increased immunity, fat stores and other essential nutrients. The baby needs very little of this during the first 2 days of life to thrive (15–30 ml with each feed). After day 3, the milk supply will increase to meet his needs and demands as long as he is allowed to nurse. It is this sucking action that will keep breast milk production to a maximum and flowing freely and plentifully. By day 4 or 5 the breasts should start feeling very full, demonstrating that the "milk production factories" are working as designed.

The baby, during the first week of life, may normally lose 5%–7% of his body weight. By 2 weeks of age he should be back to his original birth weight. Doctors do not want the baby to lose more than 10% of their birth weight.

Babies receiving adequate amounts of breast milk should have at least 1 wet diaper on day 1; 2 wet diapers on day 2; 3 wet diapers on day 3; and 4–6 wet diapers thereafter.

Your baby, during the first day of life, will pass a thick greenish black stool called meconium. Over the next 2–3 days the meconium diminishes and a more normal yellow stool will be produced. On day 1 the baby should pass one stool, 2 stools on days 2 and 3. By day 4 the baby may have a stool which is loose, yellow and seedy in nature after each breast-feeding. More or less stooling is also normal. **Green** coloured stools are fine.

If there are any problems with breastfeeding, before you reach for a supplement, my advice is to consult someone knowledgeable in breastfeeding. The most knowledgeable people are breastfeeding consultants. They can be contacted at the hospital of birth, or any hospital near you. Public Health also has consultants whom you can contact. Do not leave the hospital until you are entirely comfortable with breastfeeding and reassured that the baby is latching properly. If leaving later is not an option, ask for a follow-up with a lactation consultant the next day.

Supplemental feeding may be required, especially if the baby is losing too much weight (more than 10% of birth weight). The best supplement is expressed breast milk. The decision to supplement should be made in consultation with your family physician, pediatrician, or public health nurse or, better still, a lactation specialist. They will advise you on how to pump your breasts to obtain milk for supplementation and ensure a good milk supply. Frequent breastfeeding should not be discontinued but encouraged. Some babies may require formula supplementation for medical reasons concerning the mom, if they are not nursing well or if there are issues with milk supply. Supplementation with any iron-fortified formula is fine. About 15–30 cc (or more if he consumes it) should be placed in a sterilized medicine cup or shot glass. It should be served lukewarm. Place the cup so it is touching the baby's lower lip. Then gently tip it to allow 1 or 2 drops of formula to touch his lips. This will stimulate him to open his mouth, and start licking. With continuation of the process the baby will lap up the milk with his tongue as a cat would. Do not pour the supplemental milk into the baby's mouth, because the baby may choke and perhaps aspirate the milk into his lungs. If the baby stops drinking, do not remove the cup unless you're absolutely sure that he will not take any more. Each baby will feed at his/her own pace.

Normally, if the baby has already filled his tummy with breast milk he will no longer be hungry and therefore take no supplement. If, however, he is still hungry, give him as much expressed breast milk or formula by cup as he wants after breastfeeding (after 20 minutes of "active" sucking on each breast). If you find it difficult to feed the baby by cup you can try using a syringe or spoon. Hopefully, within 2 weeks or less, the baby will be on the breast alone without supplementation. Avoid feeding by bottle and, as well, do not introduce a pacifier until he is well established on the breast (at approximately one month of age).

Another supplemental method that may be tried to encourage your baby to breastfeed until you have a sufficient milk supply is to tube-feed him. This should be done under the supervision of a lactation specialist. With this method a syringe is filled with expressed breast milk or formula. It is attached to a tube. The other end is taped to the mother's breast with the end of the tube right beside the nipple. The syringe is placed at the level of mom's heart (slightly above the level of the baby's head). The milk will flow as the baby sucks. The baby will think he is getting milk straight from the breast and, hopefully, will start suckling vigorously once he has the taste of it. This method is continued until the reason for supplementation has resolved. In my opinion this is the optimal method to supplement a baby if it is required.

Some babies, after just a few minutes on the breast, tend to fall asleep. To wake baby up and encourage him to start sucking again, try expressing breast milk into his mouth by gently squeezing the breast. Feeding the baby while he is wearing a diaper only allows the baby to be skin to skin with mother, which stimulates suckling. The occasional flick of your fingers on his toes should get his attention to start sucking again. Changing the diaper if needed will wake him up. It is normal for babies to fall asleep between breasts and they will often wake up for the other side when they are ready. Some babies will be content after nursing on one side. As long as the baby is waking to feed, voiding, stooling and gaining weight, all is well. If you are concerned consult your physician or a lactation specialist.

To prevent difficulty weaning the baby when you wish to, I recommend that you introduce a bottle of expressed breast milk or formula 2–3 times a week after the baby is well established on the breast (8–10 weeks of age). When the time comes, weaning will be a lot easier if the baby has already learned to accept a bottle of milk. Although there is no research to support this, in my 40 years of practice I have seen this method help greatly during the weaning process.

Mother's diet should be well-balanced (remember you are now eating for two). I suggest that mothers continue to take their prenatal multivitamins during the breastfeeding period. They also should be ingesting, through diet or by supplement pill, a minimum of 600 mg of omega-3 and -6 fatty acids during the breastfeeding phase. Farmed Atlantic salmon, tuna, sardines, and anchovies are high in omega acids and should be consumed 3 times weekly or more. Other foods rich in omega-3 are fortified eggs and milk. There are a number of other choices that can be investigated.

Breast milk does not contain sufficient amounts of vitamin D, which the baby requires. After he is 1 to 2 weeks of age, begin to supplement your baby with 400 international units (IU) of vitamin D. If he is receiving only the occasional supplement of formula (1 bottle per day), 400 IU of vitamin D is still required daily. If he is receiving formula supplements after each breast feed or more than 3 bottles a day only 200 IU of vitamin D is required daily (additional amounts will be supplied by the formula). No additional vitamin D is required if formula feeding approximates 70% or more of the total breast and formula daily intake.

You may notice an orange discolouration on the diaper. This is not blood. They are urate crystals present in the urine that turn orange when they make contact with air. Usually, the presence of urate crystals is not a concern. However, if they are present after the third to fifth day, it may indicate that the baby is not taking in enough milk. Consult your physician, public health nurse or lactation consultant to ensure that your baby is breastfeeding well and to assess your milk supply. You can try to increase breast milk supply by putting the baby to each breast every 2 hours for 20-30 minutes of active nursing during the day and every 3–4 hours during the night. This should increase the amount of breast milk available to the baby. After 2 days you should be able to go back to a more realistic routine, feeding the baby every 3–4 hours during the day and every 4 hours at night. The total number of feeds per day usually ranges from 8–10. With adequate breast milk intake, the urine will become less concentrated and the urate crystals will disappear.

I do not recommend that you share the bed with your baby. Although this may be more convenient for you, the risk of the baby's suffocating is increased by 40 times. It is better for you and your baby to sleep separately – you in your bed, and the baby's bed beside yours.

The actual technique of how to breastfeed, and the manner in which to hold and latch, are well detailed in numerous books, pamphlets and websites with support information. Much of this information is made available to you at the hospital where you give birth.

Ultimately, breastfeeding for 6 months or longer is the best nutritional start at life that you can give your baby. If for any reason you have to supplement the baby while you are breastfeeding him on a regular basis, do not fret; so be it. The baby will still receive the benefit of your breast milk. For those moms who discontinue breastfeeding for whatever reason, do not feel that you have failed your child. You have tried your best and that is all that one can ask. Hopefully, you'll successfully breastfeed your subsequent children – perhaps even triplets!!

Do I Have Enough?

If the baby is frequently wetting many diapers then most likely he is getting enough milk. Ask yourself the following questions – Are my breasts full prior to feeding (do they feel full)? Are they soft after feeding (that is, the baby is getting the milk you are producing)? Does one breast "leak" milk as the baby is sucking on the other? All are signs of good milk production. The only true way to tell is by the amount of weight the baby is gaining. Your doctor will tell you if you are supplying the baby with adequate amounts of breast milk. Test weighing, whereby the baby is weighed in the doctor's office or clinic before and after breastfeeding, is sometimes done to see how much the baby has received during a feed.

Breast Care

If your baby has latched and fed well you should have little or no problems with your breasts. To prevent problems with your nipples, do not use soap to clean them. This may cause drying of the nipples with subsequent cracking. After breastfeeding express a small amount of breast milk onto your nipples. Then gently rub the milk onto your nipples and areola. Allow the milk to dry, before putting on a wireless, well-fitting brassiere.

Common Breastfeeding Problems

Poor Latch

Without a proper latch, your infant will have a problem obtaining breast milk. There are a number of problems leading to a poor latch – they can include inverted or flat nipples, poor technique in initiating latch, or, not infrequently, a crying, fussy baby who just will not latch, even though he's hungry. Normally, if you cup your breast between your thumb and fingers and gently compress the breast, it should be ready for latching. Place your nipple close to his lips, and when he opens his mouth, bringing him forward so that his mouth completely covers most of your areola. If the baby is fussy and will not latch, I suggest that you both get into a warm bath. This should relax you and the baby, making latching easier. If there is still a problem with latching please contact a lactation consultant.

Sore and Cracked Nipples

If during breastfeeding your nipples hurt, then the latch is not proper. A proper latch is when your nipple is completely in his mouth and most of the baby's lips cover your areola. The baby's lips when properly latched will be flanged, like a fish mouth. If this does not occur, you will experience pain in your nipples, with possible cracking. Check with a person who has expertise in lactation technique if the above occurs. If your nipples become cracked, apply breast milk to the nipple and areola, then air out your breasts as often and for as long as possible. After each breastfeeding express a few drops of breast milk to rub on your nipples (let the milk dry). There are breast creams that can be applied for symptomatic relief. A breast shell worn under the brassiere will prevent your nipples from rubbing against the brassiere, and thus alleviate some discomfort.

Mastitis

Inflammation of the breast, called mastitis, presents as tender areas in your breast, with the overlying skin inflamed and warm. There may be red streaks radiating up your breast toward your axilla (armpit). You may also have a slight fever. Antibiotics are required along with warm compresses. Do not stop breastfeeding.

Thrush Infection

If you have a burning sensation in the nipples, it may be a result of a yeast infection. Other than slight redness of the nipple, no rash will be noticeable. Your baby, at the same time, will most likely have the same infection in his mouth. It looks like milk curds on the gums that cannot be rubbed off. A white discolouration of the tongue alone is not thrush, but only milk residue. Medication will be required for both you and the baby – a cream for your nipples (which does not have to be cleaned off before breastfeeding) and an oral suspension for the baby. It takes a 7-day treatment and a repeat, if required. If there is no response with 2 one-week treatments, a medication change will be required.

Spitting up Blood

If the baby spits up blood, it is usually from your nipple. The baby will be fine. Treat as a cracked nipple – see above. Continue to breastfeed. If the spitting up of blood continues and there is no evidence of a cracked nipple, a visit to your doctor is suggested to rule out a ductal papilloma in your breast.

Jaundice

Most infants have a small degree of jaundice starting at day 3 after birth. This is normal physiological jaundice and will disappear within 2–3 weeks. Infants who are breastfeeding may have a degree of jaundice, which is also normal. Physiological jaundice, with added breast milk jaundice, is usually of a higher degree than for those infants with physiological jaundice who are bottle-fed alone. Breast milk jaundice may last for up to 6–8 weeks. This is the norm. Only if the child becomes dehydrated or very lethargic will the jaundice level be elevated to a point of concern. This is very uncommon. Phototherapy is rarely required for breast milk jaundice. There is nothing in particular that you have to do with an infant who has breast milk jaundice (for example, putting him near a window to expose him to the light is unnecessary).

Blocked Milk Ducts

You may experience a painful lump in one of your breasts. This is most likely due to a blocked milk duct. Because the milk is unable to pass through the duct, the milk gland becomes swollen and tender. If this occurs, use hot compresses frequently on the area. A hot shower may also give symptomatic relief. Try to massage the nodule with a motion towards the nipple. Have the baby feed on this breast first.

Engorged Breasts

You may be one of the fortunate ones who produce more breast milk than the baby consumes. Express breast milk between feeds and store for future use. See Feeding for breast milk storage. If there is a latching problem your breasts will become engorged and painful. Consult a lactation consultant.

Medications to Avoid

If a physician prescribes a medication for you, remind him or her that you are breastfeeding. With most antibiotics you may continue to breastfeed. Laxatives can be taken without problem. Many over-the-counter medications may be used safely, including those for pain relief (but avoid codeine). Most other medications will not interfere with the baby by crossing over into the breast milk. If you are in doubt, before you stop breastfeeding, consult with your pharmacist, a lactation consultant, or your doctor.

Unfortunately, because of certain medications, you may have to stop breastfeeding. If this is the case then express breast milk on a regular basis and discard it. After the medication is finished, you may restart breastfeeding in 48 hours (to give time for the medication to clear your system).

Insufficient Milk Supply

It is the frequent sucking that stimulates the breast milk production and flow. Put the baby to the breast every 2 hours for 30 minutes of active sucking on each breast. During the night feed every 3 hours. After 2 days your breast milk should be flowing to satisfy his hunger. If it is not, I suggest that you go to the health food store and buy blessed thistle and fenugreek. Take

2–3 capsules of each 3 times a day. Breast milk flow should increase within a few days. They work best to stimulate breast milk production in the first 2 weeks of initiating breast-feeding. You can continue with these herbs for as long as you wish. There are no serious side effects, either short or long-term, for either you or the baby. A medication called Domperidone (which requires a prescription), may also be used to increase breast milk production. A visit to a lactation consultant may be required to assess the quality of feeding. Post-feeding pumping every 3 hours for 10 minutes may be required.

Tongue Tie

Under the tongue there is a piece of skin that attaches the bottom of the tongue to the floor of the mouth. It is called the frenulum. Rarely, if the tissue is attached too far forward on the tongue, the infant may have problems with extending his tongue for proper latching. If your baby is able to extend his tongue to his lower lip then there should be no problem with latching. If, however, this does not occur and there is a concern that the frenulum is impeding a proper latch, then the "tongue tie" should be released. This is most commonly done by an ear, nose and throat specialist. It is a simple and quick procedure done in his office. If this is the reason for poor nursing, then the baby should have immediate improvement with his latch. Complications of this procedure are rare.

Supplemental Bottles of Milk

Once the baby is well established on the breast, supplementation with a bottle of milk (no more than once a day) is fine. Bottle supplementation may be started at around 6–8 weeks of age. By that time nipple preference (your breast) has been well established, so there is little concern that he might prefer the bottle over the breast. It is best to supplement with expressed breast milk. If there are insufficient quantities of breast milk, a powdered formula may be substituted. Giving him a bottle does have benefits. It gives you a break, especially if someone else, such as your husband, feeds the baby. It gives dad more one-on-one time to spend with the baby and helps them to bond. If you have to leave for a short period of time, you will be reassured that the baby will drink. It also makes weaning much easier (this is a real bonus).

Fathers

While your wife is breastfeeding and doing the main share of baby care, this is certainly not the time for you to be sitting around as a bystander. She needs your emotional support and as much help as you can offer. You must understand that your wife has just gone through a period of extreme mental and physical duress during her pregnancy – culminating with labour and delivery. Now there is another living being that you both are responsible for. You are the one who needs to take the initiative, to be by your partner's side and to help her; so step up to the plate and hit a homer!

For babies who are being breastfed at approximately 2–3 months of age, the stools may still be occurring daily but may be spread out with several days between each bowel movement. The stools, although infrequent, are soft and passed without pain. They are yellow/brown/green in colour. If the baby is comfortable and in no distress, and this has become his stooling pattern, it does not matter what the time interval is between stools. Nothing is broken; therefore nothing has to be fixed; no suppositories or anything else is required to induce a bowel movement. Do not listen to your "advisory staff"! In my practice, one mother waited patiently for 21 days before her baby stooled. We celebrated with a glass of champagne and an extra breastfeeding for the baby. We thought that we had broken the Guinness book of world records. Unfortunately the record, I believe, was 32 days, but we gave it a good try.

The colour of stools may change from yellow to green to brown. This is normal.

Note: All breastfeeding mothers should remain on a well-balanced diet. Continue with your prenatal vitamins, taking at least 1000 IU of vitamin D daily, as well as a minimum of 600 mg, either in the diet or by supplement, of DHA (omega 3). All breastfed infants at 1–2 weeks of age should be supplemented with 400 IU of vitamin D daily until at least 8 months of age.

For more information on breastfeeding refer to Feeding Infants.

Breastfeeding–Weaning (from Breast and Bottle)

Breast

You have successfully breastfed for long as you wanted. The baby has thrived. The time has come when you would like to wean the baby off the breast. Some infants make the transition from breast to bottle or cup with ease. For these lucky ones there are no problems in the weaning process. There are, however, many mothers who do not have it this easy. Sometimes there follows a titanic struggle between the mother and baby, which too often leaves the mother frustrated, crying and completely lost as to what to do. The baby resists to the end of his endurance, with every scream known to mankind, by constantly wiggling his head and pushing out the bottle nipple with his tongue and never giving up the "battle for the breast".

Let's step back and try to understand how the problem evolved. It would all make sense if you were to think about it from the baby's point of view. From minutes after arriving into this world he has been put to the breast. This has been his sole source of nourishment for months. He loves the milk. He loves the warmth of being snuggled with his mother. He can smell, touch and hear his mother breathe while breastfeeding. From his point of view what could be more fulfilling? Nothing! As a result he is not going to give up this security and comfort without a major confrontation.

So here we are – you against the baby. Who is going to win? I probably do not have to answer this – the baby, of course. Your intellectual instincts tell you to quit; however, your maternal instincts rule. You cannot sit by and watch the baby cry, and as a result you give in and breast-feed the baby. I fully understand and sympathize with the bind that you find yourself in.

Could the problem have been prevented? There is no scientific evidence to support its prevention. However, after nearly 40 years of practice, I do get the feeling there is a simple way to prevent difficulty in weaning or at least soften the transition period. Once the baby is well-established on the breast (4 to 6 weeks), I feel the early introduction of a bottle of expressed breast milk, water or formula once every two days or so will help in the weaning process. At this early age the baby will learn to accept a bottle. It will not jeopardize your breastfeeding and will make weaning from the breast a much more pleasant experience for you and the baby when you are ready to wean.

What can be done, however, if the problem does arise?

The most important thing that you must remember, and burn this into your mind, is that an otherwise healthy baby will drink when he is thirsty and, in fact, will drink adequate amounts so as not to dehydrate. Let me repeat that – an otherwise healthy baby will drink when thirsty. Let us say, for whatever reason, you have to leave the baby under someone else's care for a day or longer. I can practically guarantee you that when thirsty, the baby will drink. I can also guarantee that no baby has harmed himself by crying, even for prolonged periods of time. It'll have no short-term physical effects or cause any long-term psychological trauma for the baby. I do, however, also predict that the psychological trauma of weaning will be carried by you if you cannot weather this short-term absence.

Here are some helpful suggestions:

• You may have to try several types of nipples before you get the right one for your infant. If the baby is over 8 months of age you may even want to try a sippy cup.

• Have someone other than you feed the baby. After all, the baby associates you and not dad with the breast.

• Try to start with expressed breast milk. Rub some breast milk onto the nipple of the bottle so that his first taste is milk rather than the artificial nipple. You must be patient and not get upset if the formula is refused. Put the bottle down and pacify the baby. Try again. If unsuccessful, place the baby down and have a cup of tea. Try again. Do not give in. Have faith that when the baby is thirsty, the baby will drink. If this is a "battle" that you want to win then you must be ready to "fight" it. If you feel that you are failing, then you have to remove yourself completely from the baby. Go to a movie, go shopping, visit a friend, go to the library and read a book or go out for coffee. Let the father or other caregiver take care of the baby.

The advice above is for the mother who has great difficulty weaning her baby off the breast. If there is no problem I suggest the following:

There are basically 2 methods to wean the baby off the breast. The first is to stop the breast milk completely and feed the baby formula or whole milk (if over 10 months of age). If the baby accepts formula, this is fine. You probably will have engorgement of your breasts with mild to moderate discomfort. Wear a tight binder, and take ibuprofen or acetaminophen for pain. An ice pack may help. If in extreme pain, you can express a small quantity of breast milk to relieve the discomfort. There are no medications available to stop your breast milk production once it's well established. The second method is to stop 1 breastfeeding session every 3 to 4 days. Start with the supper feed and substitute the breast milk with formula or whole milk (if over 10 months of age). Every 3 to 4 days stop another feeding time, until you gradually wean the baby off the breast. With this method there should be no discomfort.

I truly sympathize with the moms who are emotionally unable to stop breastfeeding. I am sure many would continue for years if it was socially acceptable. Certainly, breast milk is the best milk and you should continue breastfeeding for as long as you wish and are able to supply the child with enough milk. Many times, however, with the mother who has too little milk to give, the child is using her as a "human pacifier". This is especially true with a breastfed infant who wakes up several times a night. To pacify him, mother puts him to the breast. The baby sucks and falls back to sleep. Mother wanders back to bed only to be aroused 2 or 3 hours later. The cycle continues all night. Until the mother is psychologically ready to stop offering the breast there is nothing that can be done. At the point in time when you are prepared to stop offering the breast, stop offering the breast. It is best for the baby and also best for you.

Bottle

The earlier you begin to wean your infant off the bottle onto a sippy cup or regular cup, the easier the transfer will be. The weaning process should begin at approximately 8–9 months of age. Start using the cup with water or juice during the learning and adjustment period. Once the child accepts the cup, start to substitute one bottle of milk a day with a cup of milk. Start with the noon feeding. Once this is accepted, substitute another bottle and replace it with cup feeding. Be persistent; do not worry if the baby may initially resist. There may be spillage and a decrease the amount of milk taken by the baby.

The last and most difficult bottle to wean the baby off is that night bottle. Here is where the "battle" begins. From his point of view, he has had the bottle for a number of months. He reluctantly gave up the bottles during the day. Now he thinks, "I really love my night bottle and I am not going to give it up without a fight." If you run into this resistance I suggest giving him only sweetened water before he goes to sleep. If he wakes up during the night and "demands" being fed again, give him sweetened water. Once he accepts this, then switch to plain water. At the same time, reduce the amount of water that you are feeding him. Believe it that he will soon realize it is not worth the struggle and he'll gradually give up the night bottle completely.

The time frame from the beginning to the complete transition from bottle to cup may vary greatly from family to family. It basically depends on how strong your infant's will is to resist giving up the bottle when compared to your will to wean him fully. It is your decision alone as to this time frame, whether it is completed by one year of age or older. Trust me, there will be no breastfeeding at your child's wedding! Remember, in the end there may be a real power struggle between you and your baby. It is a battle worth winning – be strong!

Breath-Holding Spells

Breath-holding spells are very common in children between 18 months to 4 years of age. They may also happen earlier and sometimes may occur in older age groups. They are very frightening when witnessed.

There are basically 2 types of breath-holding spells: the kind resulting in a "blue" appearance, and the type in which the child turns pale. "Blue" is much more common.

Blue breath-holding spells usually occur during a temper tantrum. The child starts to cry. As the cry increases in intensity, the breath is held. After 20–30 seconds of holding the breath, a dusky appearance to the skin occurs, most commonly around the mouth. Subsequently, the child loses consciousness for a short period of time, usually less than 10–15 seconds. During this time, the child is limp and there may be jerking movements of the limbs. When the episode subsides, the child returns to normal.

Breath-holding spells will not cause any brain damage. For the child's own protection during the episode, hold him. If the child is not held and loses consciousness he may fall and injure himself.

Investigation of these spells is not indicated. Medications to prevent them are not indicated. Children can have as few as one or they can experience numerous episodes.

At the beginning of a temper tantrum, if you can distract the child's attention before the crying begins, breath-holding may be prevented (see also Temper Tantrums).

Pale breath-holding spells usually are the result of or follow a painful experience or sudden startle. The child turns pale and quite weak. A loss of consciousness for only a few seconds may ensue.

Subsequently the child cries and then returns to his normal state. These breath-holding spells are benign in nature.

Bronchiolitis

Bronchiolitis is a viral infection of the lower respiratory tract (the lungs). It involves inflammation of the smallest airways in the lungs – the bronchioles.

Approximately 95% of cases are due to a virus called respiratory syncytial virus (RSV).

Although bronchiolitis and asthma have similar symptoms they are somewhat different diseases. However, if there is a family history of allergy (asthma, environmental allergies or eczema) then the infant with bronchiolitis has a much greater risk of developing asthma in the future. Avoidance of secondhand smoke, environmental pollutants, dogs and cats will promote a "clean" environment, which may help to delay the onset of asthma.

Bronchiolitis occurs in infants between 2–24 months of age.

For a child, the symptoms begin with a mild upper respiratory tract infection (mainly runny nose) lasting for 1 to 2 days. This is followed by a cough and then by wheezing. A wheeze is the result of difficulty getting the air **out** (expiration). Associated symptoms are fever, irritability and disruption in both the feeding and sleep patterns. As the symptoms progress and worsen, there is a noticeable increase in the respiratory rate and indrawing (pulling in) between the ribs during breathing. The distress of these children is quite obvious. They sound just as an asthmatic child would.

The diagnosis is a clinical one, which is made by the doctor and is based on the history, physical examination and, if necessary, a chest x-ray. If the child is upset during the examination and is crying, it is extremely difficult to properly assess the chest sounds. This may result in the doctor's either missing the diagnosis or coming to the wrong conclusion. The chest must be assessed while the child is quiet, no matter how long it takes to settle him down.

A culture of the child's sputum or nasal secretions most often demonstrates the presence of RSV, which conclusively confirms the diagnosis.

The presence of bronchiolitis in a family where there are numerous allergies (upper respiratory tract or asthma) is indicative that the infant is at greater risk for developing asthma in the future.

Treatment depends on the severity of the illness and therefore varies from child to child. If the case is a mild one with the child in minimal respiratory distress and appearing to drink and remain playful, then no treatment is needed except for the use of acetaminophen or ibuprofen in the case of fever. The severity of the illness usually will often peak at day 2–3. The symptoms will continue for another few days and then slowly dissipate.

Often, when bronchiolitis is confused with asthma, bronchodilators and anti-inflammatory medication (given by metered-dose inhalers) are prescribed. Unfortunately, these medications work only for asthma and will not alter the course of bronchiolitis.

Bronchiolitis is a common condition which may require hospitalization. Usually those who are hospitalized have severe breathing difficulties, fever, lethargy, poor oral intake and a pale or cyanotic (blue) complexion. An intravenous drip to maintain hydration may be required. Oxygen may also be required. Usually a trial of bronchodilators and anti-inflammatories is tried and discontinued when there is no obvious response or lessening of the symptoms. Antibiotics are indicated only if there is a complication of pneumonia as revealed by an x-ray. The vast majority of infants admitted to the hospital will be discharged within 2–3 days and optimally with no medications.

One recent advance in the treatment of bronchiolitis for an infant in a hospital setting is the use of nebulized 0.9% (normal) saline solution or 3% saline. This is given by mask every 2-4 hours. Its use seems to decrease not only the severity but also the duration, of the illness. There are many studies on the use of bronchodilators and steroids in the management of bronchiolitis. At present there is no fixed consensus as to their relative value, but most likely they do not alter the disease process. Other studies being published have shown a beneficial effect for the use of epinephrine inhalations for infants who have severe bronchiolitis. Further studies are needed. More recently, in infants with severe bronchiolitis, administering warm humidified air by nasal prongs diminished the need for assisted ventilation by intubation. The duration of hospitalization was also significantly reduced.

Each pediatric centre has similar but also somewhat different ways of managing severe bronchiolitis. It is now being more commonly accepted that the use of steroids taken either orally, by inhalation, or intravenously, plays little to no useful role in the management of bronchiolitis.

Although any child with bronchiolitis is at risk of becoming seriously ill and may require assisted ventilation, infants with chronic lung disease or congenital heart disease or who are immunosuppressed are in the highest-risk group for requiring assisted ventilation.

Outcomes, fortunately, are quite favourable in the vast majority of cases. Nevertheless, the disease process can, on rare occasion, result in respiratory failure and the child may succumb to the illness and its complications.

To put things in proper perspective, over the past 40 years I have seen numerous cases of bronchiolitis. I can count on one hand the number of children with severe enough disease to require intensive care unit admission.

Bronchitis

Acute bronchitis

I am not 100% convinced that the disease called acute bronchitis actually exists in infants and toddlers. I know that it is frequently diagnosed and treated, but I am still not sure as to what is being treated.

Whatever it is, it is viral in origin.

Any infant or toddler with a persistent cough for 2 weeks or less, whether it is loose or dry, without any other symptoms, will frequently be misdiagnosed as having bronchitis.

A chest x-ray is normal or shows only slight heaviness in the lung markings.

The diagnosis of bronchitis certainly makes it sound like a more serious illness than just a prolonged viral cough. The diagnosis, I feel, for the most part gives the doctor an excuse to treat the child with antibiotics, with or without inhalation therapy with the use of a bronchodilator and an anti-inflammatory agent.

I believe that acute bronchitis is a viral inflammation of the medium-sized airways of the lungs; an inflammation that requires no treatment and will eventually get better on its own.

Chronic bronchitis

Chronic bronchitis occurs when a cough lasts more than 4–6 weeks without relief or occurs frequently with only short periods of being cough free.

Again, the cough may be loose or dry, is often worse at night, and may be associated with vomiting, but most often the child does not appear or act ill. There is no elevation of the temperature.

A chronic cough is very concerning to the caregivers. They want a diagnosis and a "fix".

The chest is usually clear when listened to with a stethoscope.

A chest x-ray is normal. Any blood work is normal.

In my opinion, this child should be treated as an asthmatic for a period of one month. If there is no improvement, then the child does not have asthma. If there is rapid improvement in the symptoms, the diagnosis of asthma should be high on the list.

There are other causes of chronic coughs which occur less frequently.

The bottom line is most coughs, even chronic, are postviral and, in time, improve on their own.

One problem in managing a child with a chronic cough is management of the caregivers who have to listen to the cough day in and day out. This is especially true when their "advisory staff" only fuel their anxiety.

As stated elsewhere, a chronic cough is very upsetting to the patient, the caregivers, and, finally, the doctor. Parents are frequently dissatisfied with the diagnosis of a postviral cough that requires no medication. Often they will "doctor shop" until someone prescribes an antibiotic, cough suppressant or puffers. The parents' mindset is "something is always better than nothing". Unfortunately, their thinking is wrong. Medications may do more harm to the child than the illness.

Canker Sores (Mouth Ulcers)

Canker sores are also known as aphthous ulcers. Their exact cause is not known. In children (less than 4 years old), lack of adequate dental hygiene or poor diet does not play a role in the development of canker sores.

Canker sores appear on the inside the mouth. More serious sores, due to a herpes simplex 1 virus infection (cold sores), occur on the outside of the lips and not inside the mouth.

Cankers may vary in number from one to several. They may be present on the inner lips, gums or tongue. Frequently, the gingiva (area where the teeth are inserted) is inflamed and may be swollen to such a degree that the teeth may be obscured. This is called gingivitis.

Symptoms include fever, irritability, excessive drooling and food refusal. If the child is old enough, he may complain of burning in the area where the canker sore will erupt.

First, a red bump appears. This is followed by a breakdown of the surface tissue, leaving a small crater which is yellowish in appearance. Each lesion is usually surrounded by a red margin.

The entire course of the breakout lasts 7–14 days.

Treatment

There is no specific medication to treat canker sores. Topical or oral antiviral agents are not indicated. Acetaminophen and ibuprofen are used for fever and pain control.

There are numerous over-the-counter medications that contain a local anesthetic to numb the area involved. These are rubbed onto the infected areas. They require frequent applications. Generally, I do not recommend them. For the older child who can gargle and spit, gargling frequently with salt water or plain mouthwash may be helpful. A doctor may prescribe a mouthwash containing a local anesthetic, with or without steroid.

I find that mixing equal parts of an antacid (Maalox or Milk of Magnesia) with Benadryl is effective in reducing the discomfort and inflammation. Using a cotton-tipped stick, apply the mixture to all infected areas and repeat as often as necessary.

Avoid foods and liquids that are hot. Foods served at room temperature or slightly warmed are best. Spicy, acidic foods and drinks will intensify the discomfort. Jell-O, custards, puddings, applesauce, shakes, ice cream, Popsicles, warm soup and soft foods are best. Blenderizing food may create a consistency that is acceptable to the child.

Many parents are concerned that the child will become dehydrated or will suffer from lack of nutrition. In my 40 years of experience I have not encountered one child who suffered from the above. Unfortunately, the pain is felt equally by the caregiver.

Contagiousness and spread

There are varying opinions about how contagious canker sores are. Most evidence shows that there is little contagiousness. However, in my practice I have seen more than one member of the family (or daycare playmates) suffer from canker sores at the same time. In my opinion, it is always wise to play it safe.

Good handwashing technique is mandatory. The infected child should have his own kitchen utensils. He should have his own face-washing and drying materials. Sharing of utensils that can go from mouth to mouth should be avoided.

Daycare centers and schools may differ in their criteria for when the child may return. The length of contagiousness (if any) is uncertain. Most centres will only allow a child to return if evidence of the lesions has completely cleared.

Lesions may appear on other parts of the body. Refer to Hand, Foot and Mouth Disease.

Car (Motion) Sickness

Car (motion) sickness usually occurs after 2 years of age. It may last a few years or longer.

It may be hereditary. Other family members can suffer from the same symptoms. It is sensitivity to motion in the equilibrium centre, which is located in the inner ear.

The symptoms are complaints of abdominal pain, nausea, vomiting or a combination of all.

There are many different ways to try to handle your particular child's problem. It is only by experimenting that you may find the one that works best. Some suggestions are:

• Maintain the temperature of the car on the cool side.
• If possible, have the child sit in the middle of the back seat, facing forward.
• Have the child eat a light snack before the car trip.
• Keep the child occupied: talking, listening to the radio or CD, watching a video or singing songs.
• Have the child eat crackers (on short trips).
• Some children do better if they look out the front window rather than the side. Others are better with the reverse.
• Try to drive the car as smoothly as possible, without a lot of quick turning or starts and stops.

Whenever you go out in the car, make sure you have a change of clothing, lots of bags and wipes to clean up any mess.

Medications such as Gravol are only recommended for long trips. There are a number of homeopathic medications you may try. Wristbands and patches are also available. If you're using an oral medication, reassure yourself that it is safe for your child.

Car Seats

Rear-facing car seats

Your child should be in a rear-facing car seat until he weighs at least 22 lbs (10 kg) and is 1 year of age.

If your child outgrows the infant car seat before one year of age then you should purchase a convertible car seat. Use it in the rear-facing position until he is one year of age and then face it forward.

Forward-facing car seats

Forward-facing car seats may be used once the child reaches one year of age and weighs over 22 lbs (10 kg).

Forward-facing car seats should be used until the child weighs 40–60 lbs (22–29 kg) and has reached a height of 48 in. (1.2 m).

Booster seats

Once the child reaches 40–60 lbs and has attained a height over 48 inches, he may start using a booster seat. At this time, tethering the seat is unnecessary.

The standard of when a booster seat may be replaced with use of the actual seat and seat belt alone varies depending on where you live. In some places the child may have to weigh between 80–100 lbs (36–45 kg). His height should be 4 feet 9 in. (1.4 m).

Seat belts may cause injury to the child's chest, abdomen or back if there is a motor vehicle accident. Most of these injuries occur in children too small to be using a seat belt alone. When the child is 1.4 m (4 ft 9 in.) in height, he can safely graduate to using an adult seat belt.

It is extremely important, no matter what seat you purchase, that it meets the proper safety standards and, most importantly, is installed and used properly. Your child's safety is ultimately your responsibility. Do not take this lightly!!!

Carotenemia (Yellow-Orange Skin Discolouration)

When your infant starts on yellow vegetables such as carrots and squash, you may notice an orange discolouration on the palms of the hands and on the soles of the feet.

Carotenemia is often confused with jaundice. With jaundice of the skin, the whites of the eyes are always yellow. With carotenemia, the whites of the eyes remain white.

The staining of the skin is due to the pigment carotene, present in many vegetables.

Why some infants eating the exact same amount of vegetables have no carotenemia and others have enough to "glow in the dark" is a mystery.

Carotenemia is not harmful and will fade in time.

Celiac Disease (Gluten Intolerance)

The cause of celiac disease stems from an intolerance to gluten. It is considered an autoimmune disorder. Gluten is a protein fraction found in wheat, rye, barley and other grains, which are found in numerous food products. The onset of the disease typically begins some time after gluten has been introduced into the diet.

It may be of genetic origin in many cases.

The classical indicators for celiac disease are an infant who develops persistent loose yellow stools, abdominal bloating and discomfort, failure to gain weight and, instead, loss of weight. Frustratingly, many celiac patients do not have the classical presentation of these symptoms.

Celiac disease can develop and have its onset at any time of life. Why? I do not know.

Often symptoms are misleading and do not point directly to gluten intolerance.

Such symptoms include:

- Chronic constipation
- Abdominal discomfort (often diagnosed as irritable bowel syndrome)
- Persistent generalized aches and pains
- Loss of energy
- Failure to be able to gain weight
- Weak bones (osteoporosis), usually discovered by x-ray after a fracture has occurred
- Extreme weakness and fatigue
- Irritability and behavioural changes

There are blood test markers that if positive are suggestive of the presence of celiac disease.

The diagnosis is confirmed by examining a biopsy of the intestinal wall. The biopsy is done by endoscopic examination and with small children it requires the use of a general anesthetic.

The biopsy will show flattening of the lining of the intestines (normally the lining is covered with tiny, hair-like projections called villi).

If celiac disease is suspected, the diagnosis can further be confirmed if the child is placed on a completely gluten-free diet for a period of a few weeks. After that time, if the diagnosis is indeed correct, the symptoms begin to show improvement. No child, however, should be put on a gluten-free diet without the supervision of a doctor who is thoroughly familiar with celiac disease and the gluten-free diet.

The only treatment at this time for celiac disease is a strict gluten-free diet for life.

Chicken Pox (Varicella)

Before the introduction of the chicken pox vaccine over 20 years ago, 50% of children would contract chicken pox by 5 years of age, and by 12 years of age this number would rise to 90%. Up to 20% of those who developed chicken pox would later have a reactivation of the virus in the form of herpes zoster (shingles). The medical cost of chicken pox to Canada was approximately $125 million annually. Since the introduction of the chicken pox vaccine, all the aforementioned statistics have been dramatically reduced.

Many of us can remember years back when people threw "chicken pox parties". If one child in the neighbourhood developed chicken pox, parents would bring their children over to the home in which the child with chicken pox lived. By being in contact with this child it was hoped that the other children would catch the illness. The exact reason why parents did this is still a mystery to me. If they had only known about the serious complications that could ensue I am convinced that such parties would have been prohibited.

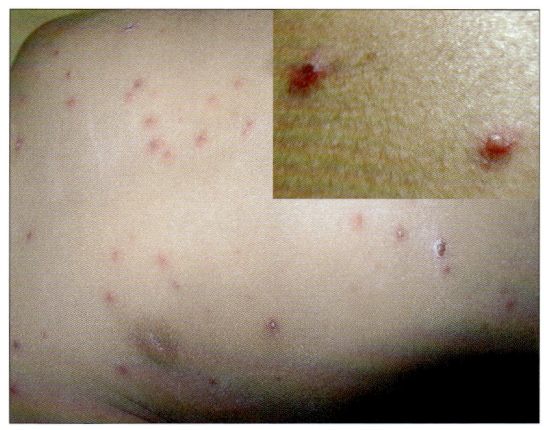

Chicken Pox

The incubation period is between 10 and 20 days.

Clinically, there are symptoms of fever and lethargy for 1 to 2 days prior to the appearance of the rash. The symptoms are similar to any other flu-like illness. Clusters of red dots begin to appear and subsequently turn into oval "teardrop" fluid-filled blisters. Each is on a red base. New crops of lesions continue to appear for 3 or 4 days. The lesions not only appear on the skin but frequently are found in the mouth, ears and mucous membranes of the genitalia and anus. The lesions are quite itchy. Most children feel better after a few days, with the lesions drying up by the 5th to 7th day. There may be as few as only 6 lesions or as many as hundreds of them.

Treatment

• keep fingernails cut short
• acetaminophen or ibuprofen may be given for fever, but NEVER give aspirin
• lukewarm baking soda baths are soothing (use one-half box in the bath water)
• calamine lotion on the lesions and an antihistamine given orally will decrease the itching and discomfort

Unfortunately, the most contagious period is during the 1 to 2 days before the rash appears and then for up to 2 to 3 days after the first lesions appear. During incubation the virus is spread by droplets from the respiratory tract. Once the lesions erupt, the patient is much less contagious and the spread at that particular time is by skin-to-skin contact with a lesion.

The virus is never spread to others by a person who has been in contact with an affected child (that is, they will not carry the chicken pox virus on their person to spread to another).

In fact, children should be able to return to daycare or school once they feel well enough to do so, despite still having lesions that are not yet dry (as long as these lesions are covered by clothing). However, most school guidelines state presently that isolation should continue until the last lesion is healed and dried. This may take up to 7–10 days. Hopefully, a statement will be forthcoming that gives new guidelines as to the duration of isolation.

Complications of chicken pox

Although the complications are uncommon they can be very serious. Complications include febrile seizures, middle-ear infections, pneumonia, encephalitis and Reye's syndrome (if aspirin is given). Eye lesions may also occur. Chicken pox is the most common cause of necrotizing fasciitis (flesh-eating disease) in children.

Chicken pox infection occurs in the epidermis (outer layer) of the skin. If it remains there until dried no scarring will result. If, however, it penetrates deeper into the dermis (inner layer), then pox scars will occur. This is the reason it is necessary to refrain from scratching the lesions. If they are scratched they may become secondarily infected and penetrate the underlying dermis, with subsequent scarring. There is a small percentage of children whose illness has a tendency to go deeper into the dermis. Unfortunately, numerous scars, which are unpreventable, will be left.

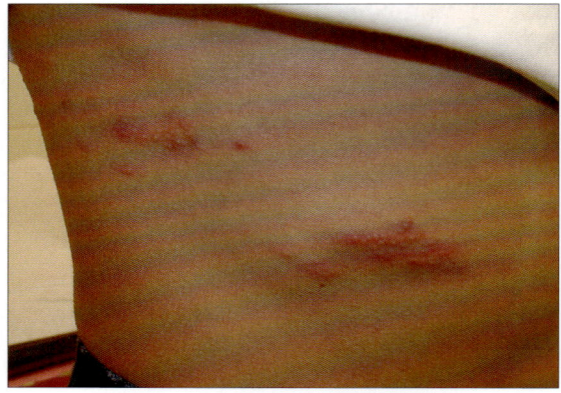
Herpes Zoster (Shingles)

Birth defects may occur in babies of women who either caught chicken pox early in their pregnancy or who have active chicken pox while giving birth. Newborns whose mothers develop chicken pox just before or after labour and delivery should be protected with an infusion of chicken pox immunoglobulin. Those individuals who are immunosuppressed for whatever reason and who come in direct contact with chicken pox are also candidates for immunoglobulin.

The chicken pox virus may stay dormant in the body for many years, only to erupt into herpes zoster (shingles). Although shingles may occur in young children it's more commonly found in adults. A person with shingles can spread the virus to others who have not previously had chicken pox (or the vaccine), resulting in clinical chicken pox. Fortunately, spread is only by direct contact with the shingles lesions early after its outbreak. Keeping the lesions covered, along with good handwashing technique, diminishes the chance of spreading the virus to others who lack immunity. Isolation, therefore, is not required as long as the above precautions are adhered to.

Chicken pox vaccine is a live vaccine. It is given to children between l2 and16 months of age, with a recommended booster at 5 years of age. Common side effects are fever and tenderness and swelling at the site of injection. Infrequently, a few chicken pox lesions may erupt approximately 2 weeks after vaccination. These lesions are not contagious.

A very small percentage of children who have had the chicken pox vaccine (which is considered only 85%–90% protective) may nevertheless develop chicken pox if they come in contact with the "wild" virus. Most often the child is not ill and only manifests a few lesions. Theses lesions, unfortunately, may not look like typical chicken pox lesions, and consequently the diagnosis is often difficult to make and frequently missed altogether.

There is a vaccine available for adults that will help protect them from developing shingles.

Child Rearing (Discipline Tips)

The good, the bad, the ugly

I do not like to use the word "punishment." Punishment can be a harsh word. I feel that it is more appropriate when dealing with toddlers and older children to use the word "consequences." Basically, the concept is the same but the word implies a logical outcome and has a less punitive tone.

What you need to remember are 4 basics: firmness, fairness, structure (in routines) and, above all, consistency. Start practicing these early and I can fairly guarantee you that there will be fewer conflicts and discipline problems to deal with. How early to start? No later than 4 months of age.

The words come easily; the doing is hard.

The Good

1. Children learn by example. Parents and other caregivers are their first role models. As such, they must set a good example. "Do as I tell you, not what I do or say" just does not work.

2. Remember the old clichés – "He is a chip off the old block" and "The apple does not fall far from the tree." Believe me, there is some truth in these sayings: more than you may think. Even young infants can be more perceptive than you give them credit for. Your child is always watching you. He is listening to you. His hearing is excellent and he can hear from distances that you cannot guess he is able to. So be very careful about what you say and how you say it.

3. Take a good look in the mirror. Not to see how you appear on the outside but to look deeper and try to expose the "inner you". Would you like your child to be taught by and perhaps emulate someone like yourself? If not, changes must be made!!!

4. Consequences must take place at the time of the misbehaviour, without delay. Do not wait until another primary caregiver comes home.

5. Whenever possible, the consequence should fit the "crime". For example, if the child will not pick up his toys in his room, the consequence should be that he stays in his room until the job is done. Here the consequence is related to and fits the "crime." "You cannot go to the movies if you don't tidy up" is a consequence that does not fit the crime. This is not fair. I recognize that very often it is difficult for the consequence to be completely suitable. However, be creative and try your best.

6. You should make the rules of acceptable behaviour and consequences very clear. Give choices of consequences whenever possible. Of course, this depends on the child's age. By doing this you will instill a sense of fairness and he will also have a feeling of empowerment by participating in the process. The consequence will thus be more readily accepted.

7. Stay firm in what you have to say, using as few words as possible. Always make eye contact to ensure the child is listening. If he is old enough, ask him if he understands and is able to repeat what you have said. If not, say it again.

8. When the child is old enough to understand consequences, they should be discussed and agreed upon ahead of time by you and the child, before the misbehaviour is committed. This is especially true if the same pattern of misbehaviour gets repeated. Reminding the child will give him a sense of fairness and empowerment and, as well, an awareness of expectations. The misdemeanour will most likely not be repeated, but if it is, the consequence will be more readily accepted.

9. Be firm and fair about consequences. They should be age appropriate. Once the event is over that is it. Do not keep blaming. Time out is one consequence that can begin at around 2-1/2 to 3 years of age – one minute per year. Set an egg timer so that the child knows exactly when time out is completed. Time out should be designated as an area where the child must sit. Sending the child to his room is not a firm consequence. There are lots of things to happily occupy him there. Some experts feel that during time out there should be nothing in that place to occupy his attention – that he ought to "reflect". (I myself am not so sure that most children are mature enough to do this). Others feel that the focus should be on the fact that the child has to sit in a specific area for a specific length of time regardless of what he is doing while he is there, be it reading or colouring.

10. I like the one, two, three method – if, after counting to 3 slowly, the child has not complied, then the consequence should be the result. The counting has to be direct and done with no hesitation between numbers. You should not be hoping that by the time you reach 3, compliance will have taken place (no "1, 2, 2-1/4, 2-1/2, 2-3/4, I'm going to say 3"). The child soon learns that you say what you mean and mean what you say – cooperation should follow. It is a lesson well learned.

11. No matter what the misbehaviour is, always remind your child that you love him but you just do not love what he has done. After a bad day, when tucking him in at bedtime, make sure that you put his world back together again. Reassure him by telling him how much you love him, then give him a big hug and whisper in his ear, "We will have a better day tomorrow."

The Bad

1. Lack of consistency is by far the most common fault in parenting. A consistent approach must be applied by all caregivers all of the time. It is a must that grandparents and babysitters or any other caregivers buy into the rules you have decided upon when providing caregiving. A child will comply with the reasonable limits set for him and be less confused if these limits are set with consistency. Another mistake is made when caregivers disagree in front of the child. There also may be lack of consistency in dealing with the same recurrent issues. One time you ignore them and another time you come down on the child "like thunder". Far too often the response to the misbehaviour is based on your mood and coping skills at that time. Inconsistency results in confusion and no lesson is taught; the misbehaviour is repeated and sometimes can escalate.

2. In fairness, try not to treat siblings differently when meting out consequences for similar "crimes". This disparity, I guarantee you, will lead to feelings of unfairness, resentment and perhaps the escalation of misbehaviour. Sibling rivalry can also escalate when one child feels that he or she has been unfairly treated. You will seldom find out who was the initiator of an altercation. Allow children to problem solve. Ultimately, if they are unable to settle conflicts, it is best to assume that both are guilty and receive the same consequence.

3. Never "shoot from the hip". What I mean by this is do not decide consequences so hastily or in such anger that later you realize they are unrealistic and impossible to impose or completely inappropriate and do not fit the crime. You put yourself in a position that is very difficult to wiggle out of.

4. Do not try to deal with multiple behavioural issues in one large sweep. This will become completely unmanageable. Start with one small problem. Hold your ground and do not give in or give up. When one goal is accomplished, move on to another issue and so on. Of course, the child may have input, but the final say is yours. Once you settle the first issue you are on a roll. Each subsequent issue will become easier to deal with and resolve. Less effort will be required for compliance.

5. Do not give in to tantrums. A tantrum is basically a child's wanting you to change a "no" to a "yes". Giving in will only encourage further tantrums and lead to their escalation. If you see a tantrum starting, try to distract the young child by saying something silly such as "Look at the frog in the sink" or "See the butterfly behind you?" This technique frequently prevents the oncoming storm from materializing. If it does not, then allow the child to have his tantrum (just

ensure that he does not harm himself). Do not make a fuss about it afterwards and just go on with your normal routine.

6. Avoid power struggles as much as possible. These will only reduce you to a child's level, which is not a very good position to discipline or teach from. For example, if you have made plans to go for a visit to grandma's or for a special outing but when the time comes the child refuses to go, *whenever possible*, it is best for you to just carry on with the plans, leaving the child at home with another caregiver. I truly empathize with those parents who have continual situations in which there is a power struggle – the "I won't," "You will," "I won't," "Yes, you will" tug-of-war. In these situations it is best to back off and allow time for the situation to fizzle out. Once your nerves have settled approach the problem again. You may have to use another strategy to achieve cooperation.

The Ugly

1. Avoid phrases which destroy self-esteem; these include:
- "You can never do anything right!"
- "I can't deal with you anymore!"
- "Why are you the bad apple in the family?"
- "Why can't you be like your brother?"

2. Worse still is threatening a child with bodily harm or saying that you're going to send him away if he does not measure up. Continually having to raise the level of your voice until shouting becomes the norm will only result in a headache and sore throat for you. The more you scream, the less the child will listen. This will have a serious adverse effect on your relationship with your child. If it becomes a recurrent pattern it will cause the child to fear you rather than respect you. What next? Spanking?

3. Do not use physical punishment or more than just a "light tap". Children, who are continually exposed to corporal punishment are more likely to become abusive themselves as adults. Always remember, treat others, including your children, as you would like to be treated yourself.

4. Do not give a reward that reinforces misbehaviour. When you say, "Be good and you can have a treat," then if the child misbehaves where does that leave you? Most of the time he receives the reward anyway. He will learn to manipulate this reward system. Now I ask you, "What lesson has been taught?

No one ever said that parenting is easy!!!

Child Rearing (How-to's)

Many books by many experts have been written about child rearing. I have raised my own children, and believe me, I do not purport to be an expert myself. I have made many mistakes, and if I had to do it all over again knowing what I know now, I certainly would have changed some things.

Nevertheless, there are 8 guidelines that I have learned:

1. The words come easily but the doing is hard work.
2. It is easier to raise someone else's children.
3. The basic principles for successful child rearing have changed little over time but the terminology is all different. **Increasingly, outside influences will challenge these principles.**
4. The greatest challenge one will ever face is to raise a child.
5. There is no greater reward than watching your child blossom.
6. Child-rearing mistakes are easily seen in other caregivers but seldom recognized in your own parenting.
7. Many behaviour problems in children are created by poor parenting skills. In such cases parent counseling is often more effective than counseling the child.
8. Child rearing is never finished. It is a lifelong endeavour.

The most obvious advance I have seen in child rearing over the past years is in the area of discipline. We are leaning away from negative reinforcement, especially via physical punishment, and gaining compliance by employing more positive methods of reinforcement. This way, we hope to achieve more acceptable behaviour. Doing this I feel we are heading in the right direction.

Most of us hope for the same qualities in the child we bring into this world. We crave the enjoyment of watching him/her grow into a physically healthy, mentally strong, and emotionally stable individual possessing a sense of independence and positive self-esteem, a good sense of humour, ability to show tolerance, kindness, charitableness, curiosity, open-mindedness, and the capability to demonstrate love, respect and kindness for himself, his fellow man and the environment.

A tall order, no? But how does all this come about? Certainly, not by some magic genie waving a wand or by wishful thinking. It only happens with effort. To some it may seem to come easily; for most it will only be accomplished through constant hard work.

Granted, we all are born with certain personality traits that are already a given and can never be altered. These are the spots that a leopard is born with, the ones that cannot be changed. Any other "spots" are acquired through the learning process. The most important ones are learned from you, the parent(s). The earlier most lessons are taught and the more strongly they are reinforced, the harder they are to will away. This goes for the "spots" that are positive – ones that you want to retain – and those that are unacceptable – ones you wish to eliminate. With determination persistence and consistency, the bad habits of the poorly acquired "spots" can be changed; but change will be difficult the longer negatives are reinforced. As soon as your baby is born you begin to mold and shape the kind of adult he will develop into.

I cannot emphasize enough how important these first weeks and months are to getting off to a positive early start.

The reality is that, as the caregiver, you have become your child's most important teacher and role model. If you, yourself have not yet learned life's lessons, how will you make a positive impact on your child? Important skills could be missed and unfortunately "bad" lessons could become ingrained.

Perhaps now it is time for you to take a good, objective look at yourself in the mirror – a good hard look. What do you actually see? Is it someone who is easygoing or tense, generally even-tempered or moody, confident or lacking self-assurance? Are you happy with what you see? Can you say, "I would like my child to be just like me?" Most of us cannot. We see things in ourselves that we do not want to pass on to our children. I would like to have met the person who coined the old clichés, "He is a chip off the old block," or "The apple does not fall far from the tree." That guy "hit the nail right on the head"! Unless you have the desire and are ready to make personal sacrifices, then you too will pass on to your child many of the undesired personality traits (qualities) you find in yourself. Changing yourself is no easy task. It takes time and a lot of effort. But in the end, becoming a more positive role model is well worth it.

We all love our children. In fact, love is the cornerstone of successful child rearing. Though each may love in his own way, this boundless feeling that we have for our children is the internal thread that binds all parents through all times. Given that love is the cornerstone, then I should again reiterate the important building blocks for successful child rearing. These are:

- an early start to effective parenting
- becoming a good role model yourself

What are some of the other building blocks?

Be firm, be fair and be consistent. We all have difficulty with these, especially the latter. Lack of consistency makes caregivers falter the most. To further complicate the issue, often there are others who would try to "parent" your child as well. These include, for example, daycare workers, extended families, nannies and, most commonly, grandparents. All have different views on and methods of child rearing when your child is in their charge. This can be very confusing for a young child.

Both parents should assume the role of "head coaches" who must set down the guidelines and ensure that they are followed by other caregivers. They need to maintain a "united front". There should not be one parent who overindulges and says yes – "Mr. Nice Guy", while the other parent does the reverse, playing "Mrs. Meanie". This gives the child mixed messages, which are confusing. The result is ineffective parenting and poorly taught lessons. Because children can't easily deal with this type of divided parental authority you will not be happy with the results.

Do not mistake giving love with giving in, giving up or just giving. You cannot over-love, but you certainly can overindulge your child.

Children thrive best with structure. Routines should be initiated very early in life and be adhered to. The more you can structure the environment with daily routines, the more secure children will feel.

Problem solving can only happen if both parents are emotionally and physically ready to attack the problem. Preferably all caregivers must be made aware of the established plan. If they are not on the same page, problems, including power struggles with regards to issues of sleep, feeding and poor behaviour, will be difficult to overcome.

Set limits for your child. The limits set should be reasonable, age appropriate and attainable. These will differ according to the values from family to family but the basic principle is the same. Set reasonable boundaries within which your child can grow. You, not the child, are the teacher and are in charge. As the child grows and is able to live within the boundaries set for him, then and only then should the boundaries be broadened.

As your child grows, the spheres of influence he is exposed to will expand. These will go beyond the other caregivers such as babysitters, nannies, and daycare providers, to include coaches, teachers, religious leaders and the formidable peer group. At some time they will meet and influence your child. A child, who has learned to live comfortably within your guidelines, set down early on in his own environment, will have fewer problems adapting to the external pressures applied by our society. The lessons that you taught him early in life and reinforced will last a lifetime. You will already have given him the tools and ability to be able to cope with life, to pick and choose what to accept and what to reject. Have faith that he will become the person you have carefully encouraged him to be.

Have realistic expectations, both daily and for the long term. If you set unrealistic goals for your child, they will become a source of frustration for both you and him. Neither of you will be a happy camper. Accept that your child is his own person. There is no greater gift. Recognize that each child has his own strengths and is unique. Encourage all the potential that is there right before your eyes. All too often, we fall into the trap of expecting too much from our children. We push and push to try to mold them into something that they may never be. We may fail to realize that they may have a very different agenda for themselves. Note, I am saying "different" and not "wrong". The friction created by nonacceptance will weaken and perhaps even erode your relationship with your child. Instead, help him to utilize his own strengths with constant support and encouragement. Remember, never compare one child to another, especially within your own family. Self-esteem rather than an "I'm not good enough" attitude should be nurtured if you want your child to have confidence and self-reliance as an adult.

As parents we always want to "rescue" our children. All too often we assume that they cannot sort out problems on their own. We think failure is not an option for our child. We don't want them to ever experience disappointment. Yet nothing can be more unrealistic. We all want our children to learn by doing. We all want our children to grow mentally and emotionally strong. We all want our children to be able to cope with all the stresses that life will heap upon them. If we do not allow children to taste some failure and disappointment this will not happen. You would be surprised at how resilient your child is and what he can accomplish if he is allowed to do things on his own. If he fails to reach his goal, an excellent learning opportunity has presented itself, one that he must accept and resolve. As it has been said, "It's not whether you win or lose. It's how you play the game". In the end, it is the effort that counts. If your child has done his best, nothing more should be asked of him. A simple, "I know how hard you tried and I am proud of you" in the long run will go much further to build his self-esteem than any badge or trophy.

On the other side, many parents see their child as the "greatest". Let's be honest, everyone cannot be the greatest. Unfortunately, if you keep repeating this message over and over, your child may come to believe it. When he enters the real world (starting as early as daycare), he will soon find out that he is not "numero uno". This may be difficult for him to accept, promoting a reaction which may be negative in nature and a feeling inside that he can never live up to your expectations. There is never an issue with praise when well deserved, but try not to over-build your child's ego to larger than it already is. Children have a great ability to recognize the truth. Let them find their own level of greatness – disappointment will thus be avoided.

Always encourage independence. This can be started early on. Allow an infant to self-feed finger foods. For a toddler encourage independence by giving choices where possible regarding his food clothing and activities, help in dressing, bathing, teeth cleaning (under your supervision), etc. Allowing your child to take part in the decision-making encourages his self-esteem and independence.

Imagination is a wonderful and creative process. Every child has it but, unfortunately, these days, I feel it is underutilized. We are caught up with electronic gadgetry that is excellent for hand-eye coordination but does little to tap into a most important resource – the imagination. How many times have you seen your child play with the box or the wrappings rather than the toy? Imagination will never allow things to become boring. It takes very little to stimulate the imagination. It is the most cost-effective way a child can entertain himself. The safe "tools" for imaginative play are all around us in every room of the house – pots and pans, spoons and boxes. All you have to do is to make them available to your child and then sit back and enjoy. Imagination is the fuel that stimulates creativity. It is creativity that stimulates future success.

By the way, are we overprogramming our children, leaving them too little free time to do what comes most naturally, to simply let them just play?

Teach your child respect. Respect not only for you, for himself, for others, and their belongings, but also for the environment. This is only accomplished if you as well show the same kinds of respect. You are the most important teacher and role model here. Set a good example and he will follow.

Be patient with your child. Remember, he is just learning. If you become frustrated this will only result in raising his frustration and anxiety – not a good situation for learning.

Use common sense and have confidence in your own decision-making. Do not allow your un-elected, self-appointed "advisory staff" to influence you to take a direction that you feel is wrong for you and your child. No one knows your child better than you. No one knows better than you what works for your child. So, if your mother, mother-in-law, Aunt Gertrude, neighbour, friend or lady at the checkout counter gives you advice, say a polite thank-you and just carry on. By the way, how often does your "advisory staff" say something positive about your parenting? Discuss all serious issues with a professional (your doctor should be #1).

Remember, communication with your child is extremely important. Communication must be appropriate for the age he is at. Eye contact ensures that you have got his attention. The younger the child, the fewer the words you need to use. Also remember that communication is a two-way street. That is, you must listen as well as talk. Listen to what is said, observe the expression on your child's face as he speaks, and take note of the tone in which he frames his words. Never trivialize your child's message to you by brushing it off lightly. It may appear as minor to you but it can be very important to him, and that's what counts.

Always be firm and fair, trying to speak in a soft voice. If your child is not listening, raising your voice will only lead him to tune you out further. Your only recourse is to raise your voice louder and louder until it escalates to screaming. You're out of control then. What is next?

I do not favour the use of the word "punishment." In my opinion it is too harsh and has too many negative connotations; not the best choice of words to use when you wish to correct the misbehaviour or lack of compliance. I do prefer the term "consequence". It sounds less threatening and puts some of the onus for poor behaviour back where it belongs – with the child.

If your child misbehaves or fails to carry out expected chores or responsibilities, then a consequence is in order. Asking your child, "Why did you do that?" puts him on the defensive. It is much better to say, "How do you think we can make things right?" Now you are on his side – a much more comfortable place for all in problem solving. A well thought-out "action plan" should be constructed and carefully put in place. The consequence should be clear, age-appropriate and understood by the child. As well, it should be reasonable and enforceable. The consequence should be agreed on by all involved (including you and the child). Whenever possible the consequence should fit the "crime". For example, if he refuses to tidy his room then he must stay there until the task is completed. Here, the consequence fits the crime. Telling him he cannot go to the circus next week certainly hurts. However, going to the circus has nothing to do with tidying up. The lesson is out of sync with the consequence. Once cooperation gets going, let it be; do not keep going over the original misdemeanour.

"Time out" is an excellent consequence that can be used if you are uncertain as to which consequence is the most appropriate one. Begin using time out at around 2-1/2 to 3 years of age: one minute per year of age. Set an egg timer so the child knows exactly when the time out is completed. The area where time out takes place should have things to occupy him, such as a book or colouring pad. The important thing is that he must remain in a specific area for a specific length of time and not misbehave while there. It is not that important as to what he is doing while he is there. It does, however, give your child quiet time to contemplate the misbehaviour. If he does not go voluntarily, take him there by his hand or by carrying him. If he leaves before the time out is over, patiently keep putting him back and reset the timer; eventually he will learn. Time out should not exceed 5 minutes. When time out is completed, the event is over and forgiven; do not dwell on it.

I also like the 1, 2, 3 method. If, after you count to 3 slowly, the child does not comply, then the consequence must be administered. The counting has to be consistent and done without hesitation between numbers – no 1, 2, 2-1/4, 2-1/2, 2-3/4 then 3. The child will soon learn that you say what you mean and mean what you say – if you don't stall, compliance will follow. It is a lesson well learned.

Never make empty threats that you don't plan to carry out. Guess what – if you continually say, "If you do this, then – if you do this one more time, then –" and you continue to harp at the child with little follow-through, I guarantee that nothing will be accomplished. Just say what you mean and mean what you say – just do it! Remember, a "no" means "no"– not a "maybe" or "we will see." Your child will have more respect for you and trust me, will become more cooperative. Power struggles will happen far less frequently – a happier and healthier environment for all.

I certainly do not condone physical punishment. Physically abused children may in all likelihood themselves become abusive adults and parents. A firm grasp of the forearm and a stern voice, if meted appropriately, should be all that is necessary. As previously stated, constantly raising your voice tends to be ineffective. The volume of your voice will have to keep rising along with your anger level to new and higher levels in order to get your message across. Soon screaming becomes the norm and is completely ineffective. What follows then? Physical punishment? This certainly is not what you want. It is much wiser for you to take a step back and have a cup of tea. Then regroup and try a more effective, calmer strategy. I would much rather you lose the occasional "battle" than lose your temper and model loss of self-control. Getting into a verbal battle with your child only reduces you to his level – not an effective place to parent from. To be more effective, never fight more than one battle at a time. Keep it to one that you feel is important for you to make your point, one that you can realistically accomplish if you are persistent.

Try choosing a small issue to begin with. Form an action plan and then go for it. A "war" is won, after all, by achieving many small victories. Do not expect instant miracles. Do not start by taking a huge leap, coming down on your child like thunder. I guarantee that this will not work, in either the short or long term. Instead, make small gains, one at a time. Initiating the first step is the hardest, no matter how small. Thereafter, each step becomes easier and easier. Future confrontations become less difficult to resolve.

Consequences should follow as soon as possible after the misdeed. Delaying them by saying, "Just wait until your father comes home!" is not a good tactic. By that time, the child will have forgotten what he has done, and therefore, the consequences are essentially meaningless.

Remember, it is easier to catch flies with honey than with vinegar. In other words, praise, encouragement and a smile can often accomplish much more than harsh words or corporal punishment. Which do you think will raise your child's self-esteem more?

When you are problem solving, always be willing to negotiate but not to compromise your principles of discipline. To compromise means someone is losing something or giving in; this is not acceptable. Reasonable negotiation, on the other hand, happens when both parties alter their stance to come to a mutually satisfying solution; here there is no loser. For example, here is such a scenario: you are concentrating on some endeavour that is important to you and your child keeps disturbing you to get attention or wants you to play with him immediately. Frustrated after giving several no's, you finally give in. Here you have compromised your authority. The wrong message has been sent. He learns that if he insists long and loud enough he will get what he wants. If, on the other hand, you were to say, "I will be finished with my work soon. If you don't disturb me and play quietly while you wait, I will be more than happy to play with you afterwards." Then, if he agrees and complies, a victory has been negotiated. There is no conflict. You are both winners. You have taught him two important lessons: that patience has its rewards, and, more importantly, he cannot have what he wants when he wants it just because he wants it. He has learned an excellent lesson that will serve him well in the real world.

Listen to your child not just with your ears but also with your eyes, and keep in touch with your gut feeling. Seemingly innocuous clues may be a warning signal of an impending storm. Catch the symptoms early and they will remain as gentle rainfall. Be aware of your child's changes in eating habits or sleep patterns, mood changes, failing school performance, lack of interest, spending more time alone, being less communicative or increased irritability. These are a few of the early warning symptoms that something may be wrong. Be sympathetic; show interest by your willingness to listen when he is ready to communicate with you. Avoid preaching – it only falls on deaf ears. If he feels that you are on his side and will be supportive, then there is a far greater chance for him to open up and dialogue with you. Then, when the problem is out in the open, you can deal with it together, guiding your child to do most of the problem solving on his own. Keep reminding him that you are always there to lend an ear and be nonjudgmental. Since the child needs to feel he owns the means for resolving the many problems he will encounter, allow him to do most of the problem solving on his own. This will produce a better result and will have beneficial long-term, lasting effects; knowing that he is in control is a powerful tool for growth. It is never too late to teach these skills. It is never too late to make changes. Seek outside help for your child if you yourself cannot provide the answers.

Never destroy a child's self-esteem by saying:

- "You can never do anything right."
- "I can't deal with you anymore!"
- "Why can't you do better?"
- "Why can't you be like your brother?"

Do not give a reward for misbehaviour by saying, "Be good and you can have a treat." If the child then misbehaves and he still receives the reward, you have contradicted yourself. I ask you then what lesson has been taught? There should never be a reward for bad behaviour.

When struggling with a particular strategy to solve a recurrent problem with your child, ask yourself, "How is it working for me?" If your answer is that it is not working at all, then you had better seek another approach.

The single most productive opportunity for resolving problems with your child is when he has been put to bed, and is settled in and the lights are out. Talk softly, going over any of the day's contentious issues and conflicts that may be upsetting to both you and your child. When you have finished, always set his world right with the reassurance that you may not like what he has done but you do love him, and that "you" as a team will have a better day tomorrow.

Always remember that you are his most important teacher and role model, starting right at birth. It is the caregiver who has the power. Giving away the power too easily to your child can inadvertently, over a prolonged period of time, only cause more child-rearing problems later on. Power issues around sleep and eating are among the most common which are usually ceded unwittingly to your child. The problem becomes not your child's, but yours. The only way to correct the situation is for you to take the power back. Some issues are non-negotiable; examples would include those around safety and personal hygiene. Many social and behavioural problems seen are the result of improper parenting and not an "improper" child. Change the environment and the child will change; it is as simple or as difficult as that.

To summarize, remember the "C's" of child rearing. These are – common sense, confidence, calm, consistency, control and a good "cense" of humour. Consistency is the most important of all and is also the one most frequently forgotten mainly because of laxness in effort on the part of the caregiver – wittingly or unwittingly.

Being a parent is not unlike being a farmer. Sow your seeds early in the spring, tend to your crops with love and care and, I guarantee, you will have a harvest to reap in the fall that will be bountiful; this despite times of storm, drought and disease. It is very hard and demanding work. Certain things are completely out of your control, but we must accept them graciously, and try to live with them and to learn from them.

Remember, we all make mistakes. This is part of the human condition. However, the people more able to learn from their mistakes are the ones who will find success.

All you can ask of yourself is to try your best, to admit when you're wrong, to be willing to change your approach if necessary and to seek help if stuck.

I know; the words come easy, but the doing is hard!!! Trust me, it is worth it.

Circumcision (Advisability – Yes or No)

To circumcise or not to circumcise: that is the question. Certainly there are religions in which circumcision is mandatory. For males not belonging to these groups, it is a personal decision made by the parents.

Arguments against circumcision

Both the American and Canadian Pediatric Societies have stated that this is an unnecessary procedure.

It is a cosmetic procedure only.

The patient has no say in the decision. It is considered a painful procedure.

Complications may occur, such as bleeding, infection or more serious damage to the head of the penis.

The foreskin enhances sexual pleasure.

The foreskin's purpose is to protect the glans (head) of the penis from trauma, irritation, the elements and infection.

For psychological reasons, all the males, fathers and their sons, in the family should be the same.

The benefits of circumcision

Phimosis (tight foreskin), paraphimosis (a foreskin that has been retracted and "strangles" the head of the penis) and balanitis (foreskin infection) only occur in uncircumcised males.

There have been no studies to confirm any adverse psychological problem if there is a difference in the penises between father and child or between two brothers.

There has been no study that shows that the foreskin enhances sexual pleasure.

Cleaning of the circumcised penis is easier than for the uncircumcised.

The incidence of urinary tract infection during the first year of life is slightly increased in uncircumcised males.

HIV, the acquisition of herpes simplex virus type II infections and penile papillomavirus infection are less common for circumcised males. This is also thought to be true for all sexually transmitted diseases.

Cancer of the penis in adult males (approximately 7000 cases in North America yearly) does not occur in individuals when circumcision is done soon after birth.

With the use of acetaminophen, a topical anesthetic, sugar water for the baby to suck on and a local penile block, the amount of discomfort the infant usually feels is minimal. However, even in the best of hands, there are some infants who do feel discomfort and cry loudly. For this, fortunately, the figure is less than 10% of infants circumcised.

Any complications are rare. Bleeding, being the most common, is easily controlled. Infection is easily treated. Damage to the glans (head of the penis) occurs rarely although it can be a very unfortunate possibility. The excess tissue removed from the glans can be surgically reattached under the best of conditions with excellent results. The decision, therefore, to do or not to do a circumcision on your boy should be made only by the caregivers and not influenced by anyone else.

Routine circumcision, if chosen, should be performed before the baby is one month of age.

Circumcision (Procedure and Aftercare)

If your baby is ill at the time of the circumcision, please inform the doctor prior to the circumcision.

If there is a family history of a bleeding disorder or any other health or risk factors that may by this procedure affect your baby, please let the doctor know before the circumcision.

Discomfort

In the preparation prior to the circumcision, EMLA cream is applied to the base of the penis to numb the skin. Acetaminophen is given to decrease any discomfort during circumcision. In addition, the use of a local anesthetic block injected into the base of the penis and also allowing the infant to suck on a high concentration of sugar water will even further minimize the discomfort. To the infant the sugar water is like a double-chocolate banana milkshake. Once he tastes this, the baby is distracted from the circumcision procedure.

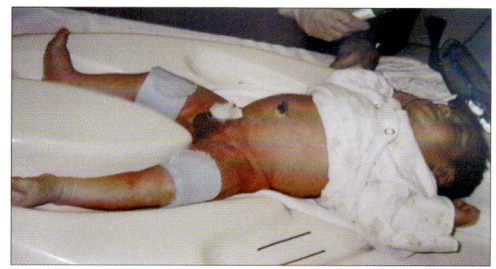

Topical Anesthetic Applied

Most infants, therefore, feel minimal or no discomfort during the procedure. However, the rare situation in which a baby cries from the time he leaves the caregivers' arms until a few hours after the circumcision sometimes arises. I have never quite understood this, since we see this procedure carried out in the same way time and time again.

The local anesthetic will last for approximately an hour and a half or two hours after the circumcision. Acetaminophen is recommended if the discomfort continues (it is usually unnecessary).

The Procedure

After the local anesthetic is given, the foreskin is freed from the head of the penis with a probe. The foreskin is then pulled forward off the head of the penis. A mogen clamp is placed behind the part of the foreskin that is to be removed (the clamp looks and works like a cigar cutter) and then closed. The foreskin is removed with a scalpel blade. The clamp is opened. The circumcision is complete. A thin piece of gauze will be wrapped around the site of the circumcision to prevent bleeding.

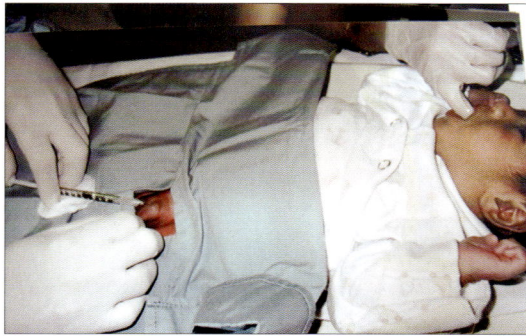

Local Anesthetic

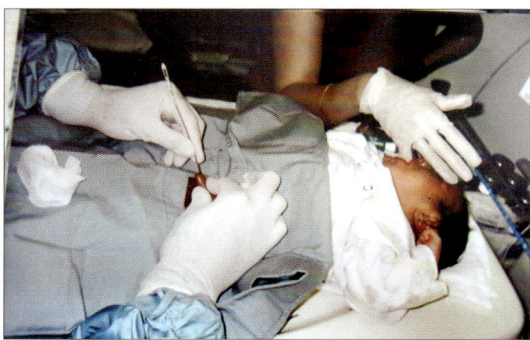

Freeing Foreskin

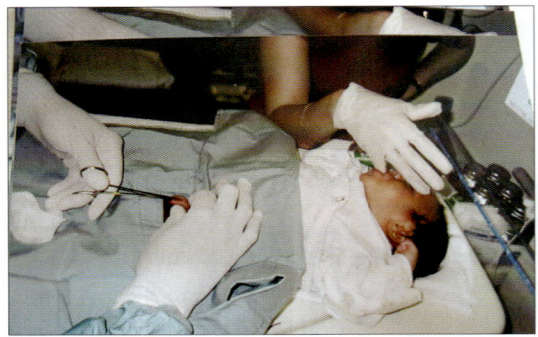
Snapping Length of Skin to Be Removed

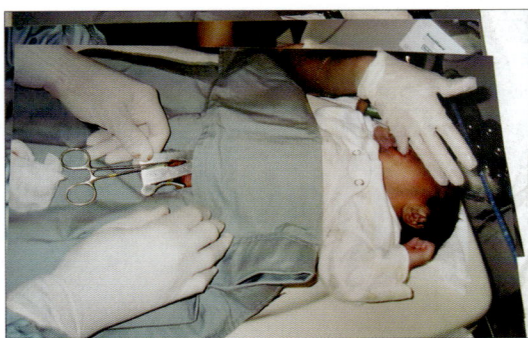
Mogen Clamp

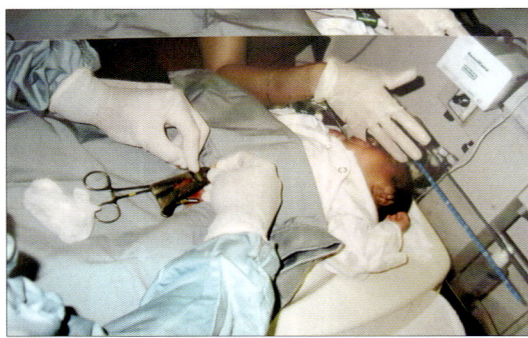
Foreskin Removed

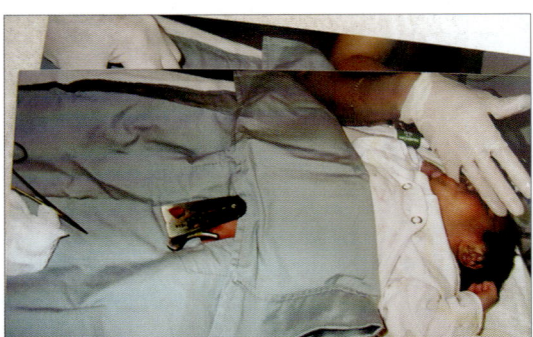
Circumcision Complete

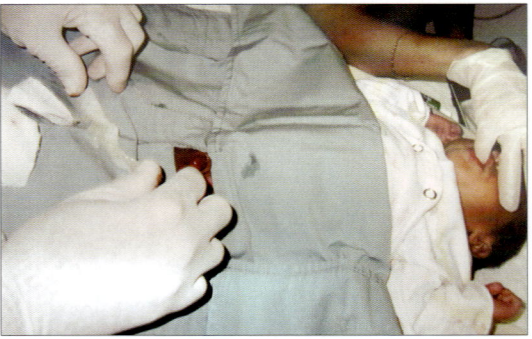
Gauze Around Site of Circumcision

Aftercare

Day 1 – With every diaper change, cover the head of the penis with a thick coating of petroleum jelly (to protect it against contact with urine or feces). The gauze will come off by itself and does not have to be replaced. You may sponge the baby but stay clear of the circumcision site.

Put the diaper on loosely to prevent any rubbing against the head of the penis.

Day 2 – Nothing is to be done. For bathing, sponge the baby only and avoid cleaning the penis.

Day 3 – same as day 2.

On the third day you may notice that at the base of the head of the penis there is a whitish colour to the skin. This is part of the normal healing process so do not worry; it will disappear in a few days.

Day 4 and thereafter – You may clean the penis as you would normally without any precautions.

Problems that may arise from circumcision

Bleeding – If bleeding occurs it usually does so within the first hour after the circumcision is completed. Measures will be taken to stop the bleeding. You and your baby will not be sent home until the bleeding completely stops. Once you are at home, a drop or two of blood on the diaper may be noticed. If, however, there is enough blood to make a stain on the diaper the size of 3 loonies on a single diaper or the same amount for more than one diaper, this is too much. The infant should be checked out by a doctor.

Infection – Here the whitish healing area at the head of the penis will turn yellowish green and probably have an odor. Infection of the wound most likely is present – if this happens you need to purchase Polysporin ointment. Apply to the site of infection with every diaper change for 5 days. If you are worried, seek medical advice.

Trauma – A circumcision is a surgical procedure. As with any surgical procedure there may be a mistake resulting in damage to the penis. Thankfully, surgical mishaps are extremely uncommon. We doctors do our best not to damage your son's penis.

Colds

Topping the list of parental concerns is the young infant who has a cold. Mom could have a cold, dad could have a cold, in fact, anyone else could have a cold and no one frets. But the baby showing just one cold symptom seems to muster up horrendous fears that there is a major health problem emerging. Why is it always the wee baby who has the severe, nasty cold and seldom the big baby who has a teeny weeny cold?

The common cold is caused by a number of viruses. These viruses are spread in several ways –by someone sneezing, coming in contact with infected tears, or touching inanimate objects, on which the virus can survive for hours to days - and then transferring the virus to the nose.

The common cold lasts for 7 to 10 days. The symptoms are usually mild in nature, consisting of a clear nasal discharge, mild congestion and feeling mildly unwell. If a fever is present it is low-grade. Complications consist of development of an ear infection or, very rarely, sinusitis. The fact that the mucus turns from yellow to green does not necessarily indicate that there is a bacterial infection requiring antibiotics. Seldom does a cold develop into anything more serious (e.g. pneumonia).

The treatment consists of waiting for the cold to disappear. Medications are unnecessary (except for saline nose drops for nasal stuffiness which interferes with feeding or sleep). In fact, children less than 6 years of age should never receive cold medication unless it is prescribed by a doctor. For these younger children, over-the-counter medication may result in side effects consisting of irritability, loss of appetite, sleep disturbance or, in rare cases, cardiovascular complications. If more than 2 medications are given to augment their effectiveness, the worsening of any side effects may occur. There is also a potential risk of medications interfering in some manner with other medication already being administered to the child for completely different reasons.

Children catch colds all year long but this happens more frequently during the winter months. This is mainly due to the fact that kids spend more time indoors, where the viruses can easily be spread from one child to another, where contact with objects such as books and crayons on which the virus has been deposited is unavoidable.

Let us go over the treatment of colds. In former days (prior to the baby boomers) there were several dastardly methods used. A mustard plaster applied to the chest to provide heat likely only damaged the hair follicles on the chest (this is probably the reason why many of my generation have hairless chests). Garlic either worn around the neck or eaten drove away friends but did little to prevent or treat the cold – viruses have no sense of smell. Vaporizers used to loosen the nasal congestion only loosened the wallpaper and did little else. Nasal aspirators removed only the mucus which was in the end of the nose. If the nose was really blocked and this interfered with sleep or feeding, the blockage was coming from higher up in the nasal passages, a place that could not be reached by using an aspirator. Steam from a hot kettle, with or without eucalyptus, would result only in first- and, occasionally, second-degree burns to the face and a good laugh for the viruses. Vapo-Rub on the chest may have smelled quite medicinal but did very little. Neither did a host of other remedies steeped in folklore and brought from the old country do much to prevent or treat the common cold. Ultimately, treating the child's cold usually makes only the caregiver feel better, because she feels, she is doing something to help even though it really does little to relieve the actual symptoms for the child.

Presently, in our "drug-hungry" modern society we have a host of remedies to prevent or treat a cold. Vitamins, even vitamin C, have been shown to have little or no effect against a cold virus. The same goes for echinacea. There is a whole array of over-the-counter medications. What do dextromethorphan hydrobromide, pseudoephedrine hydrochloride, guaifenesin, chlorpheniramine maleate, doxylamine succinate and diphenhydramine hydrochloride have in common? Give up? They are each contained in varying combinations in every cold remedy. There are decongestants, expectorants and cough suppressants – alone or in various combinations. There are nighttime as well as daytime medications. There are slow-release as well as quick-release medications. There are liquids, geltabs, tablets, capsules, drops and ones that melt in your mouth. Any of these may or may not contain acetaminophen or ibuprofen. There are nasal drops and sprays to help shrink the swollen nasal passages. By the time you figure out which one of these you need for your specific cold or that of your child, the illness will be gone. Homeopathic medications do not fare any better.

Grandma's chicken soup is the only "medicinal" treatment that I would recommend. However, saltwater nose drops may help to loosen thick nasal secretions. Elevation of the head may offer some comfort. For extremely thick nasal secretions that seem to be problematic for the child, the use of saline nasal rinses 2 or 3 times a day can be helpful (for children over 3 years of age). Vapo-Rub applied to the chest sparingly may also be helpful to relieve nasal congestion (for children over 2 years of age).

According to "Mother Nature", having a runny nose and a little bit of a cough is the best way to get rid of the virus. I certainly am not about to question Mother Nature.

There is no magic elixir that stimulates the immune system to either prevent or treat the common cold. If there were, the inventor would have won a Nobel Prize by now and be a multi-billionaire.

Cold weather does not cause a cold. Children should be allowed to play outside as much as possible – any self-respecting virus will not go outside in the cold. Not wearing a hat does not result in an ear infection: cold air entering a child's ear will not cause the ear to become infected. If you have a cold, taking a shower or bath is fine. Your child is the best barometer as to how active or inactive he wants to be. With minor sniffles, all activity should be encouraged – playing outside, swimming and participation in all sports. Dress your child appropriately for the weather, but do not overdress him just because he has a cold. If your infant or child has a cold without a fever, is eating well, is happy and has little disturbance in his sleep pattern, then the cold symptoms are likely to be bothering the caregiver more than the child himself.

The best way to prevent the spread of colds is to frequently wash the child's hands for at least 15 seconds. The use of alcohol-based hand sanitizers should be encouraged. Teach your child, when coughing or sneezing, to cover his mouth or nose with his sleeve – not his hands. The use of Kleenex is fine but often most kids do not have a tissue readily available.

Red flags

When any respiratory symptoms occur, you need to ask yourself the following questions:

- Does the child look ill?
- Does he act ill (that is, more fussy and cranky and/or more lethargic than usual)?
- Is he feeding poorly?
- Is there a significant disturbance in his sleep pattern?
- Does his breathing seem laboured (indrawing between his ribs at the top of his rib cage)?
- Is he breathing rapidly?
- Does the cough sound like a seal or dog barking – croup?
- Is he wheezing – a whistle-like sound during expiration (breathing out)?
- Are the cold symptoms which seemed to be improving suddenly worse?
- Has the cough lasted more than one week (3 days for an infant under 3 months of age)?
- Does the infant seem to be in pain and/or pulling at his ears?
- Does he have a fever?
- Is there interference with feeding? Small infants are nasal breathers. If the infant is feeding well, then the nasal stuffiness is of little concern. If the nasal passages were significantly blocked with mucus, breathing would be noticeably difficult during breast or bottle feeding. This would result in an interrupted feeding pattern.

If the answer to most of these questions is "no", then in all likelihood the symptoms of the cold are more an issue for the caregiver(s) than for the infant.

Mucus inside the nasal passages does not have to be removed. Suctioning to remove mucous that is higher up in the nasal passages is ineffective and thus will not relieve nasal congestion.

Loose, mucousy, sounds when there are none of the above red flags are of no concern. This is not a cold. The sound is created by the infant breathing through a small web of mucus in his upper airway. With your hand placed lightly on his chest you may feel vibrations. When you listen to his chest with your ear it sounds as if his chest is filled with sea water. If he was able to simply clear his throat the symptoms would disappear. Since he is unable to do this (because of his age) he will either swallow the mucus or eventually cough it up. Mucousy breathing sounds in an infant is a major concern for parents who worry that there is a health problem. Most commonly, however, the sounds bother the caregiver and not the infant – no red flags – no problem.

Remember, in the end, it is your call whether or not to seek medical advice. It is up to you to determine whether or not your child is ill – but if there is any doubt, seek your doctor's advice even if it's just for reassurance.

Use your own common sense. Your "advisory staff" more often than not will only fuel your anxiety – in their opinion a small cold soon becomes a severe pneumonia and you are neglecting your child and are an irresponsible parent.

By the way, contrary to what you may have been told, for small children do not discontinue giving milk during a cold. Milk does not significantly stimulate an increase in mucus production.

The use of antibiotics has no place in the treatment of the common cold. To sum up, please do not overmedicate your children. Too often parents will medicate a child so they themselves may be provided with a quiet night's sleep!!

Colds and Flu

Colds and flu have these 3 things in common. They're both caused by viruses, both occur for the most part during the winter cold season and early spring, and both are spread in the same manner.

Cold and flu viruses can be spread in several ways – through contact with infected tears or cough and nasal secretions, or by touching contaminated objects, on which the virus can survive for hours to days before being transferred to the nose.

The common cold lasts for 7–10 days. The symptoms are usually mild in nature, consisting of a clear nasal discharge, mild congestion and feeling only slightly unwell. If a fever is present, it is low-grade. Complications consist of middle-ear infections or, in rare cases, sinusitis. The fact that the mucus turns yellow to green does not necessarily signal a bacterial infection requiring antibiotics. Daily activities are usually not disrupted.

Catching a flu virus results in far more nasty symptoms. These include high fever, headache, severe cough, generalized aches and pains and feeling very unwell.

Flu symptoms last for 7–10 days. For most of its duration the affected person spends his time in bed moaning and groaning.

Both colds and flus are more prevalent during the winter months and early spring. This is mainly due to the fact that children spend more time indoors, where the viruses can easily be spread from one child to another or children come into contact with objects that have been contaminated by the viruses (for example, a crayon or book).

The treatment for both consists of waiting for the symptoms to disappear. Acetaminophen or ibuprofen is indicated for the control of fever, headache and aches and pains. Other medications such as antibiotics are not indicated unless there is a secondary bacterial infection. Children under 7 years of age should never be given cold medication unless it is prescribed by a doctor. Side effects of cold medications in young children consist of irritability, loss of appetite, sleep disturbance and sometimes, on rare occasions, cardiovascular complications. Saltwater nose drops may be given to loosen nasal secretions if the child has difficulty breathing through his nose. Saline nasal rinses are also effective for the removal of thick nasal secretions.

However, the bottom line is that the preceding may not always be effective or accepted by the child. Grandma's chicken soup is still the only failsafe "cold remedy."

Antiviral agents such as Tamiflu (oral) or Relenza (nasal) are helpful only if started within 48 hours of the onset of flu symptoms. They are not indicated for the common cold.

There are a few myths that I would like to dispel:

- Cold weather does *not* make one more prone to colds or flu.
- Playing outside in the winter will *not* weaken the child's immune system. In fact, it is good for it. When playing outside, children experience less crowding and therefore there is less chance of catching a virus. After all, any self-respecting virus will not go outside in the cold.
- Wearing a hat will *not* prevent an ear infection.
- Cold wind in the ear will *not* cause an ear infection.
- Stopping milk intake is *not* necessary during a cold in order to decrease mucus production.

The best way to prevent the spread of viruses is to wash your hands frequently (for at least 15 seconds). Teach your child to cover his mouth or nose with his sleeve and not his hands when coughing or sneezing. The use of Kleenex is fine but most kids usually do not have a tissue readily available.

Flu vaccination is basically recommended for all children starting at 6 months of age. The vaccine will result in approximately 80%–90% protection against severe flu and its complications.

The flu vaccine does not cause the flu. Side effects may include a low-grade fever, swelling and tenderness at the site of injection and perhaps mild aches and pains for 1–2 days. The flu vaccine has been implicated as a cause of Guillain-Barré syndrome. Its incidence after the flu vaccine is similar to the incidence in those children who do not receive the vaccine. The concern about developing this neurological disorder after flu vaccination is negligible.

Children between the ages of 6 months and 9 years require two immunizations one month apart in the first year. Thereafter, they receive the vaccine yearly.

Children over 9 years of age require only one initial immunization and yearly immunization thereafter.

Children under 9 years of age who initially received only a single immunization will require two immunizations the following year and yearly immunization thereafter.

Those children who have received only a single immunization 2 years in a row may carry on with single doses thereafter.

Remember, children between 6 months and 2 years of age are considered to be at high risk for developing the flu and its complications.

The flu vaccine contains thimerosal. Numerous studies have shown that there are no long-term ill effects from the small amount of thimerosal present in the vaccine.

There is a new flu vaccine that is administered by a nasal spray. It is recommended for children over 2 years of age and adults. Children between 2 and 9 years of age, if not previously immunized for flu, will require 2 nasal vaccinations one month apart. Those who have been previously immunized will require one dose only. Children over 9 years of age and adults only require one dose. At present, the cost of the nasal flu mist is not covered by the government but may be by some private drug plans. There is no discomfort in the administration of this vaccine. It is highly effective. Side effects include a stuffy or runny nose, nosebleed, headache, cough and occasionally fever. Side effects are uncommon and usually mild in nature.

The flu vaccine is an excellent vaccine to prevent or reduce the symptoms of a nasty illness. I highly recommend its use.

In conclusion, never overmedicate your child just to suppress symptoms. Always be wise – get immunized!!!

Colic

Infant colic is only one of the many reasons an infant cries. It occurs in healthy infants (whose growth and development are normal). Both breast-and-bottle fed infants are affected equally.

The classical definition of colic (one which I do not agree with) is of a healthy infant who has severe crying episodes for at least 3 hours a day, for at least 3 days a week, and persisting for 3 weeks. The 'worst' time for many infants is in the evening.

My definition of colic is somewhat different. Symptoms usually begin at approximately 1 to 2 weeks of age. Shortly after feeding is finished, the baby begins to cry as if in pain, the tummy may become bloated, and he draws up his legs and passes a lot of gas. Discomfort can be of a very mild nature, or such that it causes the infant to cry inconsolably. The symptoms may persist for up to 1 hour before subsiding.

The vast majority of infants outgrow colic by 4 months of age no matter which definition you use.

The cause of infant colic is unknown. Researchers have speculated that it is initiated either by the central nervous system or by the gastrointestinal system.

Infant colic is extremely worrisome for the caregiver and frustrating for the doctor. The reason is that there is no single way to manage this condition. The reality is that there is no "cure" for infant colic. Although the infant is obviously distressed, the greatest toll is most often on the caregiver.

Rubbing the baby's tummy, cuddling and rocking the baby, the use of a warm hot-water bottle and taking the baby for long walks in the stroller may be all that is necessary.

Medicinal remedies – you can try them but remember none have been proven to be successful. If one works for you, you are lucky!

Oval drops – 0.25-mL up to 0.5-mL with each meal. Not to exceed 1.5 mL per day.

Gripe water – under one month of age, 2.5 mL. Over one month of age, 5 mL – 4 times daily.

Iberogast – 6 drops 3 times daily (over 3 months of age, 8 drops 3 times daily).

Chamomile, fennel or anise tea – dilute one part tea to 2 parts water. Give 5 to 15 mLs 3 to 4 times a day.

Infantcol – 0.5 mL up to 1 mL with each feed (maximum 5 times daily).

There are a number of homeopathic medications that may be tried (for example Cocyntal – 1 mL and if necessary repeat every 15 minutes for a total of 3 doses). Are they effective? Probably not. You be the judge.

There is some evidence that probiotics may help to reduce the symptoms of colic. It may, however, take up to 2–3 weeks before seeing an effect. Because probiotics are basically harmless and inexpensive they are worth a try – for example, Bio Gaia, 6 drops once daily.

Changes in formula are usually ineffective. Knowing this, some parents nevertheless have tried formula changes to decrease the symptoms of colic. They may want to try one that is lactose free, or one that has the milk protein partially hydrolyzed (broken down) or soy formulas. Partially hydrolyzed formulas have been shown to decrease the amount of gas passed by a baby and thus may diminish symptoms of colic. All have been tried. If you are one of the lucky few for whom a formula change makes a magical difference, you are very fortunate indeed. If there is no response within 10 days, return to your previous formula.

It should be noted that hereditary lactose intolerance usually does not manifest symptoms until the baby is close to one year of age or older. Therefore restricting lactose in a very young infant is unnecessary. Saying this, I fully understand why parents may want to try a lactose-free formula, soy formula or a partially hydrolyzed one. As stated above, if it works, use it. By the way, I have had caregivers switch from one formula to another of the exact same composition. They will swear that the second formula did the trick, and that they now have a happy, contented baby. In fact, all they will have changed is the colour of the label on the can. But, if they are happy, I am happy.

For those breastfed infants with colic, I suggest that the mother try a lactose-free diet. She may still have milk and dairy but it needs to be lactose-free. This usually does not decrease the infant's symptoms because the symptoms of primary lactose intolerance do not occur until one year of age. It does, however, give the mother an action to take and as a result she feels that she is actually doing something for the baby. Cauliflower, broccoli and cabbage should be eliminated from mom's diet. If there is no improvement within 10 days, she may return to a regular diet.

Persistent spitting up with crying episodes, usually during feeding, oftentimes may mimic colic. Here the discomfort is caused by the acid of the stomach contents irritating the esophagus (swallowing tube). There may also be feeding refusal. Discuss with your doctor. An antacid may be indicated. (See also Vomiting and Diarrhea.) Celiac and milk protein allergy may present with colic.

If you become overwhelmed by the infant's symptoms, they are best discussed with your doctor rather than your "advisory staff", who will most likely, with all good intention, further confuse you.

In all the scientific studies done on colic, once again I want to emphasize that there is no single proven prevention or "cure".

Good luck, stay strong, and there is a light at the end of the tunnel. Colic usually disappears by 4 months of age.

Constipation

Constipation is defined as a passage of very hard stools associated with discomfort. The discomfort may be mild or moderate but seldom severe. The amount of time between bowel movements is not a concern as long as the stools are soft and passed without discomfort.

Breastfed babies normally have a loose, seedy yellow stool with each feeding. After a few weeks of age the frequency of stooling decreases. The infant may have a stool daily or it may be several days or longer before he has a soft bowel movement. This is perfectly normal. As long as the baby passes a stool which is soft and with minimal discomfort, no problem is present. If the stools are green in colour, this too is normal.

Bottle-fed babies may initially have 3 or 4 bowel movements daily. After a few weeks they may have only one bowel movement a day or every other day. The bowel movement is usually soft and passed without pain. This is normal. Again, a green stool is not a problem.

Often small infants under 2–3 months of age seem to have discomfort trying to pass a bowel movement. They squirm and struggle and appear to be uncomfortable for minutes or for up to an hour before passing a soft bowel movement. The problem is that the neurological coordination for contracting and relaxing the rectal muscles is not yet fully developed. This development usually occurs by 3–4 months of age, and at that time the discomfort will end. The discomfort is not due to constipation. No treatment is required.

Iron present in iron-fortified formulas does **not** cause constipation. Switching from one brand of formula to another will not relieve constipation. Soy formulas have not been shown to relieve constipation. However, some parents will contradict all of the above. If a formula change seems to be working for your infant, I am happy for you.

The consistent passage of infrequent, long, thin, ribbon-like stools with abdominal distention is of concern and should be looked at for a condition called Hirschsprung's disease. With this condition, there is a lack of nerve endings in the distal rectum. This absence of nerve endings may extend up the colon. Because of the lack of innervation, the rectum does not recognize the presence of stool. The baby's tummy may become distended. The stools that are passed are very thin and ribbon like. This diagnosis is suspected on the basis of history and the finding of an empty rectum (no stool) on rectal examination. Confirmation is made by doing a rectal biopsy which indicates the absence of nerve cells. Surgical removal of the involved bowel will be required. This condition presents itself from birth on, but may not be recognized for months or years, depending on the length of the affected bowel.

Constipation in young infants is uncommon. For breastfed babies as well as bottle-fed babies, a common cause is lack of adequate fluid intake (underfeeding). The rate of weight gain will enable the doctor to determine if this is in fact the problem. If not receiving enough breast milk results in constipation, breast milk production can be increased with the use of a medication (domperidone) and herbs called blessed thistle and fenugreek. For formula-fed babies, give as much formula as the baby wants. The bottle should never be completely emptied. If so, the baby wants more. Another cause may be that the formula is not prepared properly. If not enough water is added to the concentrate or powder formula, eventually this will lead to constipation and, as well, other serious complications in the water and electrolyte balance in the child's bodily fluids.

Constipation under 4–6 months of age: If the infant is on rice cereal this may be the factor. Switch to oatmeal or barley cereal. If this does not help, you may give prune juice (as much as needed) to soften the stool. Use on a daily basis or as needed. If the constipation persists, especially if there is abdominal distention and/or pain with passing a bowel movement, the child should be seen by his doctor.

Foods that are constipating include rice and banana. Reduce these in the diet. The ingestion of a large amount of milk – over 30 ounces per day, may lead to constipation. Reduce milk intake to 18-20 ounces per day to see if this makes a difference. Recent evidence has shown that a select group of children with chronic constipation respond within one week after the complete elimination of milk and dairy from their diet. The mechanism for this is not completely understood, but may be on an immune basis somewhat similar to milk protein allergy, but delayed in time. When cow's milk was reintroduced to those who responded, there was a relapse of the constipation. Several ounces of water daily will help. Prune juice is a natural stool softener. You cannot overdose on prune juice – give as much as is needed to soften the stool (if the infant's face becomes wrinkled like a raisin you know you have reached the maximum – a joke!). Increase the fibre in baby's diet. Fruits with the skin left on, such as raisins, grapes, blueberries, plums, and peaches, are excellent choices. Remember, leave the skin on. Try whole-grain breads. Choose high-fibre cereals rather than refined cereals. Refined cereals are not as high in fibre. Oatmeal, granola, bran, and whole-grain cereals (e.g. shredded wheat) are excellent choices.

When formula or breastfed infants are first put on 3.25% milk there may be a temporary period of constipation for 2–3 weeks. Afterwards, the previous bowel habits will return. During this transition phase try the above.

Recently, there has been evidence that a daily supplement with a **probiotic** may help in the management of functional chronic constipation.

After the first year of life, constipation may result after the infant has experienced difficulty and pain with passing of a bowel movement. To prevent more discomfort, the infant will hold the stools in for as long as possible. This only perpetuates the problem. Here again, dietary changes as stated above should be instituted. Prune juice again should be given, as much as needed. If these measures do not work then a stool softener may be necessary. My softener of choice is mineral oil. Begin with 1 teaspoon and increase by half a teaspoon every 4–5 days until you reach a dose such that the child is having a soft bowel movement passed without pain every 1 to 2 days. Whatever the dose, you may keep the child on it for a minimum of 2 months, and then slowly try to wean him off by decreasing it by half a teaspoon every 4–5 days. If during the weaning, the constipation returns, then return to the previous amount of mineral oil and use for another 2 months. Repeat the weaning process. Glycerine suppositories, as well as enemas, should only be used on the advice of your doctor. Again, if you're concerned about the constipation, seek medical advice.

Most doctors have their favourite laxative that they are comfortable in prescribing. Laxatives can work in 3 ways. They can soften the stool by mixing in with it, such as mineral oil. They can soften the stool by increasing the water content of it, such as lactulose. Lastly, they can stimulate an increase in the propulsion of stool by increasing bowel peristalsis (contractions) with laxatives such as Senokot.

For children over one and a half years of age, especially during toilet training, stressful periods such as the arrival of a new infant, starting daycare or anything that changes their environment may cause withheld stooling. This becomes a vicious cycle. Stools are passed only with a great deal of effort and discomfort. The child reacts by withholding the stools for as long as possible to prevent the symptoms, which only furthers the discomfort and difficulty in passing stools. (If the anal opening becomes overstretched by a large bowel movement, blood may be found on the stools, on the toilet paper or in the toilet water.) The rectum becomes filled with firm stool, which is often the size of a softball. Liquid stool above this mass may leak around it and stain the diaper, or the infant may pass infrequent small, pebble-like stools. The persistence of a large mass of stool in the rectum results in stretching of the rectal muscles that are used to push the stool out. With continued stretching the muscles lose their tone. They are not able to contract to push the stool out. This diagnosis is made on a rectal examination by the doctor. A glycerine suppository or a pediatric Fleet enema may be required to evacuate the stool mass. This may have to be repeated until the rectum is empty. Mineral oil is started as above and increased until the child is having a bowel movement every 1–2 days, passed without pain. Do not be alarmed if you have to increase the mineral oil above the initial dose recommended on the label for age. There is no dosage limit. The mineral oil needs to be given for 3 months (by this time the rectal muscle tone is back to normal) and then tapered off as formerly described. The child should be under medical supervision on a regular basis until this problem is resolved.

The medical term for the above is encopresis. Occasionally a parent will bring the child into the office because of diarrhea. The loose stools, however, are the result of overflow incontinence due to anal impaction with stool. The treatment for this child's "diarrhea" is to treat his chronic constipation.

For the doctor to truly determine the severity of the constipation, a rectal examination is mandatory.

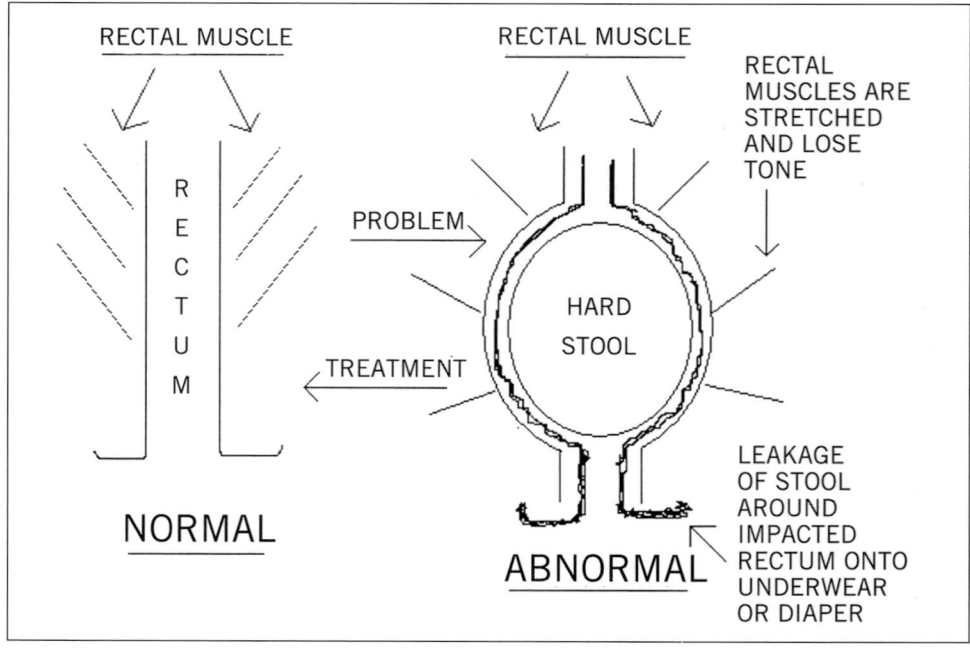

Encopresis (Severe Constipation)

Remember, negative reinforcement should not be used when the child refuses to have a bowel movement. This will only worsen the situation. If the constipation occurs during bowel training, back right off and try again in another month.

If the mineral oil does not give the desired effect or if the child refuses it, there are many other stool softeners that can be used. Discuss this with your doctor. Polyethylene glycol is my next preferred choice as a laxative for difficult cases.

There are other medical causes for chronic constipation other than those related to the diet and those that are functional in origin as reviewed above. These are uncommon but should be considered on an individual basis. Usually in these conditions, constipation is only one of the symptoms present. On history, physical examination and appropriate lab testing, the child's doctor should be able to rule out these uncommon causes or treat them appropriately. With treatment of the underlying condition the symptom of constipation will no longer be present.

Cord Blood (Storage)

There is a question every pregnant woman should discuss with her partner and the doctor before delivery. It is, "Should I save my baby's cord blood?"

In my perspective the answer should be a resounding "yes".

Although there is a cost associated with this procedure, in my opinion it is an inexpensive "insurance" that may potentially one day save the life of your child or of a close relative. The baby's stem cells, if needed for an emergency, are the most perfect match available and there is no risk of recipient rejection if they are required.

Cord blood is the blood that remains in the umbilical cord and placenta after the birth of the baby. This blood is rich in stem cells that have the capacity to differentiate into all types of blood cells, as well as into all other kinds of cells.

The cord blood is collected after the cord has been clamped and cut. There is no discomfort for the newborn.

The cord blood is frozen and, at the time of this writing, remains available for use for up to 18 years.

Cord blood stem cells have been used to treat over 70 different types of diseases. These include diseases of the bone marrow, hemoglobinopathies such as thalassemia major, hereditary immune system disorders, lymphomas, leukemias, and many others.

Currently, there are many clinical trials being done which use cord blood cells for the treatment of cerebral palsy, type 1 diabetes, spinal cord injury, stroke, muscular dystrophy, heart disease and liver disease. At present, the trials for these various disorders look promising.

The cost of preserving cord blood cells is about $1000, with a yearly maintenance fee of approximately $125 for storage of the cells.

I urge pregnant women to discuss the topic of cord blood cell storing with their family and doctor.

It is insurance that I hope that you will never have to use.

Cough

The most common reason for a caregiver bringing a child to my office with a health concern, is a cough.

Most adults with a cough carry on with their normal daily routines. They seldom see a doctor and most often do not even take over-the-counter medications. In time, the cough subsides.

With the child, however, it is a different story. Most caregivers will not tolerate a child's cough for more than a few days (or less) before seeking medical attention. Why? Because they are unsure if something serious is causing the cough which requires treatment. Could it be asthma? Could it be bronchitis? Could it be pneumonia? All of these concerns are frequently intensified by an "advisory staff" that often fuels anxiety to further heights.

This section cannot cover every cause of a cough. However, I will address the common reasons for 98% of coughs experienced in childhood.

Before going into the causes of cough, here are a few general guidelines for you to use that should alert you to when the child should be seen by a doctor. These include:

- if an infant is less than 3 months of age
- if a cough lasts over a week in a child who is not ill
- when a cough is associated with a fever for over 3 days
- when a cough is associated with difficulty breathing – wheezing (a problem with breathing out or expiration), a rapid respiratory rate (over 30 breaths per minute when not crying), indrawing between the ribs during breathing, or abdominal breathing (the tummy moves in and out during breathing)
- with a child who appears ill
- when persistent vomiting accompanies the cough
- if a cough has a significant impact on mood, eating and/or sleeping pattern
- if the child is very lethargic

- when persistent chest pain is present
- There is complaint of an earache (in an infant, pulling at his ear or excessive fussiness).

Simply ask yourself the following:

- Does my child look ill?
- Is my child acting ill?
- Does my child have a fever?
- Does my child have a major mood change, or alteration in eating or sleeping patterns?

If the answer is no to the above questions then the cough is most likely bothering the caregiver rather than the child. There is no rush to seek medical attention. Most coughs, especially those associated with a cold, last for 7–10 days.

If more than one person in the family has similar symptoms, then it is most likely of a viral nature. Medication is not required.

Complaints of chest and abdominal pain during a cough are the result of stretching of the chest and abdominal muscles during breathing. A sore throat may often accompany severe coughing.

For the first 8–10 months after entering daycare or school for the first time, many children will experience recurrent viral coughs. It is during this time that they are building up their immunity. They are also giving their own viruses to others, which helps them, in turn to build up their immunity. You can be reassured that your child has no underlying sinister illness.

Postviral coughs can last for weeks. The initial fever, which may have lasted a few days, and the accompanying stuffiness have disappeared, but the cough persists. The cough is usually loose and worse at night. There are spasms of coughing throughout the night. The child will have repeated episodes of rapid coughing spasms during which he may turn pale and after which he may vomit. No one in the household sleeps. However, during the day he seems rather well, and upon visiting the doctor (probably more than once) the child's chest is clear and a chest x-ray, if done, is normal. This child has what I call the "100-day cough". This is a post- viral cough that will not respond to antibiotics or asthma medication. Cough medicine is not advised, not only because of its possible side effects but also because the amount of medication required to suppress the cough would far exceed the recommended maximal dosage.

As a doctor, I find this one of the most difficult symptoms to deal with. It can be very hard to convince a parent that there is no treatment required. It is hard for the parent to accept that the cough will have to run its course. The cough may last for 3 months. All too often a caregiver will seek a second, third, or even fourth opinion until someone does what they really want and that is usually to have them prescribe an antibiotic. Many doctors who, unfortunately, prescribe the antibiotics all too often will add asthma puffers. The caregiver is seldom told what the doctor is actually treating.

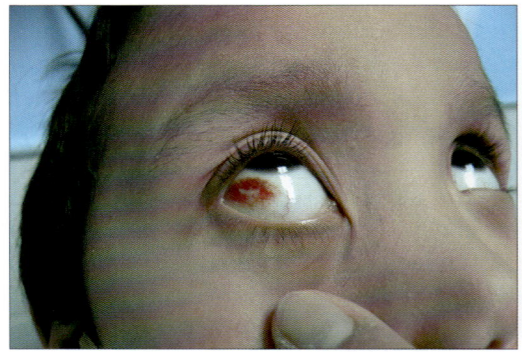
Post-Cough Hemorrhage

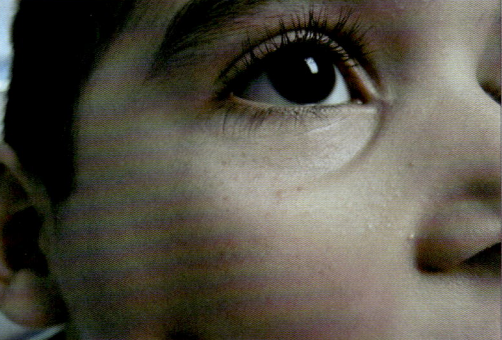
Post-cough Petechiae

The cough slowly gets better and the caregiver credits it to the use of medication and not to the fact that the disease is just running its natural course. Often the caregiver is very disappointed with the primary doctor for failing to medicate the child.

Despite receiving the primary immunizations for whooping cough, whooping cough may occur. This is not dissimilar to the 100-day cough. During the coughing spasms the child will take periodic deep inspiratory breaths (these inbreathes are the "whoops") before continuing to cough and often to vomit. The cough can be so violent that there are hemorrhages in the white of the eye and petechiae (minute hemorrhages) in the skin of his cheeks (see Whooping Cough).

A postnasal drip will often cause a cough usually when the child is lying down. The nose is also very stuffy. Treatment here consists of the use of saline sinus rinses 2 or 3 times a day until it clears. Rarely is an antibiotic required unless a diagnosis of sinusitis (see Sinusitis) is made.

Enlarged adenoids may block the normal nasal drainage of mucus posteriorly into the throat. Snoring is always present. The child always seems stuffed up. A mild postnasal drip may be present. This may result in a persistent cough, mainly at night. The problem is mechanical in origin due to the enlarged adenoids. Medications or removal of the adenoids is not indicated.

A child, who is usually over 4–5 years of age who has a persistent cough that sounds more like a dry clearing of his throat is most likely to have a habit tic. The child is not ill and there is no interference with eating or sleeping. A trigger may be found, such as starting school, home problems, bullying, etc. Deal with the trigger and the tic will slowly disappear. Asking the child to stop is like stoking the flames of a fire – the tic worsens.

Coughing due to croup, asthma, environmental causes, cold weather-induced or exercise-induced, bronchitis, bronchiolitis, pneumonia and croup are discussed elsewhere in this book.

In the end, if your child's cough is bothering you, it is always better to err on the side of caution and have the child seen by the doctor. Hopefully, at least you will have peace of mind.

Cradle Cap (Seborrhea) – Scalp

Cradle Cap

One morning you might pick the baby up out of the crib and notice a thick, flaky, yellowish-coloured crust covering the scalp. "Oh my," you remark worriedly, "some fungus is growing on my baby's scalp." Panic sets in and you are off to the doctor.

Do not fret

Close to 20% of infants will have varying degrees of cradle cap during the first year of life. It usually begins between 2 to 8 weeks of age. It ranges from a mild form, which involves minimal dryness and slight scaling of the scalp, to a thick, oily crust on the scalp that has an alarming appearance as well as an odour.

The cause of cradle cap is unknown. It is absolutely unrelated to hygiene, to breast-or bottle-feeding or to what you are applying to the baby's skin. It is not an allergy and is not contagious. It is not dangerous and if left completely alone would disappear with time. There are generally no symptoms that are associated with cradle cap except for an odour and itchiness, which causes scratching.

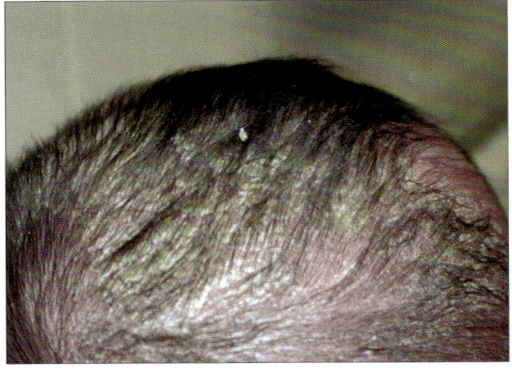
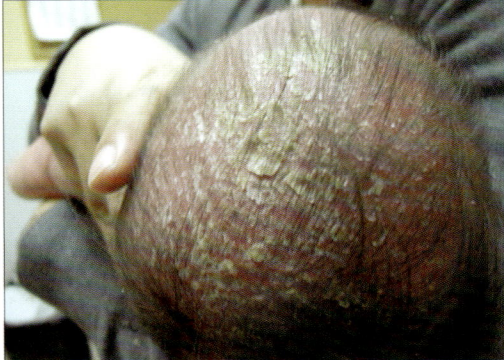

Mild Cradle Cap   *Excessive Cradle Cap*

Try the following:

1. Shampoo the hair daily with whatever shampoo you normally use on the baby's head. Be a little more vigorous in your scrubbing.

2. If the above does not work, in the evening apply mineral oil to the baby's scalp and leave it on for approximately one hour. This will soften the scales. Shampoo the hair as you do normally, using a little more muscle power. Use a soft toothbrush to gently lift off the crusts and then rinse. Do not be afraid that you will puncture the soft spot – it won't happen.

3. If the above does not work then use a medicated dandruff shampoo such as Selsun Blue or Nizoral (both can be purchased over the counter). Other medicated shampoos are available by prescription. Use one of these in step 2 instead of your ordinary shampoo. Allow the shampoo to sit on the scalp for approximately 15–20 minutes before washing it off. Use nightly and with improvement, taper off the use and use only when required.

4. For very resistant cases, a steroid lotion may be required. Leave it on the scalp overnight after step 2 is completed.

Note: The reason for treatment failure is usually related to the fact that the caregiver is too gentle about removing the scales. The pressure that is needed is the same as the pressure used when scratching an itch. Remember, you will not puncture the soft spot.

Seborrhea (Dermatitis)

Cradle cap may become part of a more generalized rash called seborrheic dermatitis. Seborrheic dermatitis of the skin usually presents itself in the first 2 months of life. A common site is behind the ears, where there is redness and cracking of the skin. It may also present as crusting on the eyelids. It is commonly found in the diaper area as well as patches on any part of the body.

The rashes of seborrhea and eczema are often confused. Eczema usually does not present itself until after the second month of life. Your doctor should be able to distinguish between the two. The basic management is similar.

The exact trigger for seborrhea is unknown. If it were left completely untreated it would eventually clear on its own. But most parents wish to have their baby's skin appear silky smooth, without any blemishes.

Repeat moisturization may be all that is necessary. Failing that, however, a mild cortisone cream will clear the problem up within one week. If the dermatitis reoccurs, reapply the cream. In the diaper area, a secondary yeast infection may occur along with the seborrhea. If this is the case, an antifungal cream is recommended in addition to the steroid cream in order to treat both conditions.

Croup (Tracheitis)

Croup is a viral illness which causes inflammation of the trachea (upper windpipe). Although many viruses can cause croup, it is usually due to a parainfluenza virus. It occurs most commonly during the winter.

Croup is most often found in children aged 18 months to 6 years, although it can equally occur at later ages. Croup can also reoccur (more than once).

Croup is spread by respiratory secretions either through a cough or from sharing contaminated objects such as straws, cups, cans, bottles and spoons.

Along with the inflammation, there is a narrowing of the airway around the voice-box area. The degree of narrowing predicts the severity of the illness. The more narrow the airway becomes the worse the croup will be, accompanied by worsening symptoms.

It usually begins as a very mild upper respiratory tract infection. Subsequently, during the night the child wakes up with a barky cough, hoarse voice and possible fever. He may have varying degrees of difficulty in breathing. Some children have very little difficulty while others have a marked difficulty with breathing in (inspiration) as compared to breathing out (expiration).

Mild Croup

For mild croup, patients do not have any respiratory symptoms other than the barky cough with or without a hoarse voice. The illness is worse at night and seems better the next day, only to return the next night. The second night the symptoms usually are not as bad as the first. During the day they are a lot better. The illness will go on for 4 or 5 days, getting better each night. It is contagious during the first 2 days of the cough.

Treatment for mild croup is controlling the fever and ensuring adequate fluid intake. Nothing more is needed. The child may prefer fluids, cold drinks, ice cream, milkshakes, Jell-O, puddings or yogurt. Do not be concerned if he does not accept solids. When there is improvement, his appetite will return.

Moderate Croup

With moderate croup the above symptoms are present but are more severe. The illness usually does not improve to any significant degree during the day. There is indrawing between the ribs and at the midline above the sternum (breastbone). This means that the airway is narrowing enough to cause respiratory distress (problems with getting an adequate supply of air). He will have more difficulty when he is trying to take air in rather than when getting air out.

Note: Your child will always seem worse when he or she is crying or upset. The only way that you can really determine if there are breathing problems is to watch the child breathing when he is quiet. If there is indrawing between the ribs, then moderate croup is present.

Children with moderate croup do not look too ill and will take an interest in normal daily activities, such as playing with toys and being read to, etc. For these children, although there is some respiratory distress, their focus is not on breathing alone.

Treatment for moderate croup is a single dose of Decadron (dexamethasone). This must be prescribed by a doctor. Rarely does it need repeating the next day. It usually requires 6–8 hours after the Decadron is given before improvement is noticed.

Many times children do not like to swallow because of the discomfort involved, so encourage, but do not force fluid intake as stated for mild croup.

If there is minimal to no improvement with the use of Decadron and symptoms seem to be worsening, then the child may be developing severe croup.

Severe Croup

With severe croup all the above symptoms have worsened. The cough becomes more frequent, a fever is usually present and there is notably a marked indrawing of the chest wall. The color of the skin may be pale or dusky. The child is focusing only on breathing. He is lethargic and just wants to lie still or be held. He will have an anxious look on his face. Respiratory difficulty will be present not only when he is breathing in but also when he is breathing out (wheezing). There is a lack of interest in anything else in the environment. Oral intake of food or drink is usually refused.

Treatment for severe croup requires intervention in the hospital emergency department. If it is needed, oxygen is given by mask. Any fever is treated. A single dose of Decadron is given. A mask of nebulized steroid and epinephrine will most likely be required. The child will then be observed in the emergency department, and if he shows improvement after 2 or 3 hours he will be sent home. A second mask may be required. If there is no improvement or further worsening, the child will be admitted to hospital. If he is refusing to drink, an IV may be required for hydration. The inhalation treatment may be repeated along with the Decadron at some point in time. In severe cases, assisted ventilation may be necessary by intubation or tracheotomy.

There are many other tools that have been used in the treatment of croup. Studies, however, have shown them to be ineffective. These include humidifiers and vaporizers, steaming up the bathroom and riding in the car with the cold wind blowing on the face. Cough medicines or decongestants should never be given for the treatment of croup, no matter what degree of severity.

Inhaled Ventolin (salbutamol) and Flovent (steroid via metered-dose inhalers) have no place in the treatment of croup. These are for the treatment of asthma only.

Bacterial Tracheitis

This illness is very uncommon but very serious. The cause is a bacterial infection of the upper airway. It begins as a mild upper respiratory tract infection with rapid progressive and increasing symptoms of croup. There usually is a high fever. The child looks toxic (quite ill). There is marked difficulty in swallowing. A severe, barky cough is present (occasionally, however, little cough is present because the child suppresses it due to pain). The child is only interested in breathing. Swallowing is extremely difficult and painful.

This condition is an emergency and the child should be taken to the hospital immediately.

The mainstays of treatment are intravenous antibiotics, fluid maintenance, temperature control and oxygen. In extreme cases, assisted ventilation (intubation or tracheotomy) may be required until the illness subsides.

Croup symptoms – starting during the day:

Viral croup usually begins during the night. If a well infant or toddler during the day has the sudden onset of a barky cough, this possibly could be the result of ingestion of a foreign body which found its way into one of the airway branches. If this occurs, then a chest x-ray is required to confirm the presence of the foreign body (if radio-opaque, it's metallic) and, if present, removal under a light general anesthetic. Non-radio-opaque foreign bodies (plastic, buttons, seeds or anything else non-metallic) will not be seen by x-ray. However, the findings on chest x-ray of shifting of the midline structures in the chest, as well as a difference in lung sizes, is diagnostic of an aspirated foreign object. Again, under a light general anesthetic it will be removed.

Crying Baby (What It Means and How to Deal with It)

Certain major events can inevitably and predictably have an adverse affect on the very fibre of family life. Such events may include, a life-threatening illness, sudden reversals in the finances of the family, or most profoundly, the death of a family member. There is, in addition, another phenomenon that is seemingly not so catastrophic. As a matter of fact, it is hardly regarded as being on the same scale as an "event". It can, however, take an equal toll on the family. Through its slow and unrelenting persistence it may thoroughly disrupt an apparently normal family; such is the crying infant.

New parents, both young and older, are frequently influenced by the quite powerful misconception that babies are not supposed to cry. After all, media images depict a Gerber baby who is always delighted, never crying. The baby on the Pampers package does not cry, nor does the cute cherub on the box of Ivory Snow. He's happy too. They're all so happy.

We need to come to the realization that all infants will cry without apparent cause and that it is quite normal. The babies have been fed and changed; no diaper pin has pierced their hip (as in the old days before disposables); they are not in discomfort from wearing tight or restrictive clothing; they have been cuddled, soothed and pampered – and yet they still may cry! The question is, "Why do they cry?"

For how long and how often during the day is it normal that an infant cry? The answer is that most infants may have up to 3 crying episodes per day: 2 short periods for less than a half an hour during the day and a more prolonged period for less than 2 hours in the early evening. The latter is the most common, constant time for crying. It is also the most distressing time for the family, because it comes when tired parents need to have their own personal downtime, to be able to unwind at the end of the day. The baby doesn't appear to be in any discomfort, the cry is not overly intense, and he usually settles when picked up or rocked. An infant whose crying pattern falls within the above range of frequency, duration and quality has no underlying sinister cause for the cry. He is just being a baby.

Crying is, in fact, the most important way in which a baby communicates his needs to you, the caregiver. Caregivers are soon able to interpret the meaning of their infant's cries. They can distinguish between the cry of hunger, the cry for attention, the cry to be picked up for a little cuddle or play, or the cry for needing a diaper change.

Again, the 3 most common causes of "normal" crying are: the infant who is hungry; the one who just wishes some extra attention and the infant who wants a diaper change. The child, once comforted, having his diaper change and being fed, will quickly settle down. In this scenario there is absolutely no medical reason for the cry.

Concerns are often raised, however, when there are changes in the infant's cry. First, there is a marked change in the infant's pattern of crying. Second, there is a change in the quality of the cry. Third, the baby becomes less easily pacified. Sometimes these changes develop slowly over a period of several days, or they may appear more quickly.

There are a number of causes for a change in the pattern of crying that have no serious underlying medical explanation. One of these is underfeeding. This leads to a hungry infant who cries until his needs are satisfied. It occurs most frequently with a breastfed infant during the first 2–3 weeks of life when the mother's milk supply may not be sufficient to satisfy his hunger. The scenario usually goes as follows. The baby seems to have a good latch. He will stay on the breast for prolonged periods of time, up to one hour or longer. During breastfeeding he may take frequent "time outs" and fall asleep for short periods before resuming his suck when prodded. After breastfeeding, he falls asleep for perhaps an hour only to wake up screaming, and is pacified only when put back to the breast. Mom then spends her days feeding the baby continually around the clock (feeding on demand). She is able to do little else; no housekeeping no time for personal hygiene, and especially no relaxing, not even to sit and have a cup of tea. Mom becomes exhausted and frustrated and her coping skills are diminished little by little. Over time, communication with her spouse (who often does not understand what is going on) becomes strained, sometimes hostile. Her whole life seems to be unravelling. Her self-appointed "advisory staff" only frustrate her further. In tears, she finally goes to her doctor to find out what is wrong with her baby. She does not realize that the cause of her problem is that she lacks an adequate quantity of milk to meet her baby's needs. After all, it seems to her that the baby nurses for over an hour and then falls asleep. Surely, he must be satisfied. She doesn't understand that the baby behaves this way out of sheer exhaustion from sucking on wind. By weighing and examining the infant, her doctor will conclude that the baby is being underfed. That being the problem, he will take steps to correct it, either by having mom see a lactation specialist or suggesting medication to increase milk production, or perhaps by recommending supplementation with formula.

The bottle-fed infant who empties his bottle completely is probably underfed. Increasing the amount of formula will stop the crying. My rule of thumb is to give the baby as much formula as he wants. However, the bottle should never be completely emptied on a continuous basis. Although it seems like a contradiction, there should be some milk left in the bottle to indicate that he has had enough.

Extended crying also occurs during the passing of hard stool pellets requiring an excessive amount of effort on the baby's part. In a small infant this too is usually due to underfeeding.

When urine or feces come in contact with an excoriated (raw) diaper rash, the infant will be irritable and cry.

Between 4 and 6 months of age, teething may begin to cause excessive crankiness. In my experience, it is best not to blame teething as the cause in every crying, fussy infant until I have ruled out other causes. And teething, by the way, does not cause fever 99.9% of the time.

Infant colic has been commonly blamed for frequent crying episodes during which the infant is usually inconsolable. Colic begins at approximately 2 weeks of age and usually subsides by 4 months. It occurs in both breastfed and formula-fed infants alike. The classical and accepted definition is an infant who cries for more than 3 hours a day, 3 days a week for 3 weeks. Personally, I do not like this definition. To me, colic occurs in an infant who feeds well, is burped, and then 5–15 minutes later begins to cry as if he is in pain. His tummy becomes bloated, his knees are drawn up to his abdomen, and/or copious amounts of gas are passed from both ends (mouth and rectum). This can last up to one hour before subsiding. It usually occurs with each feed.

Unfortunately, although there are numerous medications, including homeopathic remedies that can be tried, none have been proven to be effective. With true colic, formula changes do not seem to make any apparent difference. Limiting milk and other dairy in the diet of a breast-feeding mother is not usually successful either. Eliminating cruciferous vegetables, such as broccoli, cauliflower and cabbage, in mother's diet may help. For formula-fed infants, partially hydrolyzed milk protein formulas (milk protein has been partially broken down to ease digestion) may be tried. However, soy formula for the baby is not the answer. There are also more serious causes of prolonged crying, such as the following:

The infant who cries during feeds while arching his back, squirming and spitting out the nipple may have reflux esophagitis. This is typical especially when constant regurgitation is present. Full regurgitation may not be easily recognized with each episode. Partial regurgitation (that is, only coming up partway) still may be the cause of irritation to the esophagus (swallowing tube). To prevent the irritation, an antacid is required. To help prevent regurgitation thickening of the formula is required. The formula is thickened with rice cereal. Commercially thickened formulas without an antacid will, as well, help prevent reflux. The actual thickening process of these formulas occurs in the stomach in the presence of the acidity of the gastric contents. If an antacid is prescribed, the gastric contents' acidity is neutralized and the thickening process of a commercially thickened formula will not occur. Therefore, if the baby is on an antacid and thickening of the formula is recommended, it is best to use cereal:1 tablespoon for every 30 mL (1 ounce) of formula.

An infant who cries consistently when being moved may have a fracture, even though no trauma has been noticed. The most common sites for fractures are the clavicle, the arm or the leg. Indications of fracture include swelling, tenderness and increased crying when the area is touched or moved.

Another often-missed cause for the onset of a crying and difficult-to-pacify infant is a scratched cornea. This usually results from the infant poking his finger into his eye. Subsequently, if the infant continues to rub that eye, it can often become reddened.

Sometimes a milk protein allergy may cause an infant to cry, but he may not show any other symptoms initially. This is more suspicious, especially if there is a family history of milk allergy and, as well, some other symptoms present such as loose stools (which may be blood-streaked), abdominal distention, vomiting and poor weight gain. In the breastfed infant, breast-feeding should be encouraged for as long as possible. Mom may also try eliminating milk protein products from her own diet. A completely hydrolyzed (milk protein completely broken down) formula is necessary for the formula-fed infant.

Otitis media (middle-ear infection) should be suspected as yet another cause for extended crying, especially if the infant has a mild cold or fever.

One of the most overlooked causes of a crying infant is a urinary tract infection. Because the baby is diapered, one may not recognize that the discomfort comes during urination. Between voiding times, few or no symptoms are present. Loose stools and a low-grade fever should direct the doctor's attention to a possible urinary tract infection.

In males, irritation at the end of the penis (meatitis) or, in girls, in the vulval area (vulvitis) may also result in crying during urination.

The presence of a weak cry, especially coming from an infant who is limp, listless or pale, feeding poorly and perhaps feverish raises a huge red flag. Medical advice in this case should be sought at once. A serious infection or brain injury may be present.

Another warning symptom is the very sudden onset of a severe, painful cry, as if the infant is being hit in the abdomen by a cannonball. This could signal a bowel obstruction. This is the assumption until proven otherwise. The most common bowel obstruction in an infant would be intussusception. Other obstructions could include an incarcerated hernia, a twisted testicle, a bowel obstruction in an umbilical hernia sac or volvulus (a small bowel twisting and subsequent obstruction). All of these constitute a surgical emergency.

Infants who have suffered an "insult" to their central nervous system (such as being deprived of oxygen during the birthing process) may have prolonged times of irritability and crying. Prolonged labour, difficult delivery and low Apgar ratings may suggest the possibility of neurological factors. Observation of the infant over a long period of time may be required in order to assess his development.

Finally, there is the puzzle of the miserable little tot who just seems to like to cry. Is it his personality? (Blame it on your husband's side of the family!) There is actually nothing ostensibly wrong with him. Fortunately, on the bright side, these infants usually develop to become well-adjusted and bright, loving individuals. Ultimately, they will give their parents much pleasure, so this makes up for the early months of suffering and misery.

No infant cries without reason. All too often the reason is a puzzle and cannot be determined right away. It is frustrating for all 3 parties: the baby, the parents and the doctor. This is when the art of medicine needs to come into play in full force. It's an area, in my opinion, that is most poorly handled by some physicians. This is mainly because they do not take enough time to manage the problem. This in turn becomes a familiar reason for new parents to become disenchanted with their physician and to seek help elsewhere. Simply put, being told, "Nothing is wrong with the baby and he will outgrow it," just will not "do." By the time the baby's doctor acknowledges the severity of the problem, mom has already tried all the routine remedies suggested by her "advisory staff" and pharmacist. She has already spoken to the doctor's nurse on several occasions. In a panic, she has gone to a walk-in-clinic or the emergency ward, only to be turned away without adequate satisfaction. She may even have mentioned this to her physician during her brief office visit. Scant time is spent discussing the concern and mom is hastily "cut off" with suggestions for a formula change, colic medication or repeated and familiar reassurances. The mother is either embarrassed or afraid to express how bad the situation really is. She sees that the doctor is busy. As he exits the examining room he is saying, "Are there any problems?" She wants to cry out for help but resists the impulse. The examining room door closes. Mother is even more upset.

The cry of an infant is, unfortunately, one more stress brought to bear on a family. When added to the existing social and emotional stresses that are endured daily, the crying infant may aggravate the delicate balance of an already unstable family.

The doctor is not always privy to the various circumstances that affect the families he sees. He does not see the stress experienced by a single parent; the anxiety of the parent living in an apartment in which a crying infant may disturb the neighbours; the disorienting effect of the shift worker hours; the parent with drug and/or alcohol abuse, mental health issues or the abused parent. He does not always see the caregivers with poor parenting skills or the fact that there may be many other small children at home without adequate support systems in place for their care. Unless the physician is actually in tune with the family background as a whole he may fail to recognize the few distress symptoms; ones that are merely the tip of the iceberg. He may miss, altogether, that the parents' complaint about their crying infant is in fact their own cry for help as well.

As the mother becomes increasingly tired, frustrated, even angry, her coping skills are slowly diminished. She may go "down the tubes" both emotionally and physically and she is likely to take everybody in the family with her. The backbone of the family unit has thereby been broken. Sadly, the doctor has failed this mother. He has not picked up on the early clues because he has not listened for them.

For these moms, all I can advise is "Stand your ground!" If the doctor does not have time for you now, ask for another appointment, one in which he will be able to listen to you completely. Make a list of your concerns to bring to that appointment. If you're unable or unsure about standing up for yourself, bring a significant other with you to advocate on your behalf.

Every parent deserves to take enjoyment in his child as he grows. A crying infant with no intervention is one of those "events" which sabotages such pleasure; this is a tragedy and need not be.

Family counselling by professional counsellors may be advisable in order to support both mother and the family during this most trying time.

Daycare (Choosing)

A very difficult experience for any caregiver is to have trust in the kind of care their child will receive in a stranger's hands. Many parents choose a daycare based on the recommendations of friends who already have their children at a specific daycare and are pleased with the care. However, you may not have this luxury. You are going to have to do your own research.

Here are a few questions you should be asking to assist you in making your decision:

- Is the daycare licensed?
- How long has it been operating?
- What are the qualifications (including formal schooling, early childhood education training, first aid qualifications) of the daycare supervisor and other staff?
- What is the staff-to-child ratio?
- What is the staff turnover rate?
- Is it a safe environment?
- Does it have a clean environment with adequate bathroom and change facilities?
- What is the availability of early drop-off and late pick-up?
- What are the exclusion and return policies concerning an ill child?
- Does it have an open visitation policy?
- What are the outdoor facilities like? Are these child-friendly, clean, and safe?
- Does it have outings outside the daycare facility? How are these supervised?
- Will you be allowed to spend time observing the workings of the daycare?
- Who supervises the administration of medicine?
- What are the menu and food choices?
- How does the facility deal with food allergies and EpiPen storage?

It is obvious that financial considerations are important also. A decision also must be made as to whether you want the daycare to be situated close to home or to work, and this depends on what fits best for you, your partner and the child.

Once you are satisfied that the quality of care your child will receive at daycare meets your standards, then ask for a few references that you may phone to confirm your findings.

In the end, you must trust your own feelings and instincts to decide if the daycare is the right match for your child and you.

Daycare and Preschool-Entering Anxiety

Your child is entering daycare, preschool or junior kindergarten for the first time. Regrettably, there are a whole lot of children saying, "AYK" or "Are you kidding (me)." Why? Because they are so anxious about the prospect of taking their first leap outside of their protective environment – home.

A certain amount of anxiety is quite normal. In fact, it has its benefits. Before certain ventures, a slight degree of anxiety increases your adrenaline flow, starts the hormones churning and causes the heart to speed up. It prepares you for the challenge, whether it be jumping in the water for the first time or writing an exam.

There is a wide range to the degree of anxiety felt – from mild (which is considered normal) to extreme (not so normal). At the extreme end of the spectrum, anxiety can inhibit people to such a degree that they are unable to carry out certain seemingly ordinary functions, the vast majority of which are normally handled with ease. I am not referring to skydiving or going over Niagara Falls. For these situations, any sensible person would be hesitant and terribly anxious; this would be entirely understandable. What I am talking about here are normal, usual daily routines (such as going outside, socializing with others or riding in a car) that cannot be carried out due to a high level of anxiety. In the extreme, a person becomes immobilized by this kind of anxiety, as in the case of a panic attack.

Which children are at risk of being so anxious that going to school becomes an overwhelming and terrifying experience? First of all, it can happen with any child. Nevertheless, there are certain predictors. These predictors include: a child whose very first experience away from home is entering school; a child who has in the past demonstrated separation anxiety; a child who is generally anxious to begin with; a quiet child of anxious parents.

Think of it from your child's point of view. He has had you as his constant companions. You have always been there when you have been needed. Basically, he is totally reliant on you. To an anxious child, being sent off to school may seem like being thrown into the lion's den – a pretty scary place away from the safe place he has known.

There are some strategies that may help soften his first venture away without you. Do not try to "oversell" school. It is not the Magic Kingdom. Begin the preparation 10 to 14 days prior to the start of school. Talk to him and/or read books to him about school. Take him past his school by way of the route you intend to use. Do it 3 to 4 times. If possible, take him into the school and show him his classroom. Find out the names of his teachers and practice their names with him. If possible, plan to have another child of the same age and his parent go with you – misery always enjoys company.

Whenever possible you should encourage your child to give you his input about this new experience. It will give him a sense of empowerment that will translate into both greater self-confidence and a feeling of control. This is a much better way to start the school year. Examples of how his input could be used are: choosing his clothes on his own for the first day of school, choosing what he wants for breakfast that day (the "condemned man's last meal"), letting him decide the spot where he is to be dropped off and picked up, and allowing him to select a "security" object that he can take in his pocket to help smooth the transition (a picture of a pet, a small toy, a key, for example).

No special routine is required on the night prior to school. The less said, the better.

On the way to school, display a positive mental attitude on your part, one that conveys to your child that he will be fine. Remember to stick to the routine you have practiced in the past with him.

Now comes the moment of truth. You have arrived at the exact spot that you both have previously decided is the point of departure. Remind him that you will be right at that spot to pick him up when school is over. Ask him to be a "helper" if he sees anyone who is sad. Despite all your preparation, expect the worse. Saying, "Everything will be fine and you will be okay," will not work – forget it. If your child he is crying, although it may be the most difficult thing you ever have to do, just turn around and walk away. If he follows you, take him by the hand to a teacher (they are well trained to handle these situations) and then continue to walk away. Do not let him see you crying. Your emotions will be repeated again when he leaves for university!!

I know that you may not believe me, but you are not the first parent to face this situation. The vast majority of children do much better than their parents. Within a few minutes after you have left and he is in the classroom setting, his tears will dry (long before yours, I'm sure).

If, after the first day, he does not want to talk about his day when asked and just disinterestedly says, "It's okay," be wary that something may not have gone so well. Reintroduce the subject during some other activity: supper or bedtime. If he still does not want to talk about his experience, do not force it. Try again the next day. If this continues you may wish to speak to the teacher to determine if any problems have arisen.

In the end, I wish for you that all will go well, that he easily says "bye Mom" and off he goes, leaving only you in tears.

Remember to ensure that your child's vaccinations are up to date. The school should be made aware of any health problems that possibly could affect your child during school. Forms that give permission for the school to administer medications should be completed.

P.S.: Streetproofing should be introduced – age-appropriate, from 2-1/2 years of age on.

Daycare Syndrome

How many times have I heard parents say that their child, over the past few months, has had 4 colds, 2 bouts of gastroenteritis, 3 different rashes, 2 ear infections, pink eye and a "partridge in a pear tree?" The child was so healthy before.

My first question to the parent is, "When did he start daycare?" Nine times out of 10 they will reply, "Two weeks before he started to get ill." There is your answer.

Your child has left the protective environment of his home and you have put him into a seething pool of bugs. No, I am not talking about the other children, but I am referring to the bugs that they carry and are more than happy to share with your child and others.

Do not be upset, because your "little darling" is also spreading his share of what he has acquired at home to others.

Daycare syndrome is unavoidable. Nearly every child will pass through this when he first enters the community. Only those children who have older siblings, who over the years have brought home one bug at a time, may escape the "infection parade".

There is absolutely nothing wrong with his immunity. It is only because of the close contact he now has with other children that he catches everything.

The syndrome lasts for 8–10 months and then like magic all settles down and the child becomes well again.

If possible, do not remove your child from daycare. The importance of socialization far outweighs the viral illnesses he is receiving during this adjustment period.

When to Exclude and When to Return the Sick Child

When should a child stay home from daycare or school if he is ill and when is the right time for him to return? This seems like a simple enough question. When he is sick, he stays home and when he is better, he goes back to school. Unfortunately, the answer is just not that clearcut. There are a number of variables involved in answering the question. Your feelings about when your child is too ill to go to school or ready to go back may be different from what the child feels, what the doctor feels and, lastly, what the school feels. There are additional factors involved in the decision-making. If there is no babysitter and if you are a single, working caregiver or 2 working parents, then who stays home? Your employer will perhaps not be pleased with the amount of time that you have taken off to care for your sick child, thus placing your employment in jeopardy. If your child is not doing that well at school, any time lost from his academic studies may make it difficult for him to catch up. This could have an adverse effect on his learning – the result being that you want him to miss a minimal amount of school. In this case you would be reluctant to keep him home if he is ill and might feel pressured for him to return as early as possible – and possibly before he is ready.

Certainly common sense has to be used in your decision-making. You must remember that a child who is feeling ill will not learn optimally if sent to school. If you're using the school as a babysitter, perhaps you would be putting the rest of his classmates at risk of becoming ill. At the same time a child with a mild respiratory tract infection consisting of a stuffy or runny nose may be allowed to attend school. If we kept every child home when he had a mild cold, no one would receive a full education. The severity of the illness should dictate the absence.

If the child is missing a lot of school because of somatic (bodily) complaints such as abdominal pain or headaches, his symptoms may be related to school phobia or separation anxiety. Here the complaints are usually present in the morning before school Monday through Friday, but especially on Monday. The symptoms seldom occur on the weekends or holidays. This child has anxiety, which may not be isolated to school alone. Help is required from his teacher, the school social worker, your doctor and, perhaps, a psychologist or psychiatrist.

Although many institutions have different criteria for exclusion from attendance for a sick child, the following is the general consensus of the Canadian Pediatric Society, along with some of my own thoughts.

Any infant or child who is so ill that he or she cannot participate fully in all the daycare activities, should remain at home until well enough to return and become fully active.

Children with respiratory conditions who are well and able to participate fully in all activities may continue attending daycare.

Children with bacterial conjunctivitis (pink eye infection) may return to daycare one day after starting eye drops.

Children with impetigo may return to daycare after one day of treatment.

Children with a sore throat, as well as a positive throat swab for streptococcus, may return to daycare after one day of antibiotics being initiated. The diagnosis of a strep throat infection can only be made by having a throat swab done to confirm the presence of streptococcus bacteria. No throat swab – no diagnosis. Antibiotics should not be given without confirmation that there is indeed a throat infection due to strep.

Children with diarrhea should be excluded from daycare if:

• The stools cannot be contained in the diaper.
• The stools cannot be controlled by a previously fully toilet-trained child.
• There are symptoms suggestive of a bacterial cause of the diarrhea.

The symptoms of a bacterial infections are fever, moderate abdominal pain, and mucus or blood in the stools. These children should have a stool culture and sensitivity testing done. If it is negative they may return to daycare depending on how ill they feel. If there is a bacterial cause for the gastroenteritis and antibiotics are required, the child may return to daycare if he is well enough 2 days after the initiation of the antibiotic.

The cause of most childhood diarrhea is viral. Some of these viruses are very contagious. Only by doing viral studies on a stool sample can a contagious viral cause be determined. Unfortunately, viral studies may take up to 10 days or longer before the results are available. If there are several children in the same setting with diarrhea then one can assume that the diarrhea has a viral source – remaining at home is a must. Unfortunately, it may take several days before the stools return to normal and the child is able to return to daycare or preschool. I do understand that this is a long period for a caregiver to be absent from work.

Children with chicken pox should be allowed to return if they are not ill 2 days after the rash begins. However, most institutions will not allow a child with chicken pox to return until all the lesions are healed and dried (5–7 days).

If a child has scabies or head lice, he may return to daycare after a single treatment.

If a child has whooping cough, he may return 2 days after antibiotics are initiated.

What if a child is not really ill but running a low-grade fever? Should he stay home? This is a bit harder to answer. My opinion is that if the child does not have an infectious illness and looks and feels well, then he can probably go back to daycare or school. You must, however, inform the school of his illness. A signed note should be sent to allow the school to administer acetaminophen or ibuprofen if a stronger fever develops. If the child must take medication during school hours, in order for the school to be allowed to administer it, a note must be sent with the medication stating the child's name, the dose and when it is to be administered. The school will want to know the adverse effects of the medication and what to do if any occur. If the child becomes ill while attending daycare or preschool, it is most likely that you will be asked to pick him up and take him home. The child may return to daycare when he has been afebrile (fever free) for 24 hours.

Children who have hepatitis B and are no longer jaundiced, or who have HIV, should be allowed to attend daycare. No extra precautions are required.

As stated above, each institution may have different policies as to admission and exclusion due to illness. They are for the protection of all involved, including the daycare providers, as well as the children themselves.

Unfortunately, when a child first enters daycare he comes into contact with many other children who will be more than happy to share their "bugs". Your child, trust me, will give his share of bugs to others as well. While building up his immunity, which usually takes 8–10 months, it will not be unusual for him to have frequent viral infections, including colds and coughs, vomiting and diarrhea, various rashes and a host of other "goodies". I call it the "Daycare Syndrome". Hopefully, you will survive his early months at daycare. I am sure he will.

Your best defense from spreading illness is to use common sense, practice fastidious and frequent handwashing, properly dispose of soiled diapers, and teach your child to cover his nose and mouth with his forearm if he sneezes or coughs.

Please – spread the word but not the disease.

Developmental Milestones

I, personally, am not rigid as to the exact timing of developmental milestones. The range given in most books, I feel, is much too narrow. Over the past 40 years I have seen a tremendous variation in all developmental milestones in absolutely normal infants. In fact, one of my own grandchildren did not walk until 2 years of age. Before she turned 10 years of age she was in competitive dancing, was a competent skier, an excellent student, and all-around great kid (after all, she is my grandchild).

I've observed, over the years, that parents have not changed in many respects. They always want to compare children. They all look at the extremes of development as the rule (e.g. a child walking at 7 months of age while theirs is barely sitting). They spend so much time worrying about their child's development that the satisfaction of watching their child develop is obscured.

I am serious about the fact that one of the hardest things for me to do is to convince a parent(s) that their child is normal. Sometimes I feel that they would be more relieved if I were to tell them the one thing that they would never want to hear – that I have concerns about their child's development. I feel truly sorry for these parents, because they are missing out on all the enjoyment that the child could be giving them.

Although I could go into great detail about the numerous milestones that occur during the first 2 years of life, I do feel that this information would be more of a worry than a service to my patients. It would become very complicated and only give rise to unnecessary concerns. However, there are 2 observations that never change as to when to be concerned. The first is if the child stops progressing. The second is if the child has regression (stops doing what he previously has accomplished) in his milestones. Here are some very general guidelines:

By the first month of life

During the first month of life you should notice that your baby responds to loud noise usually with a startle or cry: for example, the slamming of a door, the start of a vacuum cleaner, or any other sudden loud noise. He will also start to move his head from side-to-side, and, all limbs will be moving as if he were in the Olympics!

By the second month of life

The baby's head will start to move toward the direction of the sound. He will be able to focus on large objects 3–4 feet away and may even be able to follow them.

By the third month of life

The baby's eyes and head will track (follow) you as you move. He will begin to smile and even laugh when being played with. Vocalization should occur – that is, cooing making "ooh" sounds. His eyes may not move together until he is close to 6 months of age. When you move his limbs, he has good tone. If you hold him under his arms, he will hang from your hands and not slip from between them.

By the sixth month of life

All the above is progressing nicely. The baby is able to recognize you and respond with a pleased expression to your voice. He is able to hold on to large objects and stare at them. He has excellent head control (when pulled up by the shoulders, his head will follow without any lag). Everything, and I mean everything, that he can grab goes into his mouth (very often even his toes). It should be noted that large babies will move at a slower pace. There is more bulk to shift around. This requires more muscle power, which they may not have at this point. This does not necessarily mean there is a concern for their developmental milestones.

By the eighth month of life

The baby should be able to transfer objects from one hand to another. He will also be able to reach out to grab whatever there is to grab.

By the tenth month of life

The baby should start to understand simple verbal requests, such as stopping an activity in response to the word "no". Many books on infant development will tell you that the infant should be rolling from his front to his back by 4 months of age and from his back to his front by 6 months of age. Personally, I have seen numerous infants who are unable to roll until 7 months (and even later) and they were perfectly normal. Any good doctor, by feeling the tone in the baby's muscles as he moves his limbs and picks him up, should be able to reassure a concerned parent that the baby is fine.

Similarly, I have seen quite normal infants delay sitting independently until close to one year of age. They may not be able to get to the sitting position on their own until 13 months of age. Normal infants may not crawl until 14 months of age or pull themselves to a standing position until 15 months of age. Walking independently may not occur until 18 months of age or even until 20 months.

Although language development will be discussed in further detail, a child should:

- coo by 3–4 months
- babble by 7–8 months
- utter a first word by 15 months (usually at least 3–5 words understandable to you)
- speak at least 10 understandable words by 18 months
- say 20 words by 20 months
- say at least 50 words by 2 years of age and start to link words together

By the fifteenth month of life

The child should be able to play with toys appropriately, for example, by rolling a car or truck the way it is meant to be rolled.

By the eighteenth and twentieth months of life

The child should be able to climb stairs on all fours. Around the same time, he should be able to walk up and down stairs with your assistance.

I am quite sure that for many readers some of the milestones I have described above would indicate a delay in motor development in their child – a delay that should be investigated. In my own defense because I work on the 'front line' I see mostly normal infants every day. I am not a tertiary-care neurodevelopment specialist who sees mostly children with delayed development, many of whom have some underlying neuromuscular or metabolic disorders causing the delay. I am not referring to these children. The children that I have described above are normal, and although their motor development may seem to be delayed even past what is considered the upper limit expected for that particular milestone, at the end of the day they will all reach the same goal – normal.

It is also normal for infants to skip milestones, for example, to sit unassisted before they are rolling both ways, to crawl before they are able to sit or even to walk before they crawl.

Not all children crawl the way you would expect – forward on their hands and knees. Some will motor backwards, some will move "commando style" – forward or backward – while others just scoot around on their bums. These are all normal patterns.

If parents have concerns about their child's motor development they should be discussed thoroughly with the child's doctor. If there is still a concern, a referral should be made for a developmental assessment. From what I have seen in the past, by the time the consultation for assessment rolls around, the child has already won his first gold medal in the "Toddler Olympics" 2-meter race. There are infant stimulation programs that the child can be referred to for the assessment of their motor development. Exercises will be taught to the parent to be used at home with their child in order to encourage and improve motor development.

By the way, politely ignore advice given to you by nonmedical persons who may try to convince you that your child has a delay in motor development. Always consult your doctor if concerned.

Ears–Middle-Ear Infection (Otitis Media)

Acute otitis media is an infection in the middle-ear compartment. Most children by three years of age will have had at least one ear infection and up to three or four. Otitis media is probably the most common infection seen in young children that may require an antibiotic.

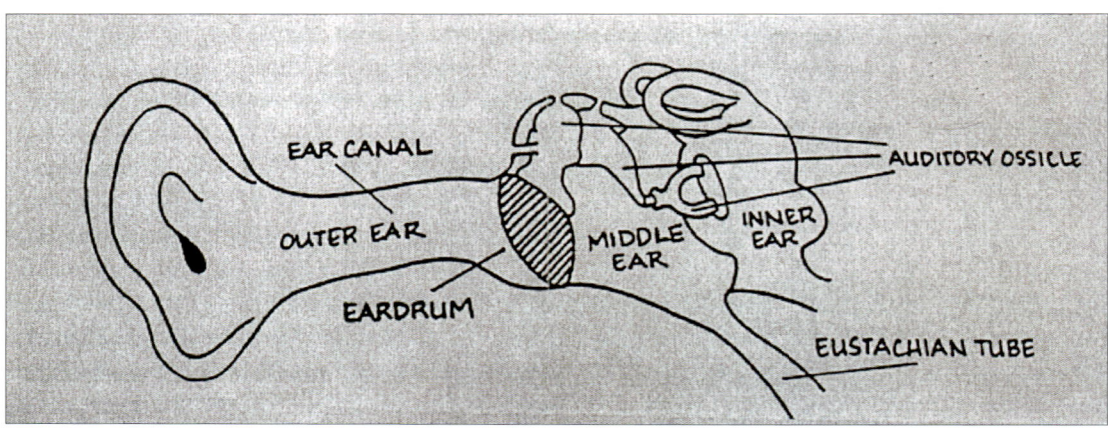

The external compartment or outer ear canal channels send sound down towards the middle-ear compartment. The middle ear is air-filled – the important parts are the eardrum and the three small bones (ossicles) which connect the eardrum to the inner ear. The middle ear is connected to the back of the throat by a hollow passage called the Eustachian tube. This passage allows air to fill the middle-ear cavity. With air present in the outer ear as well as in the middle ear, the eardrum has equal pressure on either side, allowing it to freely vibrate when sound waves strike it. These vibrations are passed through the three middle-ear bones to the inner ear. Without normal pressure between the outer and middle-ear compartment, sound waves striking the eardrum result in dampened sound vibrations. This in turn will not allow the middle-ear bones to transfer the sound waves to the inner ear. This most commonly occurs to varying degrees when there is some fluid (infected or not) in the middle-ear compartment.

The inner-ear compartment contains the organs necessary for balancing and hearing. It is here that the sound waves received from the middle ear are changed into electrical impulses, which travel to the brain for interpretation.

The steps in the development of acute otitis media

It begins with a mild cold. The lining cells of the Eustachian tube become swollen. This causes blockage to the connection between the back of the throat and the middle ear. As a result, the pressure in the middle ear becomes negative as compared to the pressure on the other side of the eardrum – the outer ear. Because of the negative pressure, the lining cells of the middle ear become swollen and fluid is drawn out into the middle-ear cavity. The air in the middle ear is thus replaced with fluid. This fluid (like swamp water) is a perfect growth medium for viruses and bacteria that may climb up the Eustachian tube from the mouth into the middle ear. The viruses and/or bacteria multiply rapidly, causing the middle ear to become infected – acute otitis media.

Symptoms of acute otitis media

Symptoms vary depending on the age of the child. In the infant or younger child they may be nonspecific – i.e. they do not point directly to a middle-ear problem. This is because the child is non- verbal and cannot say, "My ear hurts." Symptoms include the following (not all may be present at the same time) – a cold, a fever, irritability, sleep disturbance, pulling at the ear, loose stools, poor feeding and difficulty being consoled. For the older child who is able to communicate, the symptoms are usually a cold, fever, and the verbal complaint "My ear is sore."

To complicate matters, tugging at the ear may be caused by "referred" pain. This is where the problem is not in the middle ear but seemingly discomfort is transferred there from another source. Teething is a common cause for irritability and rubbing the ears. Other causes are infection in the oral cavity, dental disease or problems in the temporomandibular joint (jaw joint), inflammation or infection in or around the ear lobe, such as in a lymph gland, and infection in the outer ear (otitis externa – "swimmer's ear").

Diagnosis of otitis media

The diagnosis of middle-ear infection is made by directly examining the appearance of the eardrum. Testing for eardrum mobility with the use of air or sound may also be helpful in making the diagnosis.

Diagnostic difficulties

Doctors often encounter difficulties in visualizing the eardrum. Why?

A struggling infant is extremely difficult to examine. Any small amount of wax in the outer ear may block the view of the eardrum. This wax must be removed in order to see the drum. With a crying child, or one with a high fever, the eardrum may appear red and inflamed, which may be misleading for the doctor. A normal eardrum has many different appearances, some of which may show the typical appearance seen with middle-ear infections (this is especially true in children under four months of age). There are rapid changes that occur in the middle ear during the evolution (development) of an infection. Frequently, a child who complains of an earache may have a normal-appearing eardrum showing good mobility when first examined – no obvious infection. Yet, several hours later, the drum may appear 100% changed, even perforated and draining. So quickly does the appearance change, that two independent observers looking at the same child, within hours of one another, might see the inflammatory process at different stages and therefore come to 2 different conclusions. Many doctors who are not examining children's ears on a regular basis often do over-diagnose acute otitis media.

Treatment

The goal of treatment is to help the child feel better and to prevent any permanent damage to bone conductors in the middle-ear compartment that may lead to a hearing loss. Rare complications such as meningitis and mastoiditis also have to be prevented from occurring.

There is still much controversy over how to manage the child with acute otitis media. Treatment varies from the very infrequent use of antibiotics, as in many European countries, to the treatment of nearly every child with the diagnosis of otitis media with antibiotics as in North America. Who is treated, which antibiotic is used, the number of days that the treatment lasts, and the follow-up management may all vary throughout the medical community.

Natural course

Before antibiotics were widely available, the vast majority of ear infections cleared up on their own without any treatment. Acute complications such as mastoiditis or meningitis occurred, but rarely. Permanent degrees of hearing loss also occurred, but again those numbers were few. Why then are we using antibiotics so often for the treatment of acute otitis media? This is a difficult question to answer. The vast majority of ear infections are caused by viruses. For those infections, antibiotics are of no value. The problem is that it is very difficult to distinguish between a viral and a bacterial ear infection. Needle aspiration of fluid from the middle ear for bacterial culture would allow doctors to treat only bacterial causes, using the antibiotic that the bacteria is specifically sensitive to. This would be ideal but, unfortunately, completely impractical. Many ear infections, even those caused by bacteria, will clear up on their own without the use of any antibiotics.

The overuse of antibiotics in North America in the treatment of acute otitis media is related, in part, to public pressure that demands quick cures. It is so much easier for the doctor to prescribe an antibiotic than to take the time to explain why the use of antibiotics is unnecessary. Too many caregivers feel that not prescribing medication is "neglectful" on the doctor's part. If they don't get some from one doctor, they will go elsewhere until their "need" is fulfilled.

If antibiotics – for how long?

Decades ago, treatment lasting for 14 days was commonplace for antibiotic use. Now the course of antibiotics is given for 10 days. There is recent evidence that even this may be too long, and perhaps five to seven days of treatment is all that is required. This latter holds true for children over 2 years of age. However, in children under 2 years of age or for those who have recurrent ear infections, there would still be benefits from a 10-day course of medication. Newer antibiotics are given for three days but remain active in the bloodstream for seven days or longer. I am quite sure that, shortly, there will be a one-dose treatment that will cover most of the bacteria causing acute otitis media. For the present, however, if an antibiotic is prescribed, those under two years of age should have a 10-day course, and those over 2 years of age, a 5- to 7-day course.

Any child with recurrent ear infections, failure to respond to initial therapy, a perforated eardrum, or an immune problem should have the full 10 days of medication. Ultimately, every child who appears ill should be treated irrespective of his age.

Complimentary treatments

The use of decongestants, nasal sprays, and antibiotic ear drops (unless there is a perforated eardrum or a ventilating tube in the infected ear) has no place in the treatment of acute otitis media.

Who should receive antibiotics?

Here, again, there is no universal agreement:

1. Children under 2 years of age: Again, one may argue that the child from 6 months to 2 years of age who is not ill and has been diagnosed as having an ear infection may be treated symptomatically for fever and pain for at least 48 hours. If there is no improvement, antibiotics may be indicated.

2. Children over two years of age who are not ill (without high fever, lethargy or poor oral intake, for example) should not be treated with antibiotics. The symptoms of an ear infection due to viral origin usually last less than 48 hours. During this time symptomatic treatment with acetaminophen or ibuprofen is primarily used for pain and temperature control. If the symptoms persist longer than 48 hours, antibiotic treatment should be considered on an individual

basis. Any child, however, over 2 years of age who appears and acts ill should be treated with antibiotics without the waiting period (this should be the doctor's decision).

3. A child with chronic, recurrent ear infections (3 to 4 in an eight-month period) would most likely benefit from antibiotics.

4. The child who is under observation because of persistent fluid in his ear, and develops another infection, should be treated with antibiotics.

5. Any child with an immunodeficiency disorder, or who is on immune-suppressive medication, should be treated with antibiotics.

The above guidelines are not written in stone. There are exceptions based on each individual patient and physician decision-making. As well, the area in which the physician was educated and how current he is with the recent literature may dictate the management of a middle-ear infection.

Follow-up, with or without treatment

If a child is on antibiotics and is still symptomatic after 72 hours, consideration should be given to using a different antibiotic. If the symptoms continue to persist for a further 72 hours, the possibility of a myringotomy (surgical incision of the eardrum), with or without a ventilating tube, should be considered. The myringotomy will allow the infected fluid in the middle ear to drain. The insertion of a ventilating tube will allow any future fluid accumulating in the middle ear to drain spontaneously.

Assuming the child has improved, he should be reassessed in approximately 1 month's time. If there is no evidence of fluid in the middle ear by examination of the eardrum, (which may include testing for normal eardrum movement with the use of pneumotympanostomy, (air blown against the eardrum under pressure) or sound tympanostomy, then the episode has completely resolved. Nothing further is required.

Unfortunately, it may take up to three to four months for the fluid to naturally be reabsorbed. This is Mother Nature's way, so I do not argue. Thirty percent of children will still have fluid in the middle ear after 1 month, with or without treatment. Ten percent have persistent fluid after 2 months and approximately 4%–6% have fluid after 3 months. The child should be followed on a monthly basis. If the fluid persists after four months, the child will be referred for myringotomy and insertion of a ventilating tube. With persistent fluid in the middle ear, even though it is sterile (not infected), an infant or child may have persistent symptoms of irritability, tugging at his ear(s), loose stools, problems with sleep, behavioural issues, learning difficulties and a mild hearing loss. He is also highly susceptible to having another ear infection.

The child who has three or four ear infections (each resolving on follow-up) over a period of 6–8 months should be referred for consideration of the insertion of ventilating tubes.

The child with a persistent "stiff" eardrum, which lacks mobility, and a 20 decibel (dB) or more hearing loss as indicated by an audiogram, should be considered for the insertion of tubes.

Infants under 4 months of age

I would be cautious in the diagnosis of acute otitis media in any infant with fever under 3–4 months of age. The anatomical appearance of the eardrum at this age is different from the older infant and child. Only a doctor experienced in assessing many infants in this age group will have the expertise to diagnose acute otitis media. The fever may be from another source, for example, a blood infection, urinary tract infection, or even meningitis. If any of these sources are missed or under-treated, serious consequences result.

Preventative treatment

Breastfeeding, and eliminating the use of a pacifier, help diminish the number of ear infections. A smoke-free environment is optimal. As with other bacterial or viral infections, frequent handwashing is mandatory.

The use of long-term (prophylactic) antibiotics to prevent recurrent ear infections has been shown to be ineffective.

Aside from removing the child from an environment where he may catch cold(s) (for example, his daycare), there is really no effective preventative measure.

No homeopathic or alternative therapy has proven to be effective. If an alternative method worked, it would no longer be alternative! Chiropractic manipulation has no place in the management of middle-ear disorders.

Activity limitation

When descending or ascending in an airplane, the child with an ear infection should be drinking liquids, sucking on a hard candy, or chewing gum. Older children, if experiencing discomfort, may use the Valsalva manœuvre. This is accomplished by pinching the nose shut and keeping the mouth closed. The child then tries to forcefully blow air out of his closed mouth, trapping the air inside. The procedure may be repeated. This manœuvre will increase the pressure in the oropharynx, and this will, hopefully, force the Eustachian tube to open. Thus the pressure in the middle ear diminishes and this in turn lessens the discomfort.

Myths

• Drafts, wind, or cold weather will cause middle-ear infections.

• Water entering the ear may cause a middle-ear infection (as long as the eardrum is intact, water entering the ear may cause an outer ear infection, otitis externa. but not a middle-ear infection).

• Milk will go up the Eustachian tube, causing a middle-ear infection if the baby is fed while lying down.

• Warm oil drops inserted in the ear will improve the condition.

• The use of the pneumococcal vaccine will prevent acute otitis media (it prevents less than 10% of cases).

• A child with an ear infection should not go swimming for least 2 days (when well enough, swimming is permitted).

• Oral or nasal decongestants are useful in the management of otitis media – not true.

• Chiropractic manipulation helps treat or prevent ear infections. (This is completely unfounded, and, in fact, spinal manipulation of a young child could potentially result in a spinal cord injury!).

• Homeopathic remedies have a role in the treatment and/or prevention of otitis media – this is unfounded and never scientifically proven.

• There are medications to increase the immune system to help prevent middle-ear infections – no such "wonder medication" exists.

One of the frustrations I have as a practicing general pediatrician is what to do with children who require myringotomy and tubes. Unfortunately there may be a long waiting time before they are seen by an ear, nose, and throat specialist. This can be a distressing time for the child, the parent and the doctor. As a parent and grandparent I fully understand this. However, my hands are tied by the system. In the end, I "hold hands" with the caregiver and we try to manage the situation as best we can until the procedure is done.

Ears – Outer Ear (Otitis Externa Infection or Swimmer's Ear)

Otitis externa is an inflammation and/or infection in the outer ear canal.

Often it is called swimmer's ear because it occurs after a child has been swimming, especially if the water is not clean (high bacteria count). However, it can also occur after swimming in a pool and even after bathing. Constant irritation of the lining skin from using cotton tipped sticks (which should never be used in the ear) or earplugs may also result in otitis externa.

Water enters the outer ear and remains there. As it dries it can cause inflammation of the skin which lines the outer ear. The inflamed skin may become secondarily infected.

The symptoms are pain in the ear(s); if infected, a discharge may be noticed, as well as an odor from the infected ear(s). The child may complain that his ear feels "plugged". Presence of a fever is unusual.

Pushing on the soft skin flap in front of the opening of the ear canal will elicit discomfort. Pulling on the ear will do the same. If discomfort is present with these manipulations then otitis externa is most likely the reason.

It is treated by the instillation of antibiotic ear drops into the ear(s) for at least 5 days. Cortisone may be included in the drops to help reduce any inflammation. The child may return to swimming as soon as the symptoms disappear.

For those children who seem to get recurrent swimmer's ear, it is best to dry the ear as thoroughly as possible after swimming. A hair dryer set at a low temperature and gentle force will help dry the external canal. Pull the ear up and back. This will straighten out the ear canal. Hold the dryer 7–10 cm from the ear and blow the warm air into the ear for 2–3 minutes. BuroSol ear drops placed in the ears after swimming will also help prevent the recurrence of otitis externa.

Ear Tubes (Myringotomy)

The surgical procedure of myringotomy with the insertion of ventilating tube(s) is the most common outpatient surgery in North America.

There are commonly 4 basic reasons for the insertion of tubes in the middle ear:

• Recurrent middle-ear infections (4–6 a year)
• An audiogram that shows a 20% conductive hearing loss or more due to persistent fluid in the middle ear (fluid present for more than 4 months)
• Severe retraction of the eardrum
• A single episode of acute otitis media that is not responding to antibiotics and the child is still symptomatic (fever, feeling unwell and sore ear)

The insertion of tubes is an outpatient procedure. A light general anesthetic is required to induce a light sleep (enough to prevent struggling and discomfort). With a scalpel, a small slit is made in the eardrum. A small, hollow tube about 3 mm in length and 1-1/2 mm in diameter is placed in the slit so that half is in the middle ear and half is in the outer ear. It is then sewn onto the eardrum to keep it in place.

The purpose of the tube(s) is to allow any fluid that accumulates in the middle ear to drain out. This will protect the 3 little bones in the middle ear from any damage. It also enables the equalization of air pressure on either side of the eardrum. This is important to prevent fluid accumulation in the middle ear (with or without a subsequent infection) and, as well, allow the eardrum to have normal movement (necessary for hearing).

After surgery, acetaminophen or ibuprofen may be given to ease the discomfort. For 2 or 3 days there may be some drainage noticed that may even be blood tinged. After the fourth day, if drainage persists see the doctor.

Unfortunately, even if inserted by the best hands, the tubes may fall out too soon and have to be replaced.

If after 1-1/2 to 2 years the tubes are still in place, they should be removed to prevent a permanent hole in the eardrum, which could require surgical repair. The longer the tubes are in place after 2 years, the greater the risk of developing a permanent hole. Remind your doctor how long the tube(s) have been in place so that he/she can arrange for their removal when necessary.

Any fluid that enters the ear may pass through the tube into the middle ear, causing irritation with or without a resulting infection. In certain situations the outer ears should be plugged to prevent fluid entering the ear. Such situations occur during bathing and washing the child's hair (soapy water will easily pass through a tube), swimming or just running through the sprinkler. To protect the middle ear, I suggest using one of the following to plug the ear(s):

- A cotton ball immersed in petroleum jelly such as Vaseline
- Ear molds that can be purchased at most drugstores – they are soft and putty-like and can be molded to fit the outer ear – they are also reusable
- Custom-fitted ear molds
- An aqua band that fits around the head or a colourful swim cap – these should be worn over ear plugs while swimming

With a tube(s) inserted in the middle ear there should be no scuba diving. There are basically no other restrictions to swimming or jumping into the water.

If the tubes are functioning properly and the child subsequently acquires a cold and an ear infection, there may be no pain or fever. All that you will see is a discharge. The vast majority of these discharges clear up when ear drops are given for 7 days. Oral antibiotics are usually unnecessary.

Remember, nothing smaller than your elbow should ever enter the ear. This is especially true when there are tubes, which may become dislodged by the insertion of cotton-tipped sticks.

Ear Wax

It never fails. At least once a month I have a parent concerned about their child having "too much" wax in his ears. It cannot be good for him!

While washing a child's ears, a caregiver notices brownish wax at the entrance of the outer ear canal. With a finger in a washcloth the caregiver pokes around in the ear until it is "spic n' span" clean or stops because the child cries in pain. To do a more thorough job, if the child will allow, cotton-tipped sticks are rammed into the ears as far as possible to clean them.

I do not know where the notion ever began that wax is bad.

Wax is present in the ear to lubricate the skin and also to protect it from any external elements that may enter the outer ear canal. The colour may vary from beige to very dark brown. The consistency may vary from putty-like to flake-like to syrup-like.

Some children have very little wax while others seem to have enough wax to open a candle factory. Both are normal.

Ear cleaning

Remember, nothing smaller than your elbow should ever enter the ear canal. You may wipe the outer ear with a warm washcloth but do not enter the canal.

The continual use of cotton-tipped sticks only results in impaction of wax in the ear canal close to the eardrum. Depending on the extent of impaction there may be resulting ear discomfort or even a hearing loss.

With any earache the doctor will attempt to visualize the eardrum. If the outer canal is impacted with wax this will be impossible. The diagnosis of otitis media (middle-ear infection) will, therefore, be impossible to make. With the presence of the wax, time must be spent to remove it (impacted wax may be extremely difficult to remove). There are also degrees of discomfort inflicted by the procedure. A doctor, therefore, may take the easy way out. He may place the child on an antibiotic without attempting to remove the wax to confirm the diagnosis of a middle-ear infection. In my opinion, this is a mistake.

On a daily basis I see children in follow-up for ear infections that were treated by other physicians.

All I can see is wax. I am quite sure that was all that could be seen when they were initially diagnosed.

The diagnosis of middle-ear infection can only be made by inspection of the eardrum. If excessive wax is present it has to be removed. This is usually done by using a curette (a plastic or wire loop) to tease out the wax. Unfortunately, the procedure is discomforting. As well, because the skin of the ear canal is very vascular it can be easily traumatized as the wax is removed. Bleeding into the external ear canal will result. Blood may drip out of the ear, much to the horror of the parent. The presence of fresh blood in the ear canal will, unfortunately, render it impossible to visualize the eardrum. A decision, therefore, to treat or not to treat for a middle-ear infection will be based on the child's history of frequent ear infections, the presence of fever and how ill he is.

The parents should be reassured that no lasting damage has been done. The outer ear, if bleeding, is usually packed with cotton for 1 to 2 hours. Acetaminophen or ibuprofen may be given for discomfort. Healing occurs within 2 to 3 days.

I have to add one caveat. Removal of ear wax is a "blind" procedure. That is, the doctor is not able to visualize exactly the placement of the curette. There are case reports of damage to the eardrum, which may result in permanent hearing loss, from inserting the curette too deeply in the ear canal. This unfortunate complication is extremely rare. From my perspective, every effort should be made to visualize the eardrum in order to make an accurate diagnosis of a middle-ear infection.

To prevent a build-up of dry, hard wax, instill 2 drops of baby oil in the ear twice a day for a few weeks. Lay the child down. Gently pull the ear up and back. This will open the outer canal. Put the drops in. Have the child lay for a minute or so before getting up to have the other side done.

For older children, who cooperate, the wax may be softened and removed by waterpic spray. There is no discomfort with this procedure.

The bad news is that the ear wax will return.

Eczema (Atopic Dermatitis)

The skin is the largest organ of the body. It is several layers thick and continuously replaces itself. Its most important function is to act as a barrier, providing protection from any external threats.

Eczema is a common skin condition that can affect all age groups. Approximately 15% of cases occur before 1 year of age. Although many may outgrow it, approximately 40% will continue to suffer from eczema into adulthood. It is, therefore, considered a chronic lifetime condition.

Those who do outgrow their eczema usually have the skin condition only, without other accompanying allergies. Those whose eczema extends into adulthood frequently develop other allergic conditions, such as food allergies, asthma or environmental allergies.

Eczema occurs most often when there is an allergic family background.

The exact cause of eczema is not known. The common factor for children with eczema is a defect in the skin barrier, which results in a breakdown of the skin's integrity. Mothers who wish to prevent eczema in their child by following a hypoallergenic diet during pregnancy, will effect only minimally its prevention. Breastfeeding, however (either with or without mother eating a hypoallergenic diet), does delay the onset and, as well, can modify the severity of a child's predisposition to having eczema (high-risk infants only). Some studies have also shown that breastfeeding may even prevent the onset of eczema in an infant at high risk for allergy (strong family history of allergy). Similarly, bottle-fed babies on a completely or partially hydrolyzed (protein broken down) formula may experience the same diminishing effect and prevention as with breast-fed infants (in high-risk infants only). Soy formulas will not help in preventing or minimizing eczema. Delay in the introduction of solids has no effect on the prevention of eczema.

Food allergy seldom causes eczema. If, however, you notice that there is a continual flare-up of your child's eczema with a certain food, then discontinue it. Allergy skin testing is indicated if there is a suspicion that your child's eczema flare-ups are related to food.

Recent evidence has shown that omega-3 (DHA) as well as omega-6 (ARA) has an anti-inflammatory effect. Children with eczema would benefit from a daily dose of 100 mg to 200 mg of omega-3 and -6 either in their diet or as a supplement. Studies have shown that it decreases not only flare-ups but also the severity of the disease.

There is a cascade of events that results in eczematous lesions. It starts with dryness of the skin. This results in the skin being itchy. The child scratches the skin. The skin becomes reddened and increased itching occurs, resulting in more scratching. This cycle repeats itself until there is breakdown of the skin and the appearance of eczematous lesions.

In infancy, eczema is most prevalent on the cheeks, the neck, the body, the back of the arms and the legs. In toddlers and older children, the creases inside the elbows, behind the knees and on the wrists and ankles are the most commonly affected areas. In teenagers and adults, it is usually limited to the hands and feet, around the lips and occasionally the nipple area.

As the eczema improves, the underlying skin may lose its pigmentation. This is most visible in infants with eczema who are dark skinned. This depigmentation may be very patchy in distribution. There is no treatment and the skin will eventually become repigmented.

152

Eczema is a difficult and frustrating skin disorder for the child, the parents and the doctor. The chief reason for this is that it is a chronic and relapsing condition that has no cure.

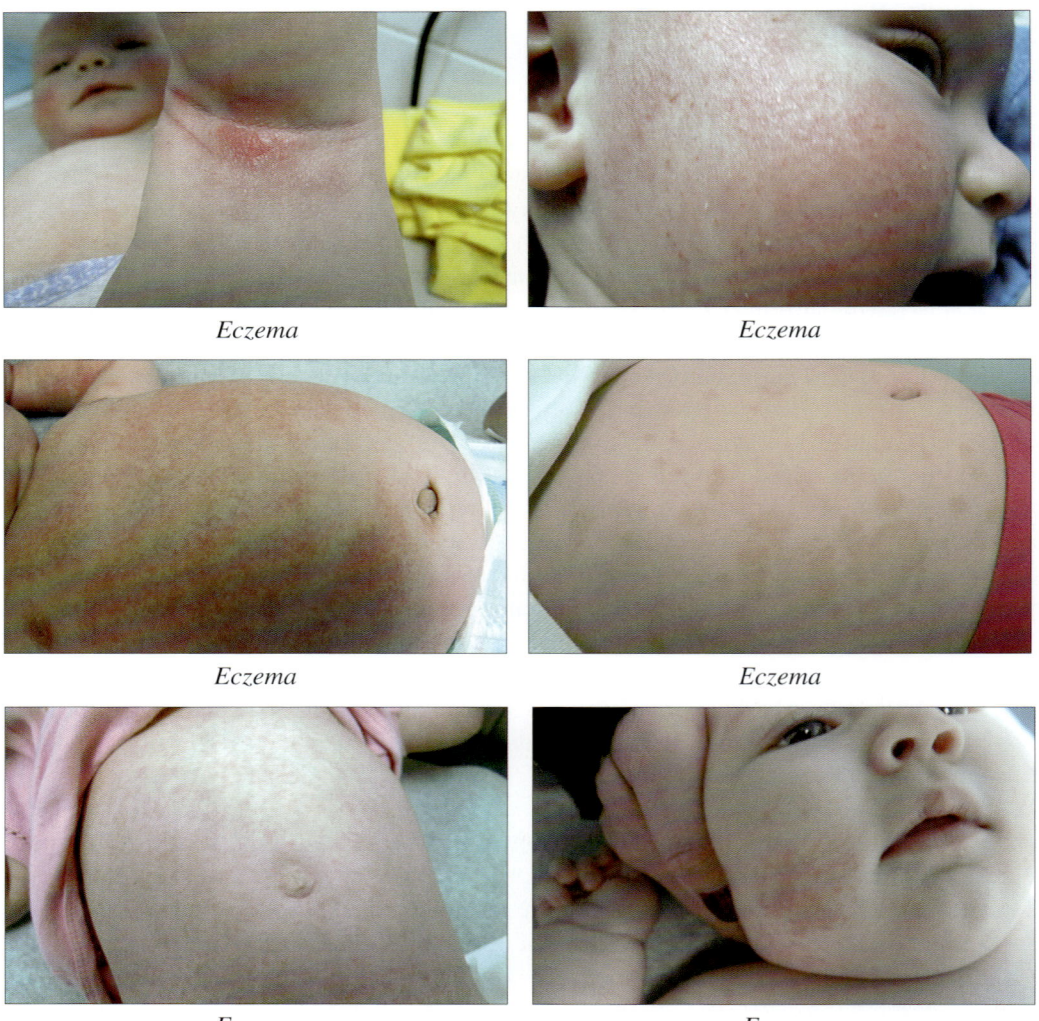

Eczema *Eczema*

Eczema *Eczema*

Eczema *Eczema*

Treatment

General Management

When washing clothing or bedding, use a mild detergent with no bleach or fabric softener. Double rinse the above.

The temperature, in the bedroom at least, should be less than 20°C. The humidity level should be between 40%–50%.

Avoid common irritants that may cause flare-ups of your child's eczema. These include:

- Dust mites
- Excessive humidity, heat, cold or dryness
- Irritants such as wool clothing or other rough fabrics
- Any known foods which cause flare-ups. The best way to discover this is by your determining what the culprit is. In the majority of infants or toddlers with eczema, food does not play a role in flare-ups. Allergy skin testing may or may not be helpful. As stated, the best test is your own observation as to whether a specific food substance continually results in eczema flare-ups. If it seems to be the case, that food should be avoided.
- Swimming pools with chlorine (if problematic, then fully rinse off the chlorine immediately after swimming)

It is a good idea to keep fingernails cut short to minimize the effects of scratching.

Specific Management

Dry Skin

Dry, itchy skin is the most common symptom for all children with atopic dermatitis. Skin dryness results in the skin being more sensitive to irritants. **For optimal improvement, the skin must be well hydrated all the time.** Cool, wet compresses will lessen the itch.

At least one or more baths in lukewarm water should be taken per day, lasting for a minimum of 5 minutes each time. A capful of unscented bath oil in the water will help the skin to retain moisture. Use a mild, unscented cleanser. Liquid cleansing agents are far less abrasive to the skin, less drying and more easily rinsed off than soaps. Bathing is better than showering. If showering, again, mild liquid cleansers are preferable to soaps.

You cannot over, moisturize the skin of a child who has eczema. The best time to apply a moisturizer is immediately after a bath when the skin is still damp. Moisturizers can be used several times a day if necessary. Creams are superior to lotions, as they are thicker in consistency. For moderate to severe eczema, emollients and ointments are preferable to creams.

Clothing

Loose-fitting cotton clothing is preferred. It is best to avoid clothing materials that may irritate the skin. These would include wool, stretch polyester or nylon. In the winter, do not overdress your child. Using layered cotton clothing is best. Make sure that hats, mittens, scarves and socks are made of appropriate materials that will not irritate or bind the child's skin.

During the wintertime there may also be problems with the feet. Feet may become scaly, dry and cracked. This can be prevented by removing the boots right away when the child comes inside so that there will be less sweating and irritation. Dry cotton socks should be used. If the child's feet are cold, avoid warming them near a heat source, because rapid temperature changes can cause itching and scratching, and a resulting flare-up of the eczema. At night, moisturize the feet well and have your child wear cotton socks to bed.

The high calcium and magnesium levels found in hard water may lead to skin irritation. Soft water is preferred.

If you clean your child's face after he eats, do not use scented wipes or those containing alcohol; do not use a washcloth. The best thing to use is a plain tissue to which you have added a moisturizer. The same combination can be used for cleaning the diaper area.

Anti-inflammatories

Topical corticosteroids are the most effective medication for controlling eczema when environmental control and diligent moisturizing are insufficient. The most commonly used is 1% hydrocortisone. This is considered to be the lowest level of strength. Topical corticosteroids range in strength from low potency (mild), intermediate potency (moderate), and high potency (high) to ultra-high potency. Well over 90% of children with eczema will require only a mild corticosteroid. It is usually applied 3 times a day before the moisturizer. It should be used sparingly but must be used regularly. If, along with all other measures, there is little or no response after 2 weeks, an intermediate-potency corticosteroid should be tried. Again, after 2 weeks if there is no response, the treatment plan should be reviewed to ensure that the parent is following the treatment regime as was directed. The oral steroid prednisone may be required to gain control of severe eczema, but only for as short of a period as possible (approximately one week). Prednisone can safely be discontinued without tapering it off. If it is needed for longer than one week, tapering off over a period of one to two weeks will be required. Once the eczema has improved, with disappearance of the rash (a little redness may persist) and no further scratching by the child, the cortisone cream may be discontinued; however, it is important to continue with moisturization.

In over 40 years of practice, dealing with large numbers of infants and children with eczema, I cannot remember ever prescribing oral steroids.

If possible, corticosteroids should not be used on the face or scrotum. Topical calcineurin inhibitors (Elidel or Protopic) are best for these sensitive areas. They are applied twice daily until effective control is achieved and then only once daily. Initially they may irritate the skin but only for the first 2–3 days. It may take 2 weeks before an improvement is noted. Do not stop the medication. Once the eczema is under control these medications may be discontinued. Reuse later if required. Calcineurin inhibitors may also be used as the first-line treatment on the body rather than steroid creams.

In Europe, cortisone is used very little for the treatment of eczema. Studies have shown that calcineurin inhibitors are very effective against all degrees of eczema, and they are commonly used for the treatment of eczema of the whole body. At present, these are the treatments mainly used (for areas other than the face) throughout Europe. This approach is just catching on in North America. Acute flare-ups are brought under control with cortisone and then kept under control with a calcineurin inhibitor. When the eczema is well under control, these inhibitors, if applied twice weekly, may prevent future flare-ups or at least decrease their severity.

Note: If the eczema on the face is severe, controlling it using a cortisone cream may be initially necessary; but then a switch back to using calcineurin inhibitors to maintain the improvement as required.

The safety profile of topical corticosteroids, when they are used appropriately, has been well documented. The common side effects, which fortunately occur only rarely, are seen mostly in teenagers and adults. These side effects include thinning of the skin, stretch marks, the appearance of surface veins (spider nevi) and rash around the lips. Prolonged usage may predispose individuals to glaucoma and/or cataracts – both are rare.

Studies have shown that growth retardation is mainly attributed to the chronic disease itself and not to the use of topical corticosteroids. There is no suppression of the immune system with the use of topical corticosteroids.

Suppression of the function of the adrenal glands, although a possibility, is extremely rare and is both temporary and reversible.

Corticosteroid phobia on the part of the caregiver can lead to noncompliance. This mindset is the major drawback of using topical cortical steroid therapy and, therefore, is the leading reason why eczema persists. This phobia needs to be overcome through education by the child's doctor.

Routine topical treatment is not effective when there is a superadded bacterial (or occasionally fungal) infection in the area of the eczema. If the eczematous lesions display more crusting than normally found, infection is most likely the cause. Antibacterial or antifungal creams and occasionally oral antibiotics are required to treat the infection. Bleach baths are helpful for recurrent infections. Use 5 ml (1 tsp.) of bleach per 5 litres (160 oz.) of bath water, 2 to 4 times per week. This is the same concentration as found in a swimming pool. Exercise caution when using bleach. After bathing, thoroughly rinse the child with warm water.

It is extremely important that at the earliest sign of a flare-up topical corticosteroids and/or calcineurin inhibitors (for the face and scrotum) be started.

Oral antihistamines may be required in order to control the itching.

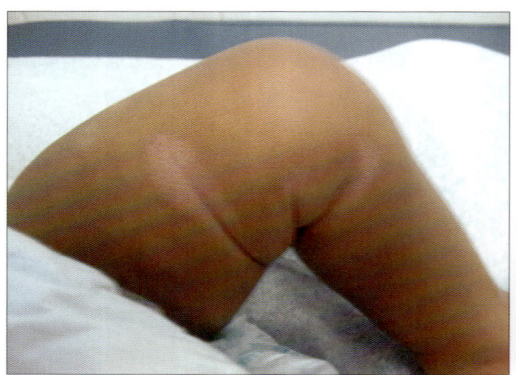
Loss of Pigmentation. Will repigment in time.

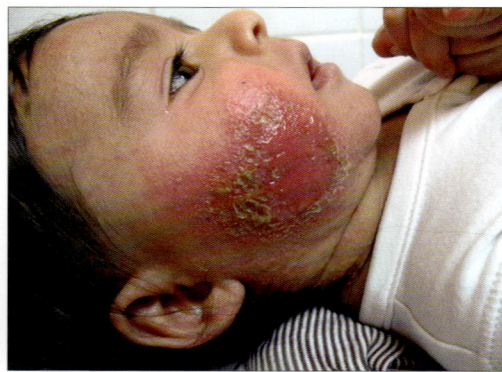
Infected Eczema

Other therapies that a dermatologist may recommend include the use of more potent steroid creams, oral steroids, immunosuppressants or phototherapy.

Recurrent flare-ups may occur despite adequate moisturization. There is good evidence to suggest that twice-weekly application of cortisone or calcineurin inhibitor to the involved area(s) when the eczema is "quiet" will significantly reduce such flare-ups.

The management of a child who has eczema is extremely frustrating and stressful for the caregiver (as well as for the child). No one likes to see a child suffer. The skin is the largest organ of the body and therefore affects the child on a grand scale. There is not a parent who does not want to see her child's skin blemish free. Closely following the child's treatment regime will ensure the best outcome. Early intervention with a treatment plan will ensure success – *Do Not Wait*. Again, if there are any doubts, discuss them with your doctor.

Suggested Moisturizers (keep in fridge and apply when cool)

Petroleum jelly applied to the skin 2 or 3 times daily (especially after that evening bath) is the least expensive and an extremely effective moisturizer.

If you're applying both a cortisone and moisturizer at the same time, put the cortisone on first.

Bath oils – Aveeno, Keri: 1 capful

Soaps – Aveeno, Cetaphil, Neutrogena, Ivory, Dove, Syndet

Lotions – Keri, Aveeno, Cetaphil, Nutraderm, Lubriderm, Nivea

Creams – Cetaphil, Glaxal Base, Lipikar, Prevex, Dormer, Impruv (excellent for use after evening bath), Dermabase, Moisturel, Eucerin, **EpiCeram**

Ointments – Vaseline, Eucerin, Glaxal Base, Nivea

Hair care – Ducray, Elution, Cliniderm

Moisturizing creams with added UV protection may be used after 4 months of age.

As mentioned previously, eczema is a lifelong condition. There is no cure. Yet with proper management, its impact on your child's daily life will be minimized. It is up to you.

Epiglottitis

Epiglottitis is a bacterial infection of the epiglottis. The epiglottis is a small piece of tissue that is located behind the tongue. Its function is to close over the windpipe during swallowing so that food is directed towards the esophagus (swallowing tube) and not down the windpipe.

Epiglottitis is due to a bacterial infection – haemophilus influenza.

Before the introduction of the haemophilus influenza vaccine, epiglottitis would be seen several times in most emergency departments each year. Since the introduction of the vaccine, epiglottitis is rarely seen and occurs only in those children who have not been vaccinated.

Epiglottitis is an extremely serious illness.

It is most common in children between the ages of 2 and 6 years.

It usually begins as a mild upper respiratory tract infection. Subsequently, a high fever develops, usually during the night. The child complains of a severe sore throat and has difficulty swallowing. Drooling of saliva occurs because of a reluctance to swallow. The child looks very ill. His complete attention is on breathing only. Indrawing of the ribcage is present. The cough, if present, is croup-like.

With the presentation of these symptoms the illness is a medical emergency.

Note: Do not offer the child anything to eat or drink.

The child should be transferred to a hospital emergency department as quickly as possible.

The diagnosis is made by history. In the emergency department the child will be kept quiet and given oxygen by mask. No attempt should be made to look into his mouth to visualize the swollen epiglottis, or to set up an IV unless an anesthetist or ear, nose and throat specialist is at the bedside. X-rays of the neck are unnecessary and only delay treatment. The attendance of the specialist is required because the child may become upset by any procedure, resulting in the epiglottis becoming lodged in the airway, causing obstruction. If this occurs a respiratory arrest is imminent. For a similar reason nothing is given to the child by mouth.

The treatment is by assisted ventilation either by intubation or tracheotomy. IV antibiotics will be required. The child will be initially monitored in the ICU.

Eyes (Blocked Tear Ducts)

Tears, when formed, drain through little ducts called tear ducts. These ducts are situated on the medial (nasal) side of the eye and drain into the nose.

In the first year of life the tear ducts may become intermittently blocked, although more commonly it begins shortly after birth. It can occur in either one or both eyes at the same time or even alternate between eyes.

The symptoms for a blocked tear duct are as follows:

1. Excessive tearing with or without swelling of the eyelid. For this there is no treatment.

2. Matter builds up in the corner of the eye. Use a cotton ball soaked in warm water to clean the eye as needed. Wipe from the nose side outwards.

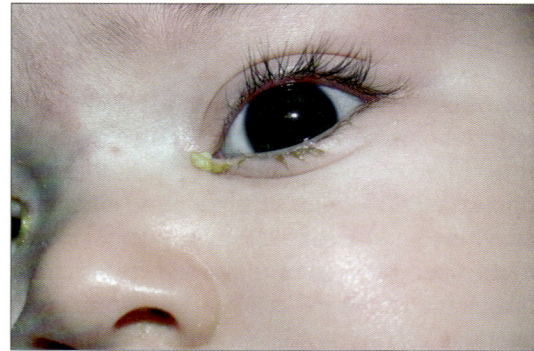

Blocked Tear Duct

3. If the eye has a thick green discharge and there is difficulty opening the eyelids, an infection may be present. Eye drops will be required. Massaging the tear duct of the blocked eye(s) twice daily may be helpful in preventing matter from building up in the eye. Place your index finger on the inner aspect of the eye and against the nose. Massage gently towards the eye and repeat several times.

By one year of age, the child should outgrow this condition. If it still persists after a year and a half, a tear duct probing may be required. This is done by an ophthalmologist.

The procedure is done in the outpatient department under a very light anesthetic. It takes approximately 10 to 15 minutes. The child may go home a few hours after the procedure.

Eyes – Pink Eye (Conjunctivitis)

Pink eye is an inflammation of the whites of the eye and the mucous membranes of the eyelids. It is usually caused by a virus or bacteria. There is also allergic conjunctivitis, a reaction to smoke or chemical vapors, and the more serious infection herpes conjunctivitis.

Conjunctivitis in the first month of life may occur in infants who have not received routine preventive eye drops at birth. The infection is caused by bacteria called chlamydia. It presents as a thick yellow to green discharge, which causes the eyelids to be glued shut. Treatment consists of antibiotic eye drops for a chlamydia infection. Chlamydia conjunctivitis should not be confused with a blocked tear duct(s), which requires no eye drops. If there is doubt, a culture should be done of the discharge to rule out a chlamydia infection.

Pink eye is very common and is very contagious. It is most often spread by transferring the droplets to another child, usually on a finger.

Often when a child has an upper respiratory tract infection he will complain of itchy eyes. They may appear red on inspection and have excessive tearing. The cause in this case is viral and requires no further treatment than warm compresses for symptomatic relief. In fact, approximately 75% of children are diagnosed with conjunctivitis that is viral in nature.

Often, it may be difficult for the doctor to differentiate between viral and bacterial conjunctivitis. Most doctors, if there is any doubt, will treat the child with antibiotic eye drops.

If the eye secretions become thick and yellow or green, then the cause may be bacterial in origin. Oftentimes the child wakes up with his eyelids stuck together.

The treatment for this type of infection is warm compresses to soften the secretions and antibiotic eye drops. When wiping the eyes, always go from the inner, nasal side outward.

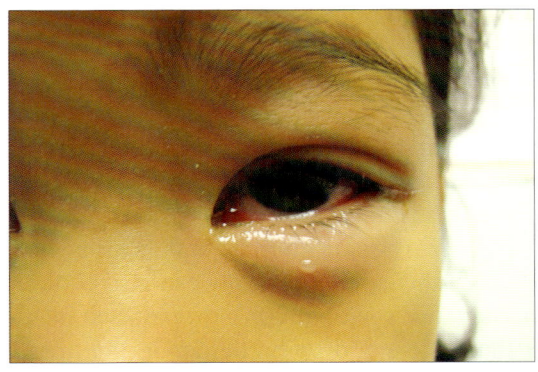

Conjunctivitis

There are many homeopathic and folk treatments for pink eye. Two examples would be the use of tea bag compresses or breast milk. Most will not help but will do no harm.

Allergic conjunctivitis presents with redness of the eyes, itchiness and excessive tearing. It is usually seasonal. It is often associated with other allergy symptoms, such as a stuffy nose, scratchy throat and cough. It is never in one eye alone.

The treatment is use of oral allergy medication. If no improvement is seen within 2 weeks hypoallergenic eye drops will be prescribed.

Herpes conjunctivitis is due to a herpes virus. Often it begins with small fluid-filled blisters on the eyelid. If this is suspected, the child should be seen by an ophthalmologist to ensure that there are no lesions on the eye itself. Antiviral eye drops will be prescribed.

The child with conjunctivitis is contagious for 24 hours after treatment is initiated. He can return to his normal lifestyle – daycare or school – after that time.

To prevent the spread of conjunctivitis, good handwashing technique must be employed by all. Your toddler daughter should use her own eye make-up. Not yours! (a joke)

Eye drops – how to use

There are a number of things that a child will not do: open his mouth to eat, open his mouth to brush his teeth, allow his teeth to be brushed, smile when you want to take his picture, take medicine and, lastly, open his eyes to allow you to put in eye drops.

Trust me, many things in life are difficult, but one on the top of the list is getting eye drops into a child's eye.

If your child refuses and struggles you are going to lose. Bribery does not work.

The bottom line is you have to do what you have to do, and whatever it takes to do it, do it!

Putting in the eye drops may require 2 people:

• Have the child lie down on his back.
• Have one person hold the child's arms over his head. Their hands should hold his arms at the level of the ears so that they can also control the child's head and arms with pressure.
• The other person drops a drop or two into the child's eye or beside it on the nasal side.
• Place the eye drop bottle down. Pry apart the child's eyelids as best as possible (as long as some of the lining of the eyelid is visible that is fine). Then roll his head to the side, allowing

the drop to enter his eye. Do the same with the other eye.

An alternative method for controlling a small child is to wrap him in a large beach towel with his arms down papoose-style (the tighter the better – less struggling). Place one of your arms over his chest to steady his body. With the hand of the same arm try to hold his head steady. With the other hand administer the eye drops as above.

When you have finished, calmly wipe the sweat off your brow. You might even compliment the child by saying "good job" or "that's a big boy" even though he has been a little monster. Guess what? If you are lucky enough to have a sympathetic doctor he will prescribe drops that will only have to be used twice a day – one down and 13 more battles to go to complete a 7-day course of drops!

Eyes – Squint (Strabismus)

When both eyes do not look in the same direction, this is known as a "squint".

Up until 4–5 months of age infants frequently appear to have their eyes intermittently not moving in a coordinated fashion. Certainly by 6 months of age eye coordination should be intact.

The presence of a squint (strabismus) requires medical attention and should be diagnosed as early as possible.

Many times when being examined by the doctor the infant is crying. It is very difficult at a time such as this to accurately judge his eye movement. If you suspect your child has a squint, try to take a picture of him to show the doctor.

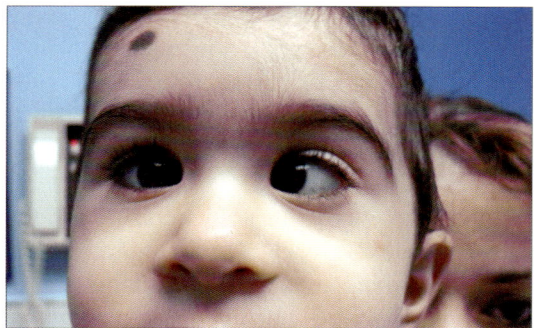

Squint (Strabismus)

Children with a wide, flat nasal bridge often appear to have "pseudo-strabismus". The eyes may not appear to be moving in a coordinated fashion. In reality the eyes are assessed as normal when examined by the doctor. No problem exists. This is especially noticed in infants of Asian descent from the Pacific coast. In time, the appearance of the eye movements will fully resort to normal.

Treatment for strabismus is performed by the ophthalmologist. Treatment options depend on the severity of the strabismus, and on the length of time it has been present.

If left untreated by 7 years of age, the vision will not be able to be corrected.

Options for treatment include:

- corrective glasses
- patching the strong eye to help strengthen the muscles of the weak eye
- surgery

The sudden onset of a squint in a previously normal child is a red flag signal. Medical attention should be sought at once.

Eyes – Stye (Hordeolum), Chalazion (Lid Cyst), Dermoid Cyst

Both eye styes and chalazions present as a bump on the eyelid. A stye is reddish in color and usually occurs at the edge of the eyelid. A chalazion most commonly presents on the middle of the upper eyelid and is non-tender.

An eye stye results from an obstruction and subsequent infection of the eyelash follicle. It most often remains tender and irritating to the child.

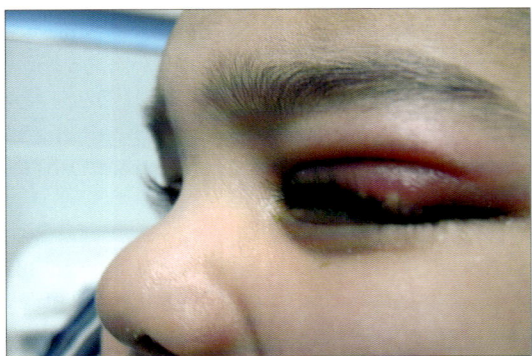
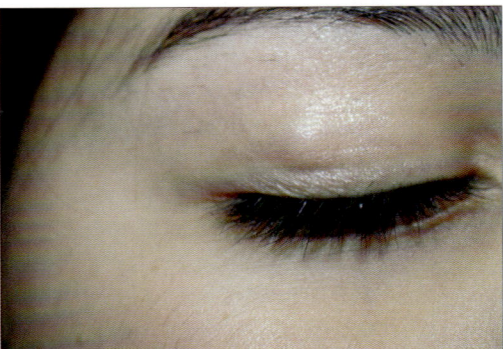

Stye   *Chalazion*

The treatment for a stye is to use a hot compress; the hotter it is, the longer left in place, and the more frequently applied, the better! In time, the material inside the stye will work its way to the surface. When this occurs, the tip of the stye will have a grayish appearance. This means that the stye is ready to drain on its own. Antibiotic eye ointment may or may not help. Do not squeeze the lesion. A hard nodule may remain for a prolonged period of time at the site of the stye.

A chalazion, on the other hand, is an obstruction in one of the eyelid's glands. It presents as a painless pea-sized lump in the eyelid. It is not an infection. A chalazion is a cosmetic problem only.

Although chalazions can spontaneously regress given time, many do not. Subsequently, the only treatment would be surgical removal for cosmetic reasons only.

A dermoid cyst presents as a soft nontender swelling above the eyelid and it may regress in time or it may require surgery to remove if it is cosmetically undesireable.

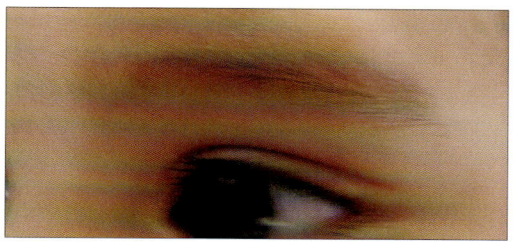

Dermoid Cyst

Feeding – Infants (Breast, Bottle, Solids)

Introduction

Over my nearly 40 years of dealing with families, my suggested infant feeding schedule is continually evolving and, hopefully, will continue to do so over the next 40 years. It is not a "bible" written in stone. There are other nutritionists, pediatricians and caregivers who will have differing views and recommendations as to what, when and how to introduce foods. My best advice is to educate yourself through the use of knowledgeable, established resources – your child's physician should have considerable input as well. Then you decide what is best for your child. Nevertheless, here are some of my own thoughts on the topic.

Over the past few decades our society has become increasingly concerned about the emotional well-being and mental stability of our children. The medical community certainly shares this concern. However we are now becoming increasingly aware of the importance of balancing this with equal concern about children's physical well-being. There must be an increase in physical activity (exercise) and proper nutrition.

It is very important to remember that "food imprinting", that is, the conditioning of food preferences, is learned early in life – in fact, it is set in motion in the first few months after starting solids. A large part of this imprinting is influenced by you – the caregiver. It is not only important to feed the child nutritious foods and introduce them in an orderly sequence, but the way you present these foods to your child is also important. We are not talking about how the food appears but how we appear to the infant during a feeding. You cannot expect an infant to accept carrots or squash if the caregiver continuously turns up his/her nose, with many facial contortions – "Eat up this yucky squash and then Mommy will give you some yummy dessert." If, on the other hand, you were to put in a little effort and enthusiasm with veggies, you mighteven teach your infant the reverse – to accept and prefer vegetables and fruits often thought of as "yucky" and to reject so-called "reward foods" or sweets. It all depends on the way you present the food to the child. Remember – there should be no such thing as a "reward food."

As adults, we are aware that being overweight is closely associated with health problems. Why then do parents consider chubby infants and children to be healthy? Good health should never be equated with excessive weight gain. This is a misperception handed down from our parents and grandparents who lived during times or in countries where food was at a premium; that is, it was very hard to come by. Remember, it is the nutritional quality of foods and not the quantity that is important.

I would like to stress that being overweight as early as 3 months of age results in a significant increase in the possibility of being overweight and even obese in adulthood. You can help prevent excessive weight gain by stopping the feeding of the baby when he or she seems satisfied. Do not "force feed" your baby.

Weight gain in otherwise normal children basically depends on three factors:

1) Hereditary background; that is, what the parents and grandparents are like physically
2) Dietary intake
3) Physical activity (exercise)

Parents have little control over the first factor but do have full control over the latter two.

"Normal" weight gain is quite variable. By two weeks of age, most infants have returned to their birth weight. At about 4 to 5 months of age, an infant will have doubled his birth weight. At one year of age, birth weight is usually tripled, and then quadrupled by two years of age. Remember however, these guidelines fluctuate a lot. When plotted on a growth chart, as long as an infant's weight gain is following a particular percentile without either tailing off or increasing excessively, then that child's weight gain is normal – whether it is following the 5th percentile or the 95th percentile.

Please do not compare the growth of one child to another, even a child within the same family. He is an individual – let him grow that way.

If you have any concerns about diet, either your own during breastfeeding or baby's formulas, or the introduction of solids, including concerns about the possible adverse effects of any particular food, then please discuss these fully with your doctor. An understanding of your child's nutritional needs along with open communication with your doctor are extremely important for optimal infant and child care.

Sterilization

The practice of sterilization may be discontinued when the baby is 3 months of age. Wash bottles and utensils as you would any other kitchen utensils. Make sure you clean the nipples well. You may have to invert them to clean out all the milk residue.

Actually, in this day and age, sterilization is probably unnecessary at any stage (but do not tell this to your mother-in-law).

Vitamins

All formulas are vitamin-enriched. Additional vitamins are unnecessary. The formula you choose should be iron-enriched as well. Contrary to a persistent myth, studies have demonstrated that the amount of iron in the iron-fortified formulas does not cause constipation or any other digestive problem. I also recommend that all formulas be enriched with omega-3 (DHA) and omega-6 (ARA) fatty acids, as well as probiotics.

Probiotics (and Prebiotics which promote growth of "good" bacteria)

Probiotics have recently been added to some formulas. A probiotic is defined as a live organism food supplement with a proven beneficial effect on human health. Copious amounts of probiotics are found in breast milk. They are extremely beneficial for keeping the "good" bacterial flora in the digestive system stable. What this means for the baby is improved immunity. Clinically, because of the improved immunity, the incidence and severity of eczema are reduced. As well, the frequency and severity of viral or antibiotic-induced gastroenteritis are also reduced.

Breastfed infants should be started on a vitamin D supplement by 1 week of age – 400 IU (1 mL) daily. It should be continued during the time the infant is primarily breastfeeding. If an infant stops breastfeeding and formula is introduced, the vitamin D should be discontinued (as it is already present in the formula). When an infant is both breast- and bottle-fed, supplemental vitamin D is unnecessary if more than 60% to 70% of the total intake of milk is from formula. Six hundred to eight hundred IU of vitamin D is recommended for toddlers, children and teens. Adults would benefit from 1500–2000 IU daily. This is necessary not only for the prevention of bone problems but also for the prevention of other health issues. This amount can be attained by diet alone. However, if you are not certain, then giving 400 IU of vitamin D on a daily basis, either alone or with other vitamins, is fine.

Mothers – Diet If Breastfeeding

While breastfeeding, mom should remember that she is now eating for 2 people. Eat a well-balanced diet. The prenatal vitamins should be continued while breastfeeding. The occasional glass of wine, alcohol or beer 2–3 times a week is fine. Smoking is prohibited. Any dietary abstinences from milk, eggs, or nuts will not delay or prevent the onset of asthma or food allergies. They may, however, delay the onset of eczema. Mothers who are breastfeeding should have adequate DHA and ARA in their diet. This will insure that there are sufficient quantities of omega-3 (DHA) and omega-6 (ARA) fatty acids in the breast milk to promote optimal vision and cognitive (brain) development. The supplement should be continued for as long as the mom is breastfeeding. If the baby is weaned before one year of age, then he should be supplemented with a DHA-fortified formula until 11–12 months of age During the mom's next pregnancy the above supplementation schedule is recommended during at least the third trimester (or earlier) as well.

The average Canadian woman's omega-3 intake is approximately 80 mg per day. This is far less than what is recommended (200 mg for adults and 300 mg for those breastfeeding) daily. Insufficient intake of DHA (omega-3 fatty acids) in a mother who is breastfeeding will result in deficient amounts being delivered to the baby through the breast milk. The increase in baby's brain growth during the last trimester in utero is approximately 260%. The increase in brain growth during the first year of life is another 175%. There is approximately a 20% increase during the second year of life. It is during these times of rapid brain growth that adequate amounts of DHA are required to ensure optimum brain development – especially from the period during the last trimester of pregnancy until the end of the first year of life.

DHA and omega-3 dietary sources:

- Milk (8 oz, DHA enriched) – up to 20 mg
- Egg (omega-3) – up to 125 mg
- Salmon (3 oz, Atlantic farmed) – 1238 mg
- Salmon (3 oz, Coho wild) – 560 mg
- Shrimp (12 large steamed) – 96 mg
- Sole (3 oz, cooked) – 219 mg
- Cod (3 oz, Atlantic, cooked) – 131 mg
- Sardines and Anchovies – very rich

If the dietary intake is limited, then daily doses of DHA and ARA in the form of supplements can be obtained from the pharmacy or health food store.

Formula Feeding

The proper amount of formula a baby requires with each feeding is that which is enough to satisfy his needs. If he continually empties the bottle, give him more. A small quantity of milk should be left in the bottle after each feeding to demonstrate that his needs have been satisfied. As a general rule, the baby should ingest approximately 90 cc (3 oz) per pound or 180 cc (6 ounces) per kilo daily until he reaches 35 pounds, or approximately 16 kg. Remember, this is just an approximation and every baby is an individual. Do not compare one with the other. As long as there continues to be an adequate weight gain, then the amount of formula ingested by your infant is fine.

As with breastfed infants, bottle-fed babies should at first be fed on demand. This will usually translate to every 3-4 hours for 6-8 feeds a day (with some babies more feedings are necessary).

You can help prevent the development of gum and dental disease. Never give a pacifier dipped in honey, corn syrup or any other sweetener. Similarly, never leave an infant or toddler with a night bottle of milk, juice or other sweetened liquids in his crib to "graze" on overnight. If absolutely necessary, leave only a bottle of unsweetened water. Best option: leave nothing at all. A bad habit will not be formed if not encouraged. For the same reason do not allow your toddler to walk around with a sippy cup of milk or juice to sip on periodically. The constant flow of sweetened liquids over the teeth will result over time in dental decay.

Dental care starts with keeping the gums clean by using a wet, warm washcloth. After the eruption of the first tooth and subsequent teeth, keep them nice and shiny – use a washcloth twice a day. Starting early with the infant toothbrush (when there are 4 teeth) will help with its acceptance later on. Only water is required; however, a non-fluoride toothpaste can also be used – just a dab, though.

Milk storage

Breast milk (freshly expressed) may be stored at room temperature for 6 hours, in the refrigerator for 3 days, in a home freezer (at the back) for up to 6 months. Breast milk previously frozen and then thawed should not be stored at room temperature (that is, use immediately when thawed, and discard any remaining). If thawed but unused, it may be refrigerated for 24 hours. Never refreeze thawed breast milk for future use.

To freeze, seal 2 ozs (60 mL) to 4 ozs (120 mL) of breast milk in each individual bag. You may add small amounts during the day to get the desired quantity of breast milk (stored in the fridge) – then freeze.

Store the milk in specially designed plastic freezer bags. Leave a little space at the top because, like most liquids, breast milk will expand when frozen.

Seal with freezer or masking tape. Date the time of freezing.

Use the earliest dated frozen breast milk first.

To thaw frozen milk, place the milk in the refrigerator the night before it is to be used. The defrosting process will take approximately 12 hours. Or place the milk in warm running water (not hot). Never microwave breast milk.

During the freezing process the fat of the breast milk will rise to the top. When thawed, gently swirl to mix.

For formula-fed infants you may prepare each bottle as needed or you can prepare a whole day's worth, which can be stored in the refrigerator. It can be kept at room temperature and reused for up to 2 hours – after that time discard it.

If you follow the above guidelines closely, the milk will retain its full nutritional value and will be totally safe for use.

Cow's milk

Cow's milk as the main source of dietary milk intake should not replace formula or breast milk prior to 8 months of age and preferably not before one year of age.

Switching to cow's milk from formula does not require weaning. Finish the formula and then start the cow's milk.

Use of homogenized (3.25%) milk, which is vitamin D–enriched, is preferred until two years of age and may be continued thereafter or substituted with 2% milk. Skim or 1% milk should not be used unless it is advised by your doctor.

When cow's milk is introduced, in addition, I advise giving a liquid multivitamin containing vitamins A, C and D – 1 mL daily until one and a half years of age. From then on, vitamin D is recommended to be taken daily at 400-800 IU until adolescence is completed. If a well-balanced diet is provided, vitamins other than D are probably unnecessary. If, however, you are concerned about adequate vitamins in the diet, then any multivitamin will do the job.

It should be mentioned that vitamins will not stimulate the appetite, will not increase growth and will not have any effect on the immune system (to ward off infections).

It should also be noted that when switching to cow's milk, constipation may result for a few weeks. During this phase-in time give extra fruit, water or prune juice to help soften the stool. A normal stool pattern will return within a few weeks.

Note: Milk intake after one year of age should not exceed 20 ounces (600 mL) a day. It is extremely important not to satisfy the child's hunger with milk alone such that he will be reluctant to take in solids. If the infant takes in too large a quantity of milk and does poorly on solids he will, within a few months, develop nutritional anemia. If you restrict the amount of milk ingested, he will be hungry enough to eat solids. If he's thirsty, give water as desired.

Bottle to cup

Between 9 to 10 months of age you may be able to switch baby from a bottle to a training cup, or better still, to a regular cup or glass, as grazing on a sippy cup promotes the development of dental caries (decay). Do not worry about larger quantities of milk dribbling down the baby's chin. The baby will not dehydrate himself. As long as he is producing 5 or more wet diapers during any 24-hour period, then fluid intake is sufficient.

There is no given time frame for this transfer. It depends entirely on both you and your infant. By 1 1/2 years of age most toddlers should be off the bottle, except perhaps the one given prior to bedtime. This is the one bottle that parents find is the most difficult to have the child give up. The bottom line is – it is your child – it is your call. Do what you feel most comfortable doing – go by your agenda and no one else's.

Soy formulas

Soy formulas are different from routine formulas in that they are soy-protein based and lactose-free.

There are only 2 common indications for the use of soy formulas – a family who wishes to keep a strict vegetarian diet or the presence of a specific type of "true milk allergy" (which is very uncommon).

There may be a limited value to using soy formulas on a short-term basis (1 to 3 weeks) after a bout of diarrhea which either relapses or does not seem to improve when baby is placed back onto a routine formula or cow's milk. During this period, any lactose-free formula, lactose-free cow's milk (if infant is already on cow's milk) or their soy-based counterparts (because they are lactose free) are more easily digested. Until there is complete healing of the inflamed small intestinal lining (2–3 weeks), the use of any lactose-free milk in the meantime can be beneficial.

To further explain this: after or during a bout of gastroenteritis there may be a temporary lactose intolerance because the inflamed intestinal wall loses its ability to absorb lactose (milk sugar). Lactose is normally present in routine formulas as well as cow's milk. The undigested lactose acts as a stool softener, which further perpetuates loose stools. Maintaining an infant on his routine formula or cow's milk, both of which contain lactose, can have the effect of prolonging the diarrhea. Restricting lactose from the diet during this healing phase will result in speedier return to a normal stool pattern.

Soy-based formulas or soy milk probably have little or no value in changing the consistency of stools or in the management of colic. Nor has it been shown that soy formulas diminish spitting up or tummy distention. Soy milk may minimally reduce fussiness and the expelling of excessive amounts of gas. There are, however, those who swear by soy formulas as the "saviour product" for their infant's digestive problems. If soy seems to be working for your baby, that is fine. Continue its use. Infants will thrive on soy-based formulas or soy milk.

Various studies have shown that up to 60% of infants who have one of the 2 types of allergy to cow's-milk protein (present in formulas or cow's milk) may also have a sensitivity to soy protein. A similar relationship is present with goat's milk. Rice milk, however, may not cross-react with cow's milk and, therefore, possibly could be substituted for cow's milk in a toddler (over one year of age) if there is a cow's-milk protein intolerance. Be sure to consult with your doctor before introducing rice milk. If an infant is on rice milk for a prolonged period of time he will require supplemental vitamins as well as folic acid and calcium. The rest of the child's diet may also have to be adjusted to meet his nutritional needs. I cannot remember any time in the past 40 years of practice that I have suggested the use of rice milk for any digestive problem. Specialized hydrolyzed milk formulas are recommended for those infants who have a cow's-milk protein sensitivity or allergy. These are available for all ages. Your doctor will advise you as to which product is best suited for your child.

Lactose-free formulas

Symptoms of an inherited lactose intolerance usually do not begin until late in the first year of life or afterward. Therefore placing an infant under 1 year of age on a lactose-free formula because of digestive problems is unnecessary. After a bout of acute gastroenteritis, an infant may have persistent loose stools because of a secondary lactose intolerance. Here a lactose-free formula may play a role in the management of the prolonged diarrhea for 2 weeks. Thereafter, the infant should be able to tolerate his routine formula. The reason for this is explained under "soy formulas."

Partially hydrolyzed formulas

These may help decrease excessive fussiness and gassiness in an infant. In a family where there is a strong history of allergy, especially eczema, using a partially hydrolyzed formula may help with prevention, delay of onset, or the severity of eczema.

Water

Whether breastfed or formula-fed, infants essentially do not require extra water. Nevertheless 1 oz (30 mL) or more may be given if desired, daily or more often. Giving water is also useful to help fill the baby's tummy if the baby is gaining weight at an undesirably fast rate.

Fluoride is extremely important for the prevention of tooth decay. If it's not present in your water it should be introduced into your infant's diet by 6 months of age. Adequate quantities of fluoride are present in most Canadian municipal water supplies. Insufficient amounts may be present in well water as well as in bottled water. If you use either of the latter two for preparation of formula, as well as the primary water source in cooking, your child may be receiving inadequate amounts of this important nutrient. Well water should be checked for its fluoride content. Enquire from the source that produces your bottled or filtered water as to the amount of fluoride present.

Your water source should have a concentration of at least 0.3 ppm of fluoride. This will supply enough fluoride for your infant from 6 months to 2 years of age and will help to prevent dental disease. If you're concerned consult your doctor.

Excessive amounts of fluoride intake, especially with the use of toothpaste that contains fluoride when it is swallowed, can cause pitting of the permanent teeth. Toothpaste with fluoride should not be used until the child is able to spit and rinse his mouth out (this ability develops at 4-1/2 to 5 years of age).

Introduction of solids

The delayed introduction of solids will not prevent eczema, other allergies or asthma.

With formula-fed infants, solids should not be introduced prior to 4 months of age unless specified by your doctor. If, prior to 4 months of age, the baby seems to be very hungry and is emptying 8 oz. bottles of formula or more with each feed, one to two tablespoons of cereal may be added to one or more bottles. This should help satisfy the baby's hunger. The opening in the bottle's nipple may have to be increased in size to accommodate the thickened formula. This can be done with a heated darning needle pushed in and out of the nipple opening. Spoon-feeding cereal one or more times a day may also be helpful (refer to section on cereal).

For breastfed infants solids are not required in the infant's diet until 5-1/2 to 6 months of age.

Foods that are prepared at home are nutritionally better for your child than any commercial (canned or bottled) counterparts. A good blender will pay for itself in no time if used to prepare infant foods. Make large quantities, blend and pour into ice cube trays, cover with plastic wrap or freezer bags that are dated and then freeze them. Use the earlier dated ones first. Keep salt and other spices, as well as sweeteners, to a minimum. Foods that are frozen will maintain their nutritional value in the frozen state for at least 3 months.

When introducing any new food to your infant, toddler or older child, it may initially be refused. Do not fret. It often takes up to 12 attempts to introduce a new food before it is accepted – so try again.

The sequence of adding foods – cereals followed by vegetables, then meat and, lastly, fruits is my own personal preference. It is merely a guideline. It has worked well for my patients for the over 40 years that I have been in practice. You may, however, wish to introduce foods in a different sequence. This is certainly acceptable.

The consistency of any food which is being served should change as the infant gets older. Start with puréed food, then "lumpier" food, followed by softened small, whole pieces of food and, lastly, more solid food. Remember, every child is different. Start introducing lumpier food at around 6 to 7 months of age. If tolerated, then gradually adjust the texture. There is no time frame medically speaking in which this transition takes place. Do not compare one child to another. Given time, all children will eat solid foods. Go by the signals your child is giving you and not by your preconceived ideas or by another caregiver's agenda.

Infants do not need teeth to "gum" softened foods. Gagging is the best indication that the texture is too thick at that particular time (refer to section on a finger feeding).

Cereals (pablum)

Cereals (pablum) – introduce at 4 months of age for formula-fed infants and 5-1/2 to 6 months for breastfed infants.

Cereal is the first solid food introduced. The role of cereal is fourfold. First, it teaches the child how to eat solids. Second, it helps to fill him up. Third, it is an excellent source of iron. Fourth, cereals are the most unlikely to cause any digestive problems. Another benefit to unsweetened cereals is that they have a very low caloric content. They are good tummy fillers, especially for the infant who seems to be gaining an excessive amount of weight. Feeding him large quantities of cereal, with as little added sweetener as possible, will slow down an otherwise undesirable weight gain. Consult your doctor.

Cereals are mixed to a paste-like consistency with formula, expressed breast milk or water. They are given twice daily, at breakfast and dinner time. The quantity given is enough to satisfy the baby's hunger. Start by mixing 1 to 2 teaspoons of dry cereal (one grain) per feeding and increase to 4 to 8 tablespoons or more if desired. Increase the amount every 2-3 days. Select a schedule that suits both you and your infant. It makes little difference whether he eats his solids first, then the milk, or vice versa or partway through formula or breastfeeding. The important thing is that he has an adequate quantity of both.

With the introduction of solids, the intake of formula may be decreased. Do not fret – 5 or more wet diapers a day (24 hours) indicates adequate hydration.

Start with rice cereal (most easily digested) and then try a different type of cereal every 3 to 4 days – oat, barley and, lastly, wheat. Soy cereals are fine. After each of the individual grains has been accepted and tolerated, then mixed cereals may be introduced.

Keep the cereals as unsweetened as possible. Try to avoid fruit-flavoured cereals.

With the introduction of cereals, some infants develop a red rash around their mouth. This is not an allergy and you may continue with the cereal. The rash will clear on its own.

If the child seems to have constipation (rock-hard stools passed with pain), then avoid rice.

At 7 months of age, cereal should be given in the morning only, and at 8 months of age it may be discontinued completely. You may substitute the infant cereal with one of the iron-fortified boxed breakfast cereals (unsweetened) at your discretion (for example, Rice Krispies, Cheerios or cornflakes). Soften the cereal with milk (formula or expressed breast milk) or water and feed with a spoon or allow the baby to use his fingers to eat right out of the bowl or from the tray.

Vegetables – introduce to formula-fed infants at 5 months and breastfed infants at 6-to 6 -1/2 months.

Vegetables should be given initially at lunchtime but may be given at supper as well (i.e., twice daily if desired). Introduce one puréed vegetable every 3 to 4 days before trying the next. Begin with one or two teaspoons and gradually work your way up to approximately 150 mL (five oz) or more if desired. Carrots, squash and sweet potatoes (the most easily digested) are to be started first and then gradually you can introduce other vegetables.

With the introduction of vegetables you may notice a yellow or orange tinge to the skin on the palms of the hands and soles of the feet and around the nose of the baby. This is not jaundice. It is due to "staining" of the skin by the carotene in the vegetables. It is of no health concern and will disappear in time.

Meats – introduce to formula-fed infants at 6 months and breastfed infants at 7 to 7-1/2 months.

Meats may be given at lunchtime and/or at suppertime along with vegetables. Follow the same routine as for vegetables. Start with lamb (the most easily digested), then chicken, followed by veal. Beef is introduced last (the most difficult to be digested).

Tofu can be started along with the introduction of meats into the infant's diet.

Fruits (including juice) – introduce to formula-fed infants at 7 months and breastfed infant's at 7-1/2 to 8 months.

As with vegetables and meats, fruits are introduced the same way. They are given once or twice daily. Use fruits as a side dish or mixed with cereal. Begin with applesauce, then banana. Then add one new fruit every 4 or 5 days. The quantity is the same as for vegetables. Fresh, peeled fruit is fine.

If constipation occurs, reduce the banana intake.

Once the infant has been established on fruits, fruit juices are introduced. Freshly squeezed, as well as canned adult juices, are fine in a 1:1 dilution with water. Juice may be given between meals or more frequently during hot weather. Less than 8 oz of juice daily is more than adequate.

Note: Fruits, because of their sweet taste, should never be used as a bribe or a treat to entice your infant to eat other solids. Fruits should be treated as just another food group necessary for good health and not as a reward. Introducing them properly may avoid having a "feeding headache" later. Do not withhold fruits as a threat to your child if he does not eat. Remember always that you are the teacher and the child is the pupil – not the reverse.

Yogurt and cheese

Yogurt and cheese may be introduced between 7 to 8 months of age – given daily is fine. Within reason, larger amounts may be given.

Finger foods

At 5 to 6 months of age start the baby on "teething biscuits." These dissolve very easily in the baby's mouth and will help in the process of his learning how to chew. When the infant is 7 months of age, try "finger foods". Start with small, soft pieces of fruit, vegetables, Cheerios, or cheese. The size of each individual piece should be approximately half that of a sugar cube. Encouraging your infant to self-feed will be a time saver for you. As well, and even more importantly, it will help build his hand-eye coordination. Once the baby is able to tolerate the above solids then you may increase the size of the pieces and the consistency – add meats last. Slicing foods such as hot dogs lengthwise will decrease the chance of choking.

Do not be concerned that he may not yet have any teeth. The baby should be able to gum the food without any concerns about him swallowing the wrong way, resulting in choking. If choking does occur, then bend him forward while he is in the sitting position and gently pat him on the back. This should dislodge any food that may be stuck in his throat. You may also put your finger in his mouth to dislodge any food. This manoeuvre may also induce vomiting, the force of which will expel any trapped food. Wait a few weeks and try to introduce finger foods again.

By the way, learning how to do the Heimlich manoeuvre and taking a first aid course to learn resuscitation (with updating every few years), is time well invested. Hopefully, neither will ever have to be used.

All of the above sounds scary and may make you hesitant to start finger foods. I understand your hesitancy. I should reassure you, however, that while the medical literature may have recorded cases of aspiration of solid foods, throughout my medical career experiences I cannot remember seeing or hearing of an infant harming himself with finger foods. In life, danger lurks everywhere and yet we go on living our daily lives without fear. Just trust yourself and try starting finger foods at 7 months of age.

Note: When starting finger foods the 25%/25%/50% rule comes into play. That is 25% of the food he picks up will enter his mouth and be ingested, 25% will be on his face and 50% will be distributed in an area 2 or 3 feet around the high chair. With age comes increased strength and improved coordination – his aim will become much more accurate – watch out!!!

Honey should not be introduced into the diet before one year of age unless it has been processed under high pressure and high temperature. Unprocessed honey may contain a bacteria called Clostridium botulinum. This can cause a serious illness called botulism.

Eggs, fish and peanuts

The medical community has been rethinking the timing for the introduction of eggs, fish and peanut butter. Many recent papers argue that these foods may be introduced earlier than previously thought (even in families with a direct specific food allergy history in either a parent or sibling). This also includes family members with eczema, asthma and environmental allergies. It is thought that there may be a "window of opportunity" when the introduction of potential "allergenic" foods could delay the development of the allergy or prevent it altogether. This window is thought to be between 6 to 8 months of age. As I write this, the medical literature is promoting the early introduction of eggs, nuts and shellfish – even despite a strong family history of allergy. If you have any concerns, however, consult your doctor before introducing these specific allergenic foods.

To be completely safe, I recommend that if one parent or sibling has a true nut, egg or shellfish allergy, the introduction of these foods should be delayed until skin testing has been done to rule out allergy. Food allergy skin testing may be done to test for any potential severe allergic (anaphylactic) problem and can be done at any age. You should know that a severe allergic reaction will never occur on the first contact with an offending food. It can only occur if there has been previous contact (whether that contact is intentional or inadvertent). This initial contact "primes" the immune system so that it may resort to an anaphylactic reaction on subsequent exposure to the offending food. Skin allergy testing will only be positive if the immune system has been previously primed. Therefore, a negative test may mean only that priming has not yet occurred and an anaphylactic reaction could unfortunately still occur with subsequent exposure.

Eggs

Egg yolks may be started at 7 months of age. Hard boil an egg, remove the white and then mash the yolk up with a little water or milk (expressed breast milk, formula or a little homogenized cow's milk). You may also use prepared yolks purchased at the supermarket. Whole egg may be introduced at 8 months of age. Eggs may be given 3–4 times weekly. Eggs are rich in iron and protein. DHA-fortified eggs are preferred.

Fish

All fish, including shellfish, can be introduced between 7 to 8 months of age. Once daily is fine. Begin with tuna or salmon before trying shellfish.

Peanuts

Peanut butter may also be introduced to the baby's diet between 7 to 8 months of age. Do not, however, introduce whole nuts prior to 5 years of age because of the possibility of small pieces being aspirated into the lungs rather than being swallowed.

Note: Good table manners are learned early. If you, the caregiver, set a good example, your children should follow suit.

If you have any concerns regarding your own diet during breastfeeding or formulas for baby, the timing and content of the introduction of solids or possibly the adverse effects (allergy) of any particular solid, please discuss this with your doctor. Open communication and understanding between you and the doctor are of importance for optimal infant and child care.

To sum up, it has been said that an army marches best on a full stomach. I would like to add that it does so only if their tummies are filled with proper nutrition!!!

Feeding (Overview)

Issues concerning feeding are the most common problems parents will present to me. These, along with sleep problems, are perhaps the most difficult ones for me to help with. The reason – the mother is usually already deeply frustrated and at her wit's end. The entire issue has already been made more difficult by all the advice the mom's "advisory staff" has given her.

When an infant chooses to refuse food, the mouth is one of the most powerful tools he can use against you. Surrounded by powerful muscles, it would take virtually the "jaws of life" to open it.

Why does this happen? Partly because you have allowed it to happen. It was done with all good intentions to entice the child to eat. His need has become a want and now is a demand. With this scenario you now have the "got you" syndrome. That is, the infant has got you. You are no longer in control and now you are paying the price. The infant has the power!

Let's put things into the proper perspective. There are 2 billion people in the world who do not have enough food – they probably could not even identify an apple or a carrot.

In all of the literature there has never been a case of an infant, who is otherwise healthy, who has voluntarily starved himself.

One thing is for certain: Children thrive on structure and routine. Add common sense and consistency by all caregivers and you now have the basic foundation for stressless child rearing. I want to repeat one word: *consistency consistency consistency consistency*. If practiced by all caregivers, problems with sleeping and feeding issues would occur far less frequently.

There are some steadfast scientific truths concerning feeding during the first year of life. These are as follows: breast milk is the best milk; all breastfed babies can benefit from having a vitamin D supplement until they are well on to solids; all baby formula should be iron enriched. The introduction of homogenized milk before 8 months of age may lead to digestive problems and anemia. If you are using bottled water or home-filtered water, they may contain insufficient levels of fluoride (which is necessary for strong teeth).

Every other element of feeding baby is up for grabs – primarily the issues of when and in what order to introduce new foods. Traditionally, cereal is the first food. Thereafter, it really does not matter which new foods you introduce. Present recommendations are: solids should not be introduced until after 4 months of age with formula-fed babies, and after 5-1/2 to 6 months with breastfed babies.

Recent European studies have shown that the introduction of peanut butter, as well as shellfish, at 6 to 8 months of age may prevent allergic reactions even for babies from families who have similar allergies.

At present, in North America, the same studies are being conducted but the results are not yet available.

MYTHS & TRUTHS ABOUT: sterilization, soy, iron, how much, appetite stimulants (vitamins), bottled water, growth grids, quantity of milk after one year of age, green stools, dental care, lactose, dessert and your advisory staff:

• Sterilization – this is probably completely unnecessary in the 21st century. A good dishwasher is all you need. Make sure that you turn the bottle's nipple inside out to clean out any milk residue.

• Soy milk – there are only 3 indications for the use of soy milk and they are: first, the family is vegetarian; second, the baby has a type of true milk allergy, third; the baby has a hereditary condition called galactosemia. A fourth reason may involve an infant or child who has gastroenteritis that lingers on, and this child could benefit from any lactose-free formula. Soy formulas are lactose-free. Numerous studies have been undertaken to show that soy milk does not improve colic or other digestive problems, including vomiting and diarrhea or gastroesophageal reflux (spitting up) or constipation.

- How much is enough – all infants under 1 year of age should be given as much milk as they will take in. After 1 year of age, limit milk intake to less than 20 oz. Other fluids may account for a few more ounces (juice and water). The major cause of creating the picky eater is over-feeding with milk. Tummies are so full that the child is no longer hungry. If this continues for more than a few months the child will develop an iron-deficiency anemia.

- Appetite stimulants – the only appetite stimulant is hunger. Vitamins do not act as an appetite stimulant.

- Bottled water – if used for making formula and cooking, it may not supply sufficient fluoride. Check with the manufacturer. There is nothing wrong with using tap water.

- Growth grids – for infants who are growing normally, their growth, when plotted on a growth grid, will parallel one of the percentiles. As long as there is no tailing off there is no concern, whether the child is growing at the third percentile or the 93rd percentile. The growth grids used are based on average heights and weights for Caucasian North American children. Infants whose ethnic background makes them generally smaller in stature and weight than many North Americans will probably graph lower when plotted on a growth grid. However, as long as they are paralleling a percentile without tailing off there is no concern.

- Stool colour – stool colour may vary from yellow to brown to various shades of green. These are all normal. Persistent pasty, pale grey stools or stools that are completely black may be of some concern. Consult your doctor.

- Dental care – this starts with the eruption of the first tooth. Clean it twice a day with a washcloth and warm water. When there are 4 teeth, a rubber finger dam can be used to clean the teeth. When there are 6 or more teeth, use a small toothbrush. Use water or toothpaste without fluoride. No matter how difficult it is to get the brush into his mouth, you must brush the teeth twice daily. If you permit him to brush his teeth on his own, trust me, he'll just chew on the brush and the teeth will not be cleaned properly. First dentist visit is by 2 years of age or earlier.

- Your advisory staff – these are all the people who give you advice even though you never asked for it. They rarely say anything positive about your parenting skills. They are very good at confusing you and fuelling your anxiety.

- Night bottle – never leave a night bottle in the crib for the infant to "graze on" throughout the night. It may help in getting him to sleep but his teeth will end up severely decayed. For similar reasons, do not use a pacifier dipped in any sweetener to help pacify the baby.

- Dessert – there should be no reward for eating except for a full tummy. Enticing an infant or child to eat by promising dessert sends the wrong message.

- Fluoride – well water, filtered water and bottled water may not have sufficient quantities of fluoride for optimal dental growth. Consult your doctor or dentist concerning the need for a supplement of fluoride. The whole question of the need for a fluoridated municipal water supply is now being questioned as to its effectiveness in preventing dental caries.

The picky eater – mealtime should never be wartime; you can try decreasing the child's fluid intake, including milk, to no more than 18–20 ozs a day, to promote hunger; give no non-nutritional foods; do not run around trying to feed the child; set time limits for meals (when the preset time is up, the meal is over); give only one small nutritious snack between meals; include your child in all aspects of food preparation (shopping, table setting, preparation of food, serving of food and cleaning up, use foods with lots of colour and try making designs so that it looks attractive; use large plates with small portions. Never force the child to eat or finish everything that is on his plate. Give him praise even for trying to eat.

Remember, since you are the teacher, the child looks to you for direction. You must set a good example. Do not give the power to your child. You should be in control – not your child.

It has been said that an army best marches on a full stomach. I agree, as long as the foods chosen are nutritionally sound. Do not give control at mealtime to the child.

Feeding – Vegetarian Diet

There are some interesting statistics on families who have no dietary restrictions. Some studies have shown that approximately 40% of children between the ages of 4 and 8 years are not receiving a nutritionally balanced diet. This figure rises to 70% in the teen years.

However, from what I have read in the literature, I believe that the statistics would seem to point to fewer numbers of nutritionally unsound choices in those who follow a vegetarian diet.

There are basically 4 types of vegetarian diets:

- Lacto-ovo vegetarian: these exclude meat, poultry, fish and seafood. Dairy and egg are included in the diet.

- Lacto-vegetarian: exclude all the above as well as eggs.

- Ovo-vegetarian: exclude all the above as well as milk and milk products.

- Vegan: exclude fish, dairy and eggs, all meat and animal products, and also honey.

Much more restrictive vegetarian diets include the macrobiotic diet and Fruitarians.

Irrespective of the type of diet you choose (whether it is vegetarian or not), it must be nutritionally sound and complete to ensure the normal development of your child. A proper diet should start during pregnancy. It is equally important for breast-feeding mothers to maintain a diet that will provide all the essential nutrients for the infant's growth and development.

During pregnancy and breastfeeding the mother must have an adequate intake of vitamin D, folic acid and vitamin B12. During lactation, if there is insufficient B12 present in the mother's diet, the baby must be supplemented during the period of lactation.

During the first two years of life there is rapid growth of your infant. He or she will double his or her birth weight by 4-1/2 to 5 months, triple it by one year of age and quadruple it by two years. During this most crucial time, brain development increases at an extremely rapid rate. Nutritional deprivation could have a profound negative effect on the development of the central nervous system.

For those infants of vegetarian mothers who wish not to breastfeed or have been weaned already from the breast, the infants should be on a commercially fortified soy formula until at least two years of age. Thereafter, soy milk, enriched with vitamins as well as calcium and iron, may be given.

Critics of the vegetarian diet find some of the disadvantages typically seen in those children raised on a vegetarian diet are iron deficiency anemia, bone problems due to lack of vitamin D and calcium, and problems due to insufficient vitamin B12 intake (which is mainly found in animal products) and zinc. Insufficient protein may lead to stunted growth as well as malnutrition. However, these same deficiencies have been documented in people who eat meat.

Many studies have shown that children raised on a well-balanced vegetarian diet have normal mental and physical growth development. In fact, in some studies it has been shown that they may even grow taller than those raised on a nonrestrictive diet.

There are other benefits to being on a vegetarian diet. There is a decreased incidence of obesity, a tendency to have fewer problems with blood pressure, fewer cardiac problems and a decreased incidence of type 2 diabetes. Studies have shown that there is a 25% decrease in ischemic heart disease and an approximately 7% decreased incidence of stroke in those who maintain a vegetarian diet, as compared with those who do not.

As for any eating style, vegetarian diets require constant attention to meal planning to ensure nutritional adequacy. The diet must be reviewed as the child grows and adjusted accordingly. Because of the great variability of dietary practices among vegetarians, individual assessment of dietary intake is, I feel, necessary. Here, a registered dietitian would play a key role in educating vegetarians about food sources, specific nutrients, food purchasing and preparation and, as well, vitamin and mineral supplementation.

Tofu, one of the main-stays of a vegetarian diet, is made from soybean curd; it is low in fat, cholesterol free and protein rich. It is an excellent source of iron, thiamine, potassium and phosphorus. When the curdling agent used to make the tofu is a calcium compound, tofu is also an excellent source of bone-building calcium. Tofu may be started at 7 months of age.

The more restrictive the vegetarian diet is the more vigilant one has to be to ensure adequate nutrition. Vegan diets occasionally are low in fat and energy foods and too high in fibre.

One problem that vegetarians may not be aware of is that while the foods they are consuming may be rich in various nutrients, these nutrients may have a low bioavailability (that is, they are poorly absorbed). This is certainly true with iron. Iron absorption can be maximized by including citrus fruit in the diet and reducing dairy intake.

Consuming french fries and drinking pop for lunch may be considered vegetarian but certainly is not healthy if done on a regular basis.

Popeye received his strength from spinach. As for me, bring on a veggie burger!!!

Again, if there are concerns about proper nutrition while following a vegetarian diet, a consultation with the dietitian is recommended.

Fever (Overview)

The baby feels warm! What should I do? Here are a few steps to follow if you feel your child has an elevated temperature.

Remember, **fever is not an illness.** It is a symptom (warning signal) that something is " wrong". Fever is one of the body's ways to help defend against a variety of infections or inflammations.

Only your doctor, on history, physical examination and, if necessary, laboratory investigations, can determine whether or not your child has a bacterial infection accompanied by fever requiring an antibiotic. **Do not insist on an antibiotic.** Let your doctor make the determination.

Most infants' elevated temperatures are due to viral infections that do not require an antibiotic. Far too many antibiotics are being prescribed to appease both the doctor and the parent. The doctor, unfortunately, may find it easier to prescribe an antibiotic for a child with a fever rather than explain why antibiotics are unnecessary at that time. Only with the documentation of a proven bacterial infection should antibiotics be prescribed and not "just in case".

Remember, teething does not cause fever. Perhaps an increase of one half a degree but no higher. High fevers should not be blamed on teething. Other reasons for the fever should be looked into.

It is extremely important to take your baby's temperature. Do not rely on touch alone.

No matter how "temperature sensitive" your palm, fingers or lips are, no family should be without a thermometer or not know how to use it. Learn how to use your thermometer before you need to use it.

Sites of Temperature Measurement

There are various areas on the body used to determine an elevated temperature. These include the ear, under the tongue, axillary (armpit) and rectal.

Ear temperature: The ear thermometer is the most recent advance in recording an infant's temperature. The advantage of this method is that it is very quick. Also the child's temperature can be taken without any discomfort, even while he is sleeping. It is quite accurate.

The disadvantages are that these devices are expensive and need replacing after a certain number of uses. It also requires practice using the proper technique to get an accurate reading. It will give an accurate measurement even through substances like wax, but unfortunately, not through fluids such as pus or eardrops.

I do not recommend the use of ear thermometers for infants under two years of age at its present level of technology.

Oral temperature: This method is quite accurate if the thermometer is held under the tongue for 2 minutes. The child must be old enough to be able to keep the lips closed around the thermometer to hold it in. A child under 4 years of age will most likely be unable to use an oral thermometer.

Axillary temperature: This method is painless and can be used on infants of all ages. It is accurate only if the thermometer is placed properly in the skin folds of the axilla at the mid-point in distance from the front to the back of the armpit. Often it is not put in far enough or is placed in too deeply, resulting in an inaccurate reading. Although convenient to use, I prefer the rectal route to give a more accurate reading.

Rectal temperature: A rectal thermometer is an excellent way of determining the temperature of an infant or child up to two years of age or older. The technique is safe, simple and accurate. Being old-school, I trust this method as being the most accurate for infants and small children. However, showing that I can change with the times, I am amenable to other readings, by other methods, as long as I am assured that they have been taken accurately.

Preferred Sites for Temperature Measurement

Less than two years of age: First choice, rectal
                             Second choice, axillary
Two to four years: First choice, ear
                             Second choice, rectal
                             Third choice, axillary
Five years and older: First choice, ear
                             Second choice, oral

Note: Other methods of recording an elevated temperature, such as fever strips or the so-called thermometer pacifiers and others, may be helpful to tell if the temperature is elevated but may not give you an accurate reading.

Methods of Taking Temperatures

Rectal Route:

First, if using a mercury thermometer, clean it with an alcohol swab and shake the mercury down so that the mercury level is below the Normal line. Dip the tip of the glass mercury thermometer into a small amount of petroleum jelly. If you are using one of the mechanical digital read-out devices, cover the tip with a lubricated sleeve provided or put Vaseline on the tip. Turn on the thermometer.

For small infants under 18 months of age, lay them on their backs and grab both feet with one hand. Bend the legs at their knees so that their knees are near the tummy. This will expose the infant's anal opening. With the other hand, insert the thermometer 1.5 to 2 cm. (3/4 to 1 inch) and hold for 1-1/2 to 2 minutes in the rectum or until the beep sounds in the mechanical read-out type.

The older infant may be placed tummy or face down on your lap. Place one of your arms across the infant's back to control movement. With the hand of that same arm, spread apart the buttock cheeks to expose the anal opening. Insert the thermometer tip with the other hand.

Calm reassurance and explanation during this procedure of temperature taking will usually relax the reluctant infant. Rectal temperatures are painless if you can get the infant to relax. **You will not puncture the rectum, even if you insert the thermometer up to 3–4 cm inside.**

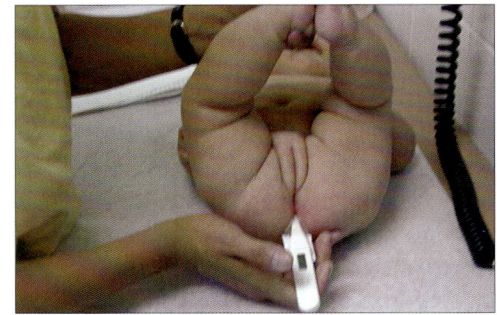

Rectal Thermometer

When finished, wipe the petroleum jelly off the thermometer and read. Then clean with alcohol and store for further use. The disposable sleeves on the mechanical devices are to be discarded.

The only concern using mercury thermometers is that if the baby is struggling a lot, the thermometer could break while inside the rectum.

If your infant is a real fighter, use either one of the mechanical rectal digital read-out thermometers or choose another site.

Axillary (Armpit) Route:

Axillary temperatures should be taken in the mid-axilla region of the armpit with the arm against the child's side. Leave the thermometer in place for 2 minutes.

Ear Route:

Turn on the thermometer. Pull ear up and back. Place tip in ear to a point halfway between the ear and eye on the opposite side of head. Click and read.

Oral (Mouth) Route:

For oral temperatures it is best taken for children who can cooperate (over 4–5 years of age). Make sure that the thermometer is kept under the tongue for 1–1/2 to 2 minutes. Lips should be closed around the thermometer.

Normal Temperatures:

Rectal – less than 38°C or 100.4°F
Oral – less than 37.5°C or 99.5°F
Axillary – less than 37.3°C or 99.1°F
Aural (Ear) – less than 38°C or 100.4°F

When to Seek Medical Advice with a Febrile Infant/Child

Using common sense is important. Only you can judge how ill your child is and when to seek medical advice. If your child is eating and is relatively playful, you can wait and see. A little crankiness is to be expected with an elevated temperature. Whether to seek medical advice in the middle of the night or not is difficult to answer. All symptoms always seems worse at night. If the infant does not seem overly distressed, try to tide him/her over until the morning before calling to see your doctor. Certainly, if your baby appears more ill than you would expect from the temperature alone, seek medical advice at once.

Any infant under 3 months of age who has an elevated temperature should be assessed as soon as possible. As a general rule, with fever, the smaller the infant, the earlier you should seek advice. Any child having a temperature of greater than 40°C (104°F) should be seen that day. Medical advice should also be sought if there is a fever accompanied by symptoms such as persistent sore throat, sore ear, pain on urination, persistent vomiting and/or diarrhea. Any cold symptoms with persistent fever lasting over 48 hours should be assessed. Other symptoms of concern are the child with a fever who is lethargic, pale, refusing fluids or limp, or who has joint pain or a rash that looks like small bruises.

DO NOT USE MEDICAL WALK-IN CLINICS OR EMERGENCY DEPARTMENTS FOR CONVENIENCE.

Look at your child; if he is not extremely ill, wait to see your family doctor or pediatrician for assessment. Generally speaking, it is not so much the height of the fever to be concerned about but rather, the total picture of the child. If the temperature is very elevated and the child does not appear or act overly ill you can wait. If however, at a low temperature the child appears and acts ill he should be assessed.

Unexplained fevers (that is, those without any other symptoms) that persist in an infant or toddler are always a concern. One common cause of such fevers is roseola. This is a viral illness occurring in infants between 6 and 20 months of age. There is a high fever for about three or four days. The infant does not appear overly ill. The fever then breaks and a faint rash appears on the trunk area of the body. The rash fades in one or two days. Never do the rash and fever appear together. That is, the fever goes and then the rash appears. If this is what your baby seems to have, do not fret. Your baby is not contagious. Let your child continue his/her normal routine.

All too often, this child is placed on antibiotics when fever first presents. The question then arises as to whether or not the child had roseola or another viral rash, or if the rash is a result of the antibiotic (which he/she probably didn't need in the first place)? Ninety-nine per cent of the time the rash is related to the viral infection and not to the antibiotic. No child should be labeled as having an antibiotic allergy unless the rash is seen by the doctor and determined to be allergic in origin. If there is doubt, allergy skin testing should be done.

A urinary tract infection is not an uncommon cause for an infant or toddler to have fever or fussiness (especially if the crying seems to indicate pain) lasting for two or three days without any other symptoms. When visiting the doctor with an unexplained fever (no other symptoms) of more than 48 to 72 hours, have the baby clean and dry in the diaper area. That is, no oils, powders or paste in this area. A urine-collecting bag may have to be applied to collect a urine specimen if the infant is not toilet trained. The sticky surface of the bag does not adhere unless it is applied directly to clean skin. Bring a bottle (milk, juice, water or a breast) with you to feed the infant. This will encourage a urine sample after a short waiting period.

There are numerous illnesses that may present with a prolonged fever as the main and even only symptom. Illnesses such as juvenile rheumatoid arthritis or inflammatory bowel disease may present with intermittent fevers for months before the diagnosis can be made only after the onset of other symptoms such as a swollen joint or diarrhea. Kawasaki's disease or leukemia are always a concern in a child with fever and little else in symptomatology. Foreign travel illnesses such as malaria should be considered on an individual basis.

Fever control: With any elevated temperature, especially of high degree (over 39°C), the baby's hands and feet may feel quite cool, lips appear purplish and, if old enough to talk, he may complain of cold feet. Shivering may be present. Do not be fooled and think from these observations that he is chilled and make the mistake of covering the child up. Leave the small infant in a diaper and undershirt with a light top only. When he sleeps, cover with a light blanket. **Remember, we want the heat to go out and not keep it in.** Cool sponge baths or alcohol rubdowns are not necessary. If your baby is willing to eat, this is good, so encourage plenty of fluids, milk being acceptable. Acetaminophen or ibuprofen is available in drops, liquids and tablets.

Dose of Medications for Fever Control

- 15 mg per kg (7 mg per lb) of acetaminophen may be given every 4 hours for a total of 5 doses in a 24-hour period.

- 8–10 mg per kg (4–5 mg per lb) of ibuprofen may be given every 6-8 hours.

Do not use any household teaspoons, which can differ in size, to measure medicine. Only use the dropper, measuring cup or measuring spoon supplied to ensure that the proper dosage of medicine is administered.

Note: the fever may return before the next dose of medication is recommended. If this is the case you may wish to try alternating acetaminophen and ibuprofen. Alternate each every 4 hours. That is, acetaminophen, then 4 hours later ibuprofen, then 4 hours later acetaminophen and so on.

If the child refuses or vomits his fever medication, then acetaminophen is also available in suppositories. The dosage is according to the infant's weight rather than age. Acetaminophen may be repeated every four hours up to five doses per day. Ibuprofen may be repeated every eight hours up to 3-4 doses (every 6–8 hours) per day. Follow the dosage schedule listed on the bottle according to weight. Acetaminophen suppositories may be used if the infant or child refuses to swallow the acetaminophen or ibuprofen.

Medication for fever control, whether it be acetaminophen or ibuprofen, may be continued for as long as the fever persists. There is no upper time limit.

If your infant or child vomits the medication within 20 minutes after it has been taken, it may be repeated. After this time, if vomiting occurs, wait for next dosage time.

With the first primary immunizations your infant receives, he may experience fever and irritability, as well as localized inflammation at the site of injection, for a period of 24 to 48 hours. Acetaminophen or ibuprofen is not required before immunizations. They are administered only if symptoms of fever and irritability occur afterwards. You should inform the doctor if the infant has inconsolable crying, persistent fever of over 40°C when temperature is taken rectally, a febrile seizure or persistent lethargy and vomiting after any immunization.

Because an immunization may be given directly into the muscle that area may become tender, warm, red and swollen. Apply ice for five minutes at a time and repeat as often as necessary. Acetaminophen or ibuprofen may be given for pain. Within a few days, the inflammation will resolve. Afterwards, a lump may be felt deep in the muscle. It may feel as big as a plum pit. There may be a dimpling in the skin over the site of injection. In time, that is, a few months, it will resolve. It occurs because during the immunization the needle pierced one of the small blood vessels deep in the muscle. There is some bleeding into the muscle at that site. In time, the blood is replaced with fibrous tissue, which feels like a firm lump. The lump will slowly resolve.

Fever (Febrile Seizures)

Many children who develop a high fever may become very agitated, delirious, seem frightened and may even hallucinate. Although the symptoms are very alarming to the caregiver they are not dangerous. The symptoms are not considered seizure activity.

There are 2 types of seizures associated with fever. They are called typical and atypical.

Typical Febrile Seizures

Typical febrile seizures are much more common than atypical. To qualify as a typical febrile seizure the following criteria must be met:

- A fever
- A seizure lasting less than 20 minutes
- The seizure is uniformly present on each side of the body from start to end
- The child is neurologically normal thereafter
- Occurs between 6 months and 5 years of age

A seizure may have several different types of clinical presentation. There is always a loss of consciousness – this is a marker for all febrile seizures. The eyes may roll back. The child may be very limp. Some children have jerking movements of all limbs.

Typical febrile seizures are quite common. A child may experience many. There is no medication that can prevent them. Putting the child on seizure medication in order to prevent recurrent febrile seizures is not indicated. By 5 years of age the child will outgrow them.

There are no resulting long-term neurological problems irrespective of the number of seizures that have occurred. There is no increased incidence of seizure disorder in the future, either with or without fever.

Some people believe that it is the degree of the fever that counts. Others feel it is the rate of the rise of fever. Still others feel that there is a "hypersensitivity" in that particular child's central nervous system, which makes him more prone to febrile seizures even at a temperature only slightly above normal.

Emergency Management

Emergency treatment consists of checking to make sure there is nothing around the neck which could affect breathing. Remove anything from the mouth. Turn the child on his side, preferably with his head below the level of his legs. Remove all clothing and cover him with towels soaked in cool water. Have the child assessed medically.

For typical febrile seizures no investigations are required.

Again it is important to remember that antibiotics are not required for every child with a fever. They are required only if there is a bacterial source as the cause of the febrile illness.

Atypical Febrile Seizures

These are less common than typical febrile seizures and have the following features:

- Occur in an age group outside of the typical febrile seizure age
- A seizure that is one-sided only or spreads from one side to the other
- Seizure lasts longer than 20 minutes
- Neurological symptoms and/or signs (detected on examination) after the seizure
- More than one seizure in a 24-hour period

These seizures are often more difficult to control at first. Seizure medication may be required and is given under the tongue, rectally or intravenously to control the seizure.

This child will require an EEG. A CT scan of the head and/or an MRI will be necessary if the EEG shows a focal area as the probable source of the seizure. With atypical febrile seizures, there is a potential for future afebrile (no fever) seizures. Depending on what is discovered, further investigations may be required in order to determine how it will be managed best.

If the EEG is normal, depending on the specific case, medication may not be initiated unless a second seizure occurs. If an abnormal EEG is found, medication will be required for a minimum of 3 years after the last seizure. If the child is doing well on medication, the EEG will probably be repeated 1 to 2 years after the initial one. If the child remains seizure-free for 3 years, tapering off his medication will be considered on an individual basis.

Depending on which anticonvulsant medication is used, periodic blood levels will need to be done to ensure that the concentration of the medicine in the blood is within the therapeutic zone. Other blood tests may also be required.

Fever – Fifth Disease ("Slapped Face Fever")

Fifth disease is caused by parvovirus B19. It occurs most often in the wintertime and spring. By adulthood, up to 80% of individuals have been infected with this disease. Approximately 50% have symptoms while the others are completely asymptomatic.

The incubation period from time of exposure to the first symptoms is from 4 to 20 days. There may be a brief illness involving fever, headache, and muscle aches, which occurs approximately 1 week before the appearance of the typical rash. The rash appears on the cheeks and looks as if the cheeks have been slapped – thus the name "slapped face fever." A few days later a red, lace-like rash appears, first on the arms and then on the trunk. The fever may last for a few days; the rash may fluctuate in intensity for up to 3–4 weeks.

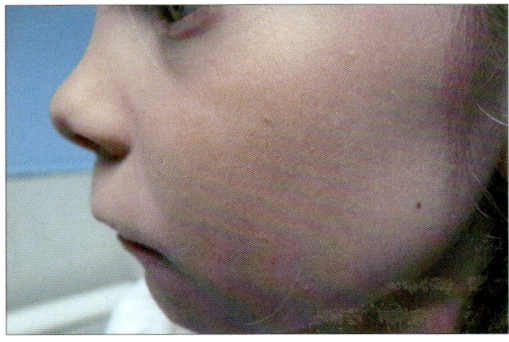

Slapped Face Fever

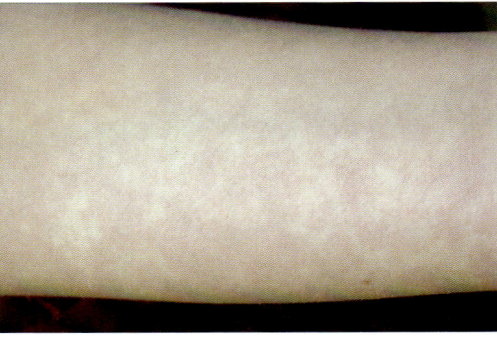

Lace-like Rash

It is spread by droplets containing the virus via coughing or sneezing.

There is no treatment except for fever control.

Fifth disease is contagious during its incubation period and until the appearance of the rash. Once the rash appears, the child can return to normal activity (he is no longer contagious). In adulthood, symptoms are as above, but also may include painful joints which can last for a few months.

If your child has fifth disease, he should avoid contact with any woman who is in her first trimester of pregnancy while he is in the contagious stage. Unfortunately the diagnosis is not usually made until after the typical rash appears, which is after the time when the child is contagious. A woman who has not been previously infected by this virus, and subsequently becomes infected with the parvovirus for the first time in her first trimester of pregnancy, has an increased risk for spontaneous abortion. Try to recall if your child was in contact with any woman in her first trimester of pregnancy when he/she was in the contagious period. Such women should be contacted and evaluated by their doctor because of their possible exposure to the parvovirus.

Fever – Kawasaki Disease (Mucocutaneous Lymph Node Syndrome)

Kawasaki disease in my opinion is a sneaky illness, which if not recognized and treated appropriately, can cause serious or potentially lethal results. I used the word "sneaky" because each of the symptoms by themselves mean very little. However, when added up and clustered, a potentially serious illness is indicated. There is no known cause for Kawasaki disease, the onset of which may be preceded by a mild cold or by nothing at all. It is most likely an autoimmune disorder.

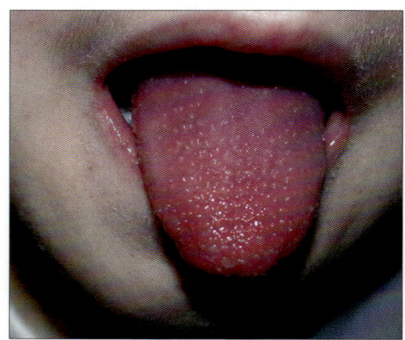

Strawberry Tongue

Possible symptoms:

- A high fever persisting for more than 5 days
- Reddened eyes
- Cracked, dry lips
- A reddened tongue (has a strawberry appearance)
- Enlarged neck lymph nodes
- Slight swelling of the hands and feet, with reddened soles and palms
- Peeling of the skin of the fingers and toes – this is a late symptom
- Other uncommon symptoms can include joint swelling, abdominal pain and headache

The child with Kawasaki disease most often looks ill and acts ill. This is a very important feature of this illness.

Kawasaki disease is a multisystem disorder. It may involve inflammation of the heart, the lungs, the liver, joints and central nervous system. There are no specific diagnostic tests for Kawasaki disease. The white blood count may be slightly increased. The platelet count may be moderately increased. The ESR is always elevated. An ECG may show abnormalities suggestive of a cardiac problem. The child with Kawasaki disease will be hospitalized. He will be treated with intravenous gamma globulin and acetylsalicylic acid (aspirin). A 2-D echocardiogram will be done of the heart to rule out coronary artery disease. The follow-up management will depend on the presence, absence or severity of coronary artery disease.

Fever – Pain and Fever Control

Tylenol and/or Tempra = acetaminophen, every 4 hours (15 mg/ kg/dose)
Advil = ibuprofen, every 6 to 8 hours (10 mg/kg/dose)

To ensure proper dosage, medications should be measured by using the supplied dropper, medicine cup or marked syringe. Do not use kitchen spoons.

Acetaminophen and Ibuprofen Dosage Chart

WEIGHT		CONCENTRATED DROPS		SUSPENSION		CHEWABLE TABLETS	CHEWABLE TABLETS
lbs / kg		Tempra Tylenol **80 mg/mL**	Advil **200 mg/5 mL**	Tempra Tylenol **160 mg/5mL**	Advil **100 mg/5mL**	Advil Jr. **100 mg**	Tempra Tylenol **160 mg**
6-8	2.5-3.9	.5 mL	.75 mL				
9-11	4.0-5.4	.75 mL	1.0 mL				
12-14	5.5-6.4	1 mL	1.25 mL		2.5 mL		
15-17	6.5-7.9	1.25 mL	1.5 mL		3.0 mL		
18-20	8.0-9	1.5 mL	2 mL	4.5 mL	3.75 mL		
21-23	9.1-10.9	1.75 mL	2.5 mL	5.0 mL	4.5 mL		
24-35	11-15.9	2 mL	3 mL	5.5 mL	6 mL	1 Tablet	1 Tablet
36-47	16-21.9	3.5 mL		10 mL	7.5 mL	1.5 Tablets	1.5 Tablets
48-59	22-26.9			12.5 mL	10 mL	2 Tablets	2 Tablets
60-71	27-31.9			15 mL	12.5 mL	2.5 Tablets	2.5 Tablets
72-75	32-45.9			19 mL	15 mL	3 Tablets	3 Tablets

Note: If fever returns before time of next dose you may alternate acetaminophen and ibuprofen every 4 hours. That is, give acetaminophen, 4 hours later give ibuprofen, 4 hours later give acetaminophen, and so on.

NORMAL TEMPERATURES:

Rectum – 38°C or less (100.4°F)
Armpit – 37°C or less (98.8°F)
Mouth – 37.5°C or less (99.5°F)
Ear – 38°C or less (100.4°F)

RECOMMENDED SITE FOR TAKING TEMPERATURE

Age	Rectum	Axilla (Armpit)	Mouth	Ear
Less than 2 years	First choice	2	–	–
2-5 years	2	3	–	First choice
Over 5 years	–	3	2	First choice

• If the child VOMITS the medication, you may repeat the dose if the vomiting has occurred less than 15 minutes after taken.

• If child REFUSES oral medication or REPEATEDLY VOMITS use acetaminophen suppositories (120 mg strength):

```
12–14 lbs    5.5–6.4 kg    =  1/2
15–17 lbs    6.5–7.9 kg    =  3/4
18–20 lbs    8–9 kg        =  1
21–23 lbs    9–10.0 kg     =  1-1/2
24–35 lbs    11–15.9 kg    =  2
36–47 lbs    16–21.9 kg    =  2-1/2
```

Note: Temperatures that are taken by forehead fever strips, temperature pacifiers or any other non-thermometer technique may be inaccurate and thus misleading.

Flat Head (Plageiocephaly)

Due to the risk of sudden infant death syndrome (SIDS), the recommendation for placing infants down to sleep is to put them on their backs until 8 months of age. An infant's head is heavy and the skull is soft and very malleable. Because the baby is repeatedly placed in this position, over time there may be flattening on one or both sides of the back of the head to varying extents.

The flattening of the back of the head, if it occurs at all, is benign in nature, as eventually the skull will round itself out. There will be no brain damage.

To prevent flattening of the head, when the baby is awake, no weight should be placed on the back of his head. The baby should be put into position either on his tummy or sitting. To prevent flattening of one side of the head, alternate the position in which the baby sleeps, with his head facing one way and alternating it in the other direction the next day. This will encourage the baby to move his head to the direction whereby he can see the world around him rather than having to look at a blank wall. A mobile hanging on the crib rail will also encourage him to look outward.

It is the rare occasion that an infant will require a specially fitted helmet to wear when asleep to prevent further flattening of the head.

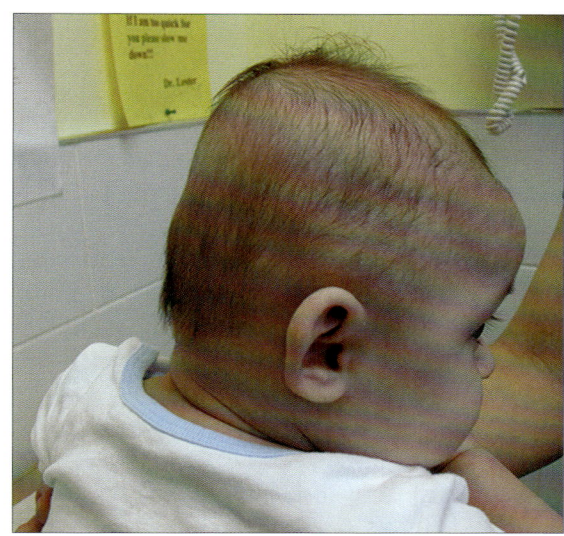

Flat Head

Unfortunately, there are some infants who just will not sleep on their backs. They prefer to sleep on their tummies. Once they are able to roll from their back to their tummy, they will do so. There are devices that you can purchase that will discourage the child from rolling. However, where there is a will there is a way. The bottom line is, if your infant will only sleep when on his tummy, then accept it. Infants who are able to roll from back to front are neurologically advanced enough that SIDS is unlikely to occur. Unfortunately, there are no monitors in our present technology to detect the possible onset of a SIDS or near-SIDS episode.

Fragile X Syndrome

Fragile X syndrome is one of the leading known causes of inherited mental retardation. It affects approximately 1 in 4000 males and 1 in 7000–8000 females.

The syndrome is the result of a mutated (defective) gene on the X chromosome. Males, who only have one X chromosome, tend to have more severe symptoms than females, who have two X chromosomes (one is affected and the other is normal).

Approximately 5% of autistic children have fragile X syndrome as the genetic underlying cause of the autism.

The symptoms of fragile X syndrome can be variable. Early symptoms usually include a delay in the development of speech and language. Poor social skills are often present, such as poor eye contact. Intellectually, there may be only a mild learning disability, attention deficit hyperactivity disorder (ADHD) or varying degrees of mental retardation. As stated, females may have softer symptoms that may even go unnoticed. Females are often shy, have problems with spatial concepts (e.g, reading maps) and executive functions (e.g., making a plan and carrying it out).

Some of the physical features which may appear as the child ages are an elongated face, large or protruding ears, flat feet, enlarged testicles in males, hyperflexible joints (fingers and wrists) and decreased muscle tone.

Children who should be tested for fragile X include those with symptoms suggestive of the diagnosis, those who have symptoms where there is a family history of fragile X syndrome and, lastly, those where there is a family history of undiagnosed mental retardation in the close family network (siblings, uncles and aunts or first cousins).

The diagnosis is confirmed by a chromosomal analysis.

Management depends on the severity of the symptoms. Very little may be required for some children with fragile X syndrome. Others may need special education or management for ADHD. Those with severe symptoms of developmental delay will require more intensive intervention..

Giardiasis – bowel

Giardiasis is a gastrointestinal infection due to a parasite called *Giardia lamblia*.

It is spread either by drinking contaminated water or through hand-to-mouth transmission. It is a very common infection among all age groups. The incubation period is 2–6 days.

Most children are entirely asymptomatic. If symptoms are present, they are loose and watery diarrhea, abdominal distention and discomfort. A fever is not usually present. The symptoms continue for a few days and then there is gradual improvement.

The diagnosis for giardiasis is made by a stool sample sent to check for ova and parasites.

The treatment, with metronidazole, is given only if the child is not already showing signs of improvement by the time the stool report is obtained. If the child is asymptomatic at that point then treatment is unnecessary. A repeat stool check for ova and parasites should be done again in one month's time.

Giardiasis has also been implicated as a cause for chronic abdominal pain, chronic diarrhea and poor weight gain.

My first recollection of coming across this illness was when I was in medical school. I was asked on a test to write a short paragraph on *Giardia lamblia*. I had absolutely no clue as to what it was. Since I had some time left on the exam I did write a short paragraph. I said that *Giardia lamblia* was a great general in Marco Polo's army. He led his troops in many a battle. Even Attila the Hun feared him.

I received an 'F 'on that question for being very 'funny'.

Giardia can be found in the stools of many of our population who are entirely asymptomatic. No treatment is required.

Growing Pains (Legs – Night Pain)

Growing pains are very common and usually occur in children between the ages of 3 and 6 years.

They characteristically take place during the night only. Growing pains do not occur during the day.

The child usually wakes up from sleep complaining of pain in one or both shins. Deep muscle pain in one or both calves may also be present. The pain may be severe enough to cause crying. It tends to last for 10–30 minutes and will disappear spontaneously.

Growing pains are consistent in that they never occur in one limb alone. Both limbs may be involved in succession. Pains could begin with the left limb or the right limb or both but **never** do they occur in isolation or in **only one limb** all the time.

The cause of growing pains is unknown and, in fact, this is a misnomer. They do not have anything to do with growing.

During the day the child is pain free and fully active – no limp.

There is no way of preventing or curing growing pains.

Rubbing the involved areas gently may help the child to relax and go back to sleep. Some may require ice while others may need heat applied for relief. The occasional use of acetaminophen or ibuprofen may be necessary, but it usually is not required because of the short duration of the symptoms.

No investigations such as blood work, x-rays or bone scans are needed.

Growing pains are seen to be entirely benign. Your child will "outgrow" them. There are absolutely no long-term side effects or association with any future muscle or joint problems.

Growth and Weight Gain

Parents always seemed to be concerned that a child is too big or too small; mainly, however, it is the latter variation that bothers caregivers most.

There are a number of factors that affect patterns for growth and weight gain. The most important one is the child's genetic background. Other factors include any underlying chronic illnesses, such as asthma or heart disease. To a lesser extent, diet plays a role as well.

We must remember that no two children are alike. So try not to compare one with the other (even within the same family).

When plotted on a growth grid, the readings for both height and weight will usually parallel a percentile. Concern arises only if there is an acceleration or deceleration of growth and/or weight gain when the plotted graph line crosses over 2 or more percentiles. For the first few months of life the percentiles are usually higher and then at about 6 months the height and weight will begin to parallel a percentile.

When gauging weight, the baby should regain his birth weight by 2 weeks of age. He should double his birth weight by 5 months, triple it by a year and quadruple it by 2 years. Remember that these parameters are not written in stone.

With height the rate of growth normally parallels that for weight. What is most important in the pattern for height is that its acceleration should parallel a percentile. Here I have to make a confession. Accurately measuring the length of an infant on an examining table can be a challenge; it depends on where you assume the top of the head to be, and how much you stretch the child out. A struggling infant is extremely difficult to measure. The tape measure is placed along the examining table from the top of his head to his heels. Occasionally I have had a child appear to "shrink" because of a mismeasurement – a real no-no in the eyes of the parent. I have had several medical students measure the same infant. Measurements have varied by up to 2 or 3 centimetres! There are available very accurate measuring devices that are used for a child who is either lying down or standing. Most pediatric offices do not have these. The devices are mainly used in specialized clinics dealing with growth problems.

How tall will your child be? You can estimate best by looking at the parents and grandparents. There is actually no accurate formula for predicting eventual height.

An educated guess is best. There is, however, one formula that is used and it goes as follows:

• Females – subtract 13 cm (5 in.) from the father's height and add this to the mother's height. Then divide by 2.

• Males – add 13 cm (5 in.) to the mother's height and add this to the father's height. Then divide by 2.

In over 40 years of practice, I have never heard a parent complain that her child will be too tall.

More often, I have encountered short parents who do not understand the fact that their child will rarely, if ever, be able to dunk a basketball (unless he is standing on a ladder).

Hand, Foot, and Mouth Disease

This is an enterovirus (viral) infection characterized by symptoms which include a general feeling of unwellness and fever, followed by red spots on the hands, feet and in the mouth that often blister. The lesions also may be found in the region of the buttocks. Often the lesions are most prominent in the mouth with few or none elsewhere.

Although cases may occur in isolation, affecting only one child at a time, more often they occur in clusters of children at daycare or school.

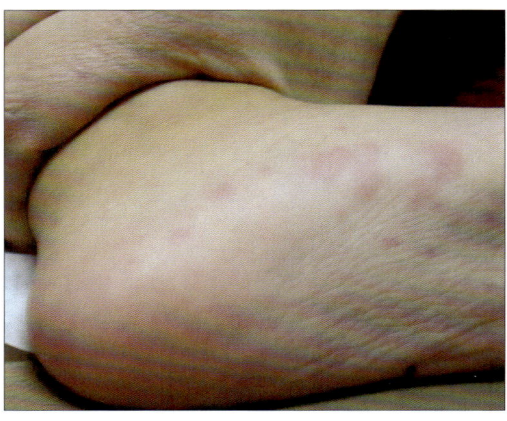

Rash on Foot

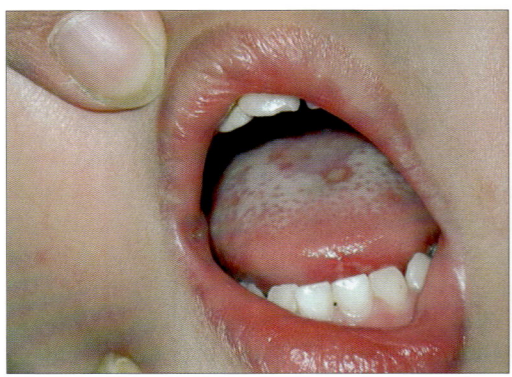
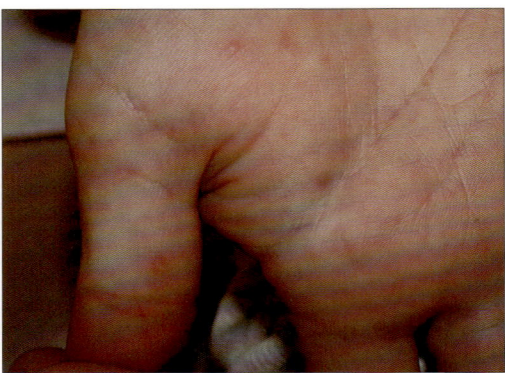

Mouth Lesions   *Rash on Hand*

Although it is more commonly found in preschoolers, it can occur at any age. Treatment is symptomatic only. Acetaminophen or ibuprofen is given for pain or fever. The child should be encouraged to drink to maintain adequate hydration. The appetite may become suppressed to varying degrees for 3 or 4 days. "Neutral" foods such as Jell-O, puddings, yogurt and other soft foods are preferred and more accepted than spicy foods. Food should not be served too cold or too hot. It is best served at room temperature or slightly warm.

Antibiotics or antiviral agents are not indicated.

As long as the child is urinating 4–6 times a day, then proper hydration is being maintained.

Isolation should be undertaken for a minimum of 4 days after the onset of the lesions.

There are no long-term complications from this illness.

Head Injury (Concussion)

If an infant falls and the actual fall is unwitnessed, do not automatically assume that he has hit his head unless there are signs or symptoms of a head injury. Parents frequently assume that there is a head injury when one has not occurred. If the doctor focuses only on the head because of the history given, trauma elsewhere on the body may be completely missed.

A child who has a head injury and who does not show any other symptoms except crying most likely has not suffered a concussion. This child should be monitored for a few hours and then, if he is not demonstrating further symptoms, he should be allowed to participate in normal activity. Watching him for a more extended period of time is unnecessary.

However, it can happen that after a seemingly minor head injury a child may vomit once or twice, have a headache, feel drowsy or even fall asleep. Despite the apparently minor nature of the head injury, as a precaution, the child should be examined by a physician as soon as possible. These symptoms are those of a concussion (brain injury).

The child with a concussion should always be observed for a full 24 hours after the injury. During the night, the child must be woken up every 2 to 3 hours to ensure there is a full level of consciousness. If you cannot rouse the child from sleep, seek medical help at once.

As a precaution, after a concussion, there should be no contact sports allowed for a minimum of two weeks beginning *after* there are no further symptoms present. The injured brain tissue takes time to completely heal. A subsequent concussion incurred before this healing process is completed could result in permanent brain damage. The more serious the symptoms, the longer the child should desist from activities in which a head injury is a possibility (for example, hockey, soccer, football, skiing and rodeo bronco-busting).

Symptoms for concern – serious concussion

1. Swelling under the skin at the site of the injury. This is most serious if the injury and swelling are in the area just above the ear. The skull in this area is at its thinnest and, therefore, is more susceptible to fracture.
2. Disorientation or confusion as to time and place, and inability to remember the event.
3. Blurred or disturbed vision (for example, double vision)
4. Difficulty in waking the child up
5. Blood or clear fluid leaking from the nose or ears
6. Stiffness of the neck
7. Pupils of the eyes appear unequal in size
8. Persistent vomiting
9. Loss of consciousness
10. Convulsions
11. Sudden or gradual change in personality, school performance, vision or speech

As stated, a concussion, although seemingly minor in nature, can signal an "insult" to the brain. Although the initial symptoms can disappear within 24 hours there may be long-term implications for even a single "minor" concussion. The symptoms may not manifest themselves for years. Multiple concussions have a cumulative affect. The symptoms for the injured party may be quite variable, from initially persistent headaches to underachieving at school, having poor memory, **forgetfulness** or showing personality changes, and possibly even progressing to the early onset of dementia.

One of a doctor's greatest concerns is the presence of a chronic subdural hematoma. After a concussion, there may be bleeding under the skull. This blood lies between the skull and the brain. Although it often resolves spontaneously, resulting in no health problems at all, there is a possibility that it will not. As more blood accumulates, there is an increasing amount of pressure put on the brain. Symptoms of a chronic subdural hematoma may not surface until weeks or months after the injury.

Localized chronic headaches at the sight of a previous concussion may be the only symptom of a chronic subdural hematoma. However, sometimes there are also nonspecific symptoms which may be present (by this time the head injury that previously occurred may have been entirely forgotten). These general symptoms include: poor school performance, personality changes, lethargy, behavioural issues, and loss of interest in surroundings, among others.

As parents, it is our responsibility to protect our children the best we can from all injuries, especially ones to the head. From this pediatrician's point of view, if the child has suffered more than 2 minor concussions or 1 serious concussion, he should never be permitted to partake in any contact sport for which further concussions are a possibility – ever. I know this sounds harsh, but as a parent, you do not want to be responsible for your child having a permanent impairment.

It goes without saying that proper head protection is of prime importance. Impractical and as farfetched as it may seem, ideally a helmet could be worn all the time, because a child may fall off his bed or a couch or slip on a wet bathroom floor and strike his head anytime without warning.

Helmets do help to prevent skull fractures. Unfortunately, they do not entirely prevent the "jiggling" of the brain inside the skull that occurs during a head injury. It is this movement of the brain inside the skull that may result in a concussion (brain injury).

We all love our children – let's protect them as best we can.

Head Lice

Here is everything you wish you didn't have to know about head lice.

Lice are reddish brown in colour and about the size of a sesame seed. They are wingless. They cannot fly or jump, but only crawl. They live for approximately 1 month on the human host (pets are never affected), surviving by sucking blood from the scalp skin. They survive approximately one day off the scalp at room temperature.

A head louse egg is called a nit. Nits are "glued" to a hair shaft. It takes approximately 10 days for them to hatch and another 10 for the female to mature and begin laying her own eggs. An egg found on a hair shaft more than 1 cm from the scalp skin surface has already hatched. Those closer to the scalp are still viable and have not hatched.

Nits can survive a number of days off the host.

The diagnosis of an active infestation can be only made by identification of a living louse in the hair. The presence of nits alone is not an indication of an active infestation. Nits are often mistaken for dandruff or sand. The latter can be easily removed from the hair by pulling the hair shaft between your thumb and forefinger, whereas nits stick firmly and are difficult to remove. The "head hunt" should be done in a well-lit room. Magnifying glasses may help. Divide the hair into sections and look carefully, one section at a time. Pay close attention to the areas behind the ears and at the nape of the neck.

The initial symptom of infestation is usually a scalp itch. However, approximately two-thirds of infestations are entirely asymptomatic. Itching may not develop for over a month after eggs have hatched. Unfortunately, the onset of infection is usually 4 weeks before its detection.

An individual's socioeconomic status or personal hygiene is not related to the likelihood of developing a lice infestation.

Spread occurs through close head-to-head contact. It can also occur by coming in contact with inanimate objects where lice have been deposited, for example, by sharing scarves, head bands, hats, brushes or combs.

Treatment: there are new, safe, "designer" products available that have been designed to kill lice. They can be purchased over the counter (environmentally friendly, please). Follow the instructions exactly as directed. Side effects are uncommon and usually consist of a mild rash on the scalp, which may be itchy. It will disappear within a day or so.

Today, many lice have become resistant to over-the-counter products. Some now have to be applied at least 3 times before success. Many do not work at all. In communities where resistance is low, products such as 1% permethrin or pyrethrins are preferred and repeated 9 days after the initial treatment.

The manual removal of nits immediately after treatment is not necessary.

Treat all members of the family in which live lice have been found. Only those members with nits alone, more than 1 cm from the scalp need not be treated. Each member of the family should be checked on a daily basis. If a live organism is found, then, and only then, treatment is required. Check daily for 10 to 14 days.

Treatment of inanimate objects which may carry lice: everything that can be treated, such as clothing, linens and towels, etc., should be washed in hot soapy water. Thereafter, dry on the hottest cycle for at least 20 minutes. For items that cannot easily be washed, such as stuffed animals, pillows and comforters, place in the dryer at the hottest cycle for at least 20 minutes. Alternatively, they may be enclosed in plastic bags in a cold setting such as the garage for two weeks or dry cleaned. Smaller items that cannot be washed in hot water, for example, woolen hats, head bands and scarves, may be placed in a plastic bag in the freezer for 24 hours. Brushes and combs can be covered with any of the above-mentioned pediculicides for 10 minutes and then left in hot water for 30 minutes. As an alternative, they may be soaked in a disinfectant solution such as 2% Lysol for one hour. All areas where infested shedded hair may lie should be cleaned and vacuumed.

"Natural" products and numerous alternative "cures" have been tried but have never proven to be as effective as the above. These include mineral oil, coconut oil shampoo, tea tree oil and petroleum jelly, just to name a few.

The most common reasons for failure are not using the products properly, not repeating the procedure in one week's time, incomplete removal of live nits (those within 0.5 in. of the scalp), failure to treat inanimate objects properly, resistance to the product being used, and lastly, and most commonly, reinfestation. Another problem is not using an adequate amount of the medication, especially for children with long hair. As a general rule of thumb the amount that should be used in children with long hair is about 120 mL (4 ounces) for every 13 cm (6 inches) of hair.

The single most effective preventative method for avoiding lice infestation is early detection. This can only be accomplished by checking heads on a regular basis for lice and nits. They may not be present today but visible a few days later.

There are professionals whose job it is to manage lice infestation. They can be consulted if you have a problem. Check the phone book.

If your child is in daycare or nursery school you should inform staff that he has a lice infestation. They will closely check and monitor the other children. Fortunately, the contagiousness of head lice in the classroom setting is low.

Each child centre may have different criteria concerning when your child may return. Your child should be able to return the day after the initial treatment.

New medications are coming on the market frequently to help combat resistant lice strains. To quote an old adage – check a head to avoid a spread!!!

Headaches

Intermittent headaches are always a real "headache" for the child, the parent and, as well, the doctor.

Intermittent or chronic headaches may be defined as those which happen repeatedly over a period of at least one month.

Often the child will state only that, "My head hurts." Because he lacks communication skills, we assume, therefore, that he is having a headache, although this may not always be the case.

Just as adults have headaches, so do children. Unlike adults, their headaches are not due to stress or anxiety. Psychosomatic headaches in children less than 5 years of age are extremely uncommon (but it is not so for teenagers).

Most often the possible origin for the headaches is only discovered with the history taken. The physical examination of the child by the doctor usually produces no findings. Unfortunately, an accurate history is difficult to elicit from a young child. This makes it difficult for a doctor to decide how to proceed.

Red Flags

- A headache that is severe enough that the child stops what he is doing
- The child is woken up at night by strong headaches
- The child experiences vomiting in the morning
- A preceding concussion of the head
- The child favours one side of his body during activities
- Personality changes in the child
- Increasing fatigue and decreasing appetite
- Any problem with vision
- Any developmental regression – in self-care, self-feeding or increased clumsiness are examples of developmental regression
- Regression in speech or printing, diminished accuracy in colouring or in any other fine or gross motor skills

When any child complains of a sore head, the first thing that enters a parent's mind is that he has some scary disease. All doctors understand this.

One of the major problems a doctor has is when there are no red flags present. Will he be able to convince anxious caregivers through reassurance that, at this particular point in time, investigations are not indicated? Very difficult. The parent's worst imaginings are further fuelled if some other member of the family has had a brain tumor or intracranial bleed which was "missed" for a period of time. The parents do not want this to happen to their child. Horror stories related by their "advisory staff" will only heighten their concerns.

The basic investigation ordered to rule out a space-occupying lesion in the brain is either a CAT scan or an MRI. With children less than 6 years of age this may require a general anesthetic.

If you are in doubt and are not reassured by your doctor that waiting a little while to see if the headaches disappear is valid or if red flag symptoms subsequently appear, then request an MRI or CAT scan. A pediatric neurological consultation may be required.

There is an old saying, "Horrible imaginings are worse than present fears." That is, if you were reassured by an MRI that a space-occupying lesion was not present, you would be more prepared to wait and see what could evolve with your child's headaches – the anxiety would ease.

By the way, young children may experience the same kind of migraine headaches that adults do.

Hearing

We have five senses. These include the senses of hearing, sight, touch, smell and taste. Some say that intuition is the sixth sense. I feel there is a "seventh sense" as well – common sense. In fact, many of life's problems, including child rearing, involve varying degrees of deficiencies of this seventh sense. In this section, however, I will address only the sense of hearing.

In many communities, all newborn infants receive a hearing screening to verify that the infant has no hearing problems that may have developed in utero during the mother's pregnancy. Possible causes for loss could include, for example, a hearing loss resulting from medication given to the mother, rubella syndrome, or hereditary hearing loss.

Initial newborn hearing screening is performed in the hospital before the infant is discharged. Sound frequencies of 2000, 3000 and 4000 Hz are directed at the eardrum. The sound is transmitted through the middle ear into the inner ear. If the cochlea (the organ of hearing in the inner ear) responds to the sound, it is recorded. A responding cochlea means that hearing is present. If there is no response, the test will be repeated in approximately one month. If there is still no response a brainstem audiogram will be done. If there is a family history of hearing loss, irrespective of the newborn hearing screening results, a brainstem audiogram will be performed at 4 months of age. Even if the brainstem audiogram is normal, the child will be followed with periodic audiograms over the next few years. Follow-up for infants would include monitoring the child's response to sound using a more frequency-specific method than that used for the newborn screening. For older children who are able to communicate and demonstrate that they hear the sound, routine audiometry will be performed.

There are developmental milestones that should occur in every infant to ensure that there is no hearing impairment:

• By 3 months of age – startles to loud sounds
• By 5 months of age – turns head to source of sounds, watches your face as you talk and, most important, starts to vocalize by cooing

If these are not present, an audiogram is mandatory.

An audiogram basically measures a child's ability to hear sounds of different frequencies (pitch) at various degrees of intensity or loudness. Wearing earphones, the child responds when he is able to hear the sound and this response is recorded. The frequency of the sound is measured in hertz (Hz). If you were to picture the keys on a piano, the ones to the left represent the low-frequency sounds while the ones on the right are the high-frequency sounds. The loudness parameter is measured in decibels – from quiet to very loud.

The more severe the hearing loss is, the greater will be the impact on a child's ability to communicate using speech. Early detection and intervention of a hearing loss will maximize this ability.

As previously mentioned (see Ears – Otitis Media), there are many causes for acquired unilateral (one ear) or bilateral (both ears) hearing loss. These include exposure to certain drugs such as gentamicin, diseases such as meningitis or encephalitis and damage to the ear from ear infections or noise. Not uncommonly, parents who constantly clean their children's ears with cotton-swab sticks will unwittingly pack the outer ear with wax. As a result, sound waves will be prevented from reaching the eardrum, where the processing of sound begins. A degree of temporary hearing loss may occur.

A "selective hearing response" may cause a parent to be concerned about their child's hearing. This response may result from lack of attention paid rather than from an actual hearing problem. The child may be so involved in what he is doing that he just does not "hear". Or he may just be tuning the parents out because he does not want to hear what they are saying. An example of this: he may not wish to hear the words "come to bed" and therefore does not respond. Yet he will always respond to "let's go for a treat." Nevertheless, there are some aspects of selective hearing which may also be due to a level of hearing impairment. Any child who displays selective hearing should always have an assessment by an audiologist to rule out an actual hearing loss, particularly one affecting the higher frequencies (e.g., he misses sounds such as the 's' in the word *sun*). This frequency range is where many of the critical sounds for understanding speech occur.

Persistent presence of fluid in the middle ear after a single or multiple ear infections may result in a significant hearing loss. If fluid is found in the middle ear for more than 4 months and there is a 20 or more decibel hearing loss on an audiogram, the child will require a myringotomy (a surgical procedure) and the insertion of ventilating tubes. This will allow for the drainage of any accumulated fluid at the actual time of surgery and thereafter as long as the tubes remain functional. Fluid, if left too long in the middle-ear compartment, may turn into a glue-like substance and result in varying degrees of damage to the 3 small bones in the middle ear. Proper functioning of these small bones is necessary for the transmission of sound from the eardrum to the inner ear. Depending on the extent of the damage, this can result in varying degrees of permanent hearing loss.

With the increased use of portable music devices, both children and adults are becoming more and more susceptible to potential premature hearing loss. The louder the noise and the longer the exposure, the greater is the potential for damage. This kind of hearing loss is cumulative.

Here are a few examples for the loudness of certain sounds as measured in decibels. Normal breathing is just audible and is 10 dB. Normal conversation is 60 dB. Average city traffic noise registers at 80 dB. Subway, motorcycle and lawn mower noise is 90 dB. A power saw or rock music band is 110 dB. Close proximity to thunder clapping or discotheque sounds is 120 dB. The firing of a shotgun or listening within 200 feet of a jet taking off rates 130 dB. The threshold for ear pain is about 125 dB. Repeated close exposure to sounds greater than 90 dB for more than a few minutes at any one time may result in hearing loss.

When listening to music with earphones many individuals attempt to block out the surrounding noise by turning up the volume. As a general rule, if you cannot hear surrounding noises then the music is too loud. If other people can hear what you are listening to while you are wearing earphones, it also is too loud. Turn down the volume.

The first side effect of constant exposure to loud noise is tinnitus (ringing or buzzing in the head}. Hearing loss may follow.

Select proper headphones – Earbud headphones are more damaging than the ones worn over the ear (although, unfortunately, the latter are not as "cool").

Limit exposure time – If you just cannot turn it down, turn it off for awhile. For every volume increase of 3 dB, listening time should be cut in half.

Even a mild hearing loss may have a profound effect on your child. Fragments of speech may be misunderstood. Hearing loss may result in a problem with hearing at distances as close as 5 ft. The child is likely to have delayed or disordered grammar, limited vocabulary, imperfect speech production and a flat voice quality. Intervention by way of sound amplification may be required. A personal FM system to overcome extraneous noise, plus preferential seating in the classroom, is often necessary. With the use of personal hearing aids alone, the child's ability to learn effectively in the classroom is still highly compromised.

For the child, there are psychological effects that may accompany a hearing loss. These can include poor socialization skills with peers, lower self-esteem, a feeling of rejection, frustration or being subject to ridicule, and increased fatigue from the greater effort it takes to listen. The child may appear to be inattentive (as if he is daydreaming). A team approach is required in order to prevent these problems from happening. The team should include the parents, the teacher, the doctors, the audiologist and the speech-language pathologist.

If there is a profound hearing loss due to a sensorineural problem (for example, post-meningitis or congenital) the child will require hearing aids and/or a cochlear implant. Cochlear implants are not indicated when hearing loss is due to a conductive (middle ear) problem. Hearing aids would benefit the child with a conductive hearing loss.

As an aside, have you ever been sitting in your car at a red light and all of a sudden your car starts to vibrate from the sound coming from another car? You open your window and hear the "boom boom boom" sound coming from that car. Trust me, that person (usually young) will have a hearing loss which will slowly increase each time he enters that "hostile" environment.

Hearing loss in many cases can be prevented – think about it – do something about it.

Stop – Look – Listen.

Hepatitis A

Hepatitis A is a mild viral inflammation of the liver. It is spread through the oral fecal route by the contamination of food or water.

The incubation period is between 2 and 6 weeks.

Over 95% of individuals who develop this illness show no symptoms.

There is a 100% recovery rate leaving lifelong immunity to the hepatitis A virus.

A person with chronic hepatitis B or C who subsequently develops a hepatitis A infection may experience further damage to the liver. This is the one potential serious problem with hepatitis A.

Hepatitis A vaccine may be given to infants after one year of age to induce immunity – 2 or 3 immunizations over one year will be required for lifelong immunity.

Hepatitis B

Hepatitis B is a viral inflammatory disease of the liver. It is transmitted through blood, bodily fluids and contaminated instruments (i.e., reused needles, reused razor blades, unsterilized, reused manicure instruments).

The incubation stage lasts from several weeks to several months.

Symptoms can range from few or none at all, but may include decreased energy, decreased appetite, nausea and vomiting, low-grade fever, jaundice (mostly noticed in the whites of the eyes which turn yellow), mild abdominal discomfort, especially on the right side underneath the ribcage and lastly, lightening of the stool colour.

The illness usually runs a course of approximately 3 weeks and then slowly improves.

It is most contagious during the jaundice phase.

Approximately 95% of adults who contract the disease recover fully. Less than 50% of children who acquire the illness will fully recover. The younger the child, the greater the risk there is for developing chronic hepatitis and subsequent cancer of the liver. Unfortunately, less than 5% of newborns who acquire the disease will fully recover.

A significant number of individuals who develop hepatitis B will become hepatitis B carriers. These individuals act as a reservoir to pass the virus to others. The number of hepatitis B carriers in North America is increasing at a steady rate.

The risk of passing the disease on to her newborn from a pregnant woman who is a hepatitis B carrier is approximately 25%. As stated, infants affected are in the highest risk category for developing severe hepatitis B, chronic hepatitis B and subsequently, cancer of the liver.

Fortunately, the disease can be prevented in the newborn by the use of IM gammaglobulin and by initiating a hepatitis B vaccination program for the baby. Treatment should begin within the first day after birth.

Because the risk of developing chronic hepatitis after an acute infection is much greater for young children, there is now strong evidence to support the idea that all children should receive hepatitis B vaccine starting at birth. This program is being carried out in many countries, including the USA.

As stated, hepatitis B vaccine can be initiated at any time in life. For complete immunity 3 doses are required. After the initial dose, a second dose is given one month later and a third dose 6 months after the initial dose. Immunity develops approximately 3-4 weeks after the initial immunization. For lifetime immunity to occur all 3 doses are required.

Hepatitis A and B vaccines in combination are available as well. These combined vaccinations can be administered only after 1 year of age.

There is still a controversy as to when the hepatitis B vaccine should be initiated. As stated above, many countries initiate vaccination at birth. The reason is that the chance of hepatitis B becoming a severe active disease, then a chronic disease, and eventually turning into cancer of the liver is much higher in infants who acquire the disease, compared to those who develop the illness when they are older.

Others are of the opinion that giving the vaccination in the newborn period may not result in lifelong immunity. When tested for antibodies to the hepatitis B virus as teenagers, a large number of children who had received vaccination in the newborn period had no detectable antibody level in the blood. Does this mean they did not have protection from hepatitis B? There are numerous studies that have shown that even without detectable antibodies in the blood, when challenged with a hepatitis B antigen, there is a quick antibody response. This is quite suggestive of excellent immune memory and that there is protection against hepatitis B despite low or zero antibodies in the blood in those immunized during infancy.

Who should receive the vaccine?

• All infants born to a mother who is a hepatitis B carrier, or if other carriers are in the home
• Everyone who is travelling to an area in the world where hepatitis is prevalent

The question of timing of the vaccine administration to the general population is difficult to answer. In an otherwise perfect world it would be most beneficial if given early in infancy. However, one problem exists. This problem is the various very vocal "anti-immunization" groups. Adding a vaccine that may contain thimerosal and requires 3 doses is a "hard sell". Is it safe? Yes. There are no long-term side effects.

In children 2 years of age or older, only 2 immunizations are required, 6–12 months apart.

Hernias (Hydroceles, Umbilical, Inguinal, and Granuloma)

Hydrocele

A hydrocele is a "water sac" around one or both testicles. They are usually present at birth. They vary from being barely felt to the size of a plum. They are more common in premature infants. There are no symptoms. For the vast majority of boys with hydroceles, the condition will disappear by 8 to 12 months of age. If they are present for more than a year and a half, surgical correction may be indicated. This is an outpatient procedure done under a very light general anesthetic.

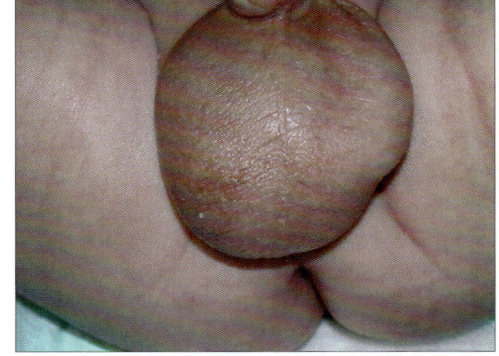

Right Hydrocele

Hydroceles can be associated with inguinal hernias. Moms – try to refrain from informing your husband about the presence of the hydroceles; most fathers are usually quite proud of their newborn baby boy's endowment. Don't tell him it is just water!

Umbilical Hernia

An umbilical hernia is a protrusion of bowel through an opening midline at the site of the belly button. They can vary from being very small to as large as a plum. They are more common in premature infants and those of African descent.

If you were to push on it with your finger it would be soft and you would feel it and perhaps hear a "squishy" sound. If you were to push further with the tip of your finger you would probably be able to feel the opening in the abdominal wall through which the hernia protrudes.

Most umbilical hernias disappear by 8 to 12 months of age. If it is still present at one year of age, it will probably not go away on its own. It can be surgically corrected. This is an outpatient procedure done under a light general anesthetic. Large umbilical hernias, which are of concern to the doctor, may be repaired early in life (less than one month old). For most, however, it is better to wait until the child is older (more than 18 months). At this age and weight your child will be better able to handle a general anesthetic.

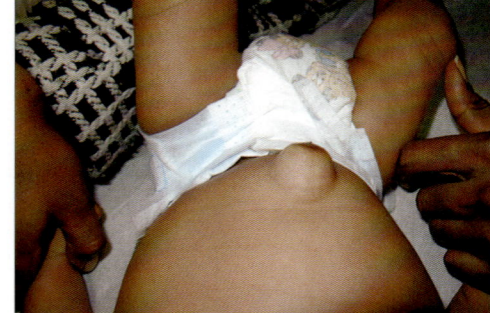

Umbilical Hernia

Home remedies, such as taping the hernia down, have been shown to be ineffective.

A word of caution – very rarely, the bowel inside the hernia sac may become twisted. The baby will howl in pain as if he has been hit in the abdomen with a cannonball. He may vomit and obviously will be in discomfort. If it is very firm and you are unable to reduce (push) the hernia sac into the abdomen then an obstruction is probably present. This is a surgical emergency. The child requires immediate surgical correction if the hernia cannot be manually reduced by the doctor.

Inguinal Hernia

An inguinal hernia presents itself as a lump which is normally soft and nontender just above the groin area. It can be either on one side or on both. It is more common in boys than in girls and in premature infants. It is often more noticeable when the infant cries or strains. There are no symptoms.

Many inguinal hernias resolve completely on their own. However, some will require surgical correction. The procedure is done as an outpatient under a light general anesthetic. The timing of the surgery depends on the size of the hernia and the age of the child (usually 6 to 24 months of age).

Inside the hernia sac is a small section of the bowel. Very rarely it becomes twisted and causes obstruction of the bowel. If this occurs, the infant will suddenly scream loudly and be in great discomfort. He may vomit. When you feel the hernia, it is no longer soft and may be tender. It does not disappear with pressure. If this occurs, it is a surgical emergency. If the doctor cannot manually reduce the hernia, the child will require immediate surgical correction.

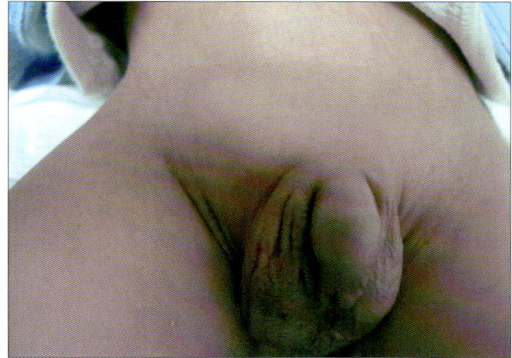

Right Inguinal Hernia

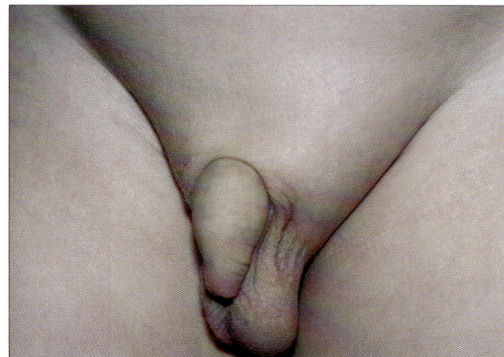

Left Inguinal Hernia

Umbilical Granuloma

An umbilical granuloma is the protrusion of the soft tissue of the belly button stump outwards. It usually is first detected after the cord has fallen off. It may be moist and stain the infant's undergarments.

No treatment is required initially. Most umbilical granulomas fully retract and disappear by 6 to 8 months of age. If by that time it is still present, it can be removed either by cauterization or surgery.

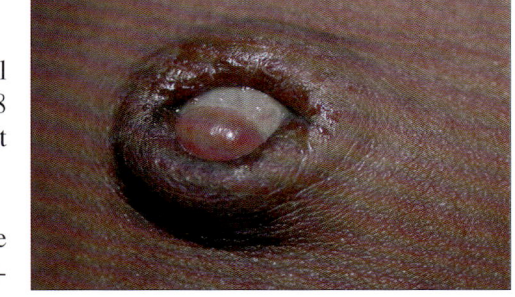

Occasionally it may become infected. The discharge will turn yellow to green and have an odor. An antibiotic cream will be prescribed.

Umbilical Granuloma

Hives (Urticaria)

Red flag

Hives may be associated with anaphylaxis (see Allergic Reaction–Severe, Anaphylaxis).

Urticaria is an immune response to some internal or external allergen (e.g., food or an antibiotic) or to a non-allergen (e.g., a cold virus).

Hives have distinct margins with slightly raised pink/red patches of varying size and shape. They may occur anywhere on the skin. They most often are very itchy. Hives can come quickly and disappear just as quickly. They may also spread to other areas of the body.

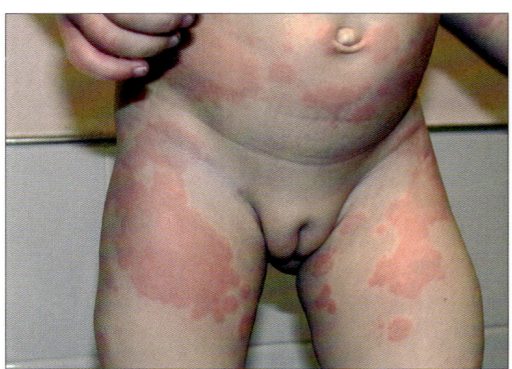   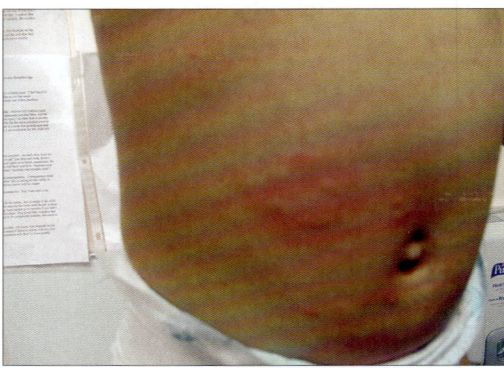

Hives   *Hives*

Urticaria most frequently is a "scratchy" problem (that is, it will often have you scratching your head!). It is perplexing for the parent as well as for the doctor. Unfortunately, in many cases there is no known trigger that can be identified.

In young children, hives are most often found following an upper respiratory tract viral infection. The urticaria, which is an immune response, is a response to the virus.

Be it an ingested substance, inhaled or the result of contact with the skin it may precipitate a reaction that results in hives. There are times when a thorough history is taken that the culprit can be determined. Unfortunately, more often it cannot be discovered.

The treatment for hives is avoidance of the trigger, if it is known, and by the use of antihistamines. Since hives are a reaction located under the skin, topical creams are essentially of no use.

An acute case of hives may last for a few weeks before disappearing. Chronic recurrent hives may last for months.

Every parent wants to know why their child has hives. As stated, the "why" is most often difficult to determine. Unfortunately, this conclusion is frequently unacceptable to parents. They may demand blood testing or allergy skin testing to determine the cause – their thinking goes, "The cause must be found, doctor."

There are millions of potential triggers which can cause hives. Allergy skin testing can only identify less than 30 potential allergens. Since many of the triggers show no reaction to skin testing, skin testing often will yield no productive information as to the cause. There are no specific blood tests to determine any allergic cause.

The result of this failure to source the cause, unfortunately, is an unhappy child with unhappy parents and a beleaguered doctor: one who usually has great difficulty convincing the parents to take a "wait and see" approach to the problem.

Close to 100% of children with recurrent or chronic hives do not have any serious underlying disorder pointing to a potential health problem.

Close to 100% of children will outgrow their hives, given time.

Antihistamines may be required on a regular basis to be given as needed. Leukotriene inhibitors (e.g., Singulair) given on a daily basis may be useful for treating chronic hives until the problem resolves.

Frustrated, parents often will turn to alternative methods of management. There have been no conclusive scientific studies showing that naturopathic investigations and treatment for chronic hives have been successful. The bottom line is: it is your child, it is your penny. From my point of view both patience and time are the best allies – now if only I could convince the parents!!!

Holidays – Halloween

When a child dresses up in his costume, he enters a world of magic. The goal: fun and bounty.

With imaginations in a heightened state children become more uninhibited – thoughts of safety become blunted.

Parent's responsibility – to ensure this magic time is also a safe time.

Remember that young children may be frightened by not only their own costume but also by those of others. Be sensitive to this. Nightmares may occur.

At school some groups exclude their children from the Halloween ritual – Seventh-Day Adventists and some Muslims, for example. Children should be made sensitive to this fact.

Your house

- Path well lit – especially if there are steps on the walkway

• To lessen fire hazards, consider using battery-powered alternatives to candles in pumpkins for lighting

Before the adventure

- Have supper
- Explain the rules of safety
- No running across lawns from house to house or running through hedges; respect others' property
- Remind children of their manners – a thank-you is always appreciated
- Dress them according to the weather
- Make sure they go to the bathroom before you put on their costumes

Costumes

- Should not restrict your child's normal gait
- Should not be too long to prevent tripping
- Fire-resistant fabrics are a must!
- Avoid masks that obstruct vision
- Light reflectors should be taped onto costume
- Attach an envelope with your phone number to your child's costume – carry a cell phone
- Take along extra bags – the loot becomes heavy

En route

- Keep your eyes on your children at all times – this is not a time for socializing.
- Keep in mind that after a short time, you will be carrying your child's hat, mask, sword or wand and extra candy collected.
- Don't travel a distance farther from your home or car than you have the strength to carry a very exhausted child or two.

At home

- Discard anything that is not wrapped and sealed.
- Divide up the loot as you see fit – there are no right or wrong rules. In the spirit of giving, consider giving extra candy to a nursing home, food bank, breakfast club or hospital learning centre: showing communal responsibility at a young age will stay with your children for the rest of their lives.

As to how much candy they consume – anything goes as long as it doesn't spoil their mealtimes. Remember to reinforce careful teeth brushing after consuming so many sweets, and don't you get caught stealing their chocolates!

By the way, if you're planning a Halloween party, make sure you speak to all the parents of your guests regarding any food allergies (nuts, soy, etc.).

Although I may be "old-school" and believe that children should always be respectful, this is the one time of the year that saying "Trick or treat, smell my feet or give me something sweet to eat" goes.

Do not forget about your pets. They too can be "spooked" on Halloween night.

I suggest the following:

• Pet costumes should be reasonable for the pet
• Provide a safe and quiet environment for your pet
• Pets may react aggressively with all the noise – ensure that they are on a lead and away from the door
• A small child may be frightened by your barking dog no matter how harmless you know him to be
• Ensure that all the "loot" gathered is out of reach of your pet

Holidays – March Break

Although I am going to use the old cliché "Today ain't like the old days," I think a very important point has to be made. Certainly the influences and pressures on parents have changed over the years, but the basic principles that my parents and their parents used to bring up their children can still apply today.

Sixty years ago I was only 10 years old. I lived with my two brothers and parents in a small house on the east side of Toronto. I shared a bedroom with one brother. In those days we were very fortunate. We had a phone in the kitchen, a phone in my parent's bedroom and 3 radios. We also had our dog Pat. Both my parents worked. During school that was fine. However, it was challenging during a school break time. When I think back, those were the best years of my life. My two brothers and I would make up games, play in the basement or backyard or go and hang out with our gang of friends. We always had something to do. We were never bored. We could spend the whole day entertaining ourselves.

Let's fast-forward 61 years to 2011. A similar family lives in a house with 2 or 3 children and perhaps a pet. So what is different? The first is that there are many more material things that are part of daily life now that were not dreamed of when I was a kid – TV, cell phones, iPods, many electronic gadgets to play with, computers, and so on. The second is that kids today are not like they were in the past. They have become accustomed to instant gratification and parental leniency has increased in response.

But there is a contradiction; although we "give in" more often, today we are afraid even to let our children play in the backyard or walk the streets for fear of their being snatched or harmed in some other way. Outside the confines of our homes they require our constant vigilance. This fear has fuelled an anxiety that causes us to overprotect our children. We hover over them like helicopters, always supervising, and thus limiting their social growth and a healthy sense of self.

What has all this to do with March break? Here is my point: when I was a kid and looked out the window on a cold, frosty morning during March break, I didn't just see a backyard full of snow. I saw an opportunity for fun and adventure – snowballs, snow forts, a snowman and making angel wings. I am afraid today too many of our children look out the window and just see snow. They have been given fewer opportunities to develop their imaginations and creative thinking – not only to abandon their "gadgets" but also to invent games with a few props. They have become too reliant on gadgetry. They expect others to entertain them – after all, this is the way that is has been since early infancy.

Although you cannot give too much love, you can give too many things or give in too often. While our children are overprotected, they are at the same time overindulged. Our children are being brought up in a world where very little effort is required to receive rewards. Our children lack opportunities to use their imaginations, to use the many ordinary things that surround them for creative play. They just do not have to use their creativity, because some thing is always there to operate, switch on, plug into, or watch.

What would happen if we let our children entertain themselves during the March break? If we disconnected all gadgetry? We must teach them to use their inventive natures; to not expect rewards without some effort or deserving behaviour; to explore nature in their own backyards. How long do you think they could survive without "dying" from boredom. If we have taught our children coping skills and how to deal with challenges and adversities, then this will be less problematic. They will have learned to demonstrate independence and creativity. We will have provided them with the necessary desire to adapt. We would have prepared them for life.

Our children are a direct reflection of how they are brought up.

They will survive the March break if we give them the right tools.

Hygiene **(General)**

There is an old cliché that states: "Cleanliness is next to godliness." If this be true, then from my observations some people are far off the mark; some are to the right of the mark, while others sit to the left.

The case in point: In the old West, cowboys, after spending 2 or 3 months on the range driving cattle, would finally arrive at their destination. During the cattle drive they would seldom or ever wash, brush their teeth or change their clothes. It is hard to understand how anyone could bear to stand downwind from them. When the cattle drive was over, they would ride into town to celebrate. A few would have a bath, some just doused themselves with toilet water, while others skipped the clean-up altogether and headed straight to the saloon.

In the old cowboy movies no one seemed to mind each other's odor. Although it was only Hollywood's portrayal, these characters were obviously far off the mark. There the "hygiene pendulum" had swung far to the left.

Some are too close to the opposite extreme. Despite the fact that there is a theory called the "hygiene hypothesis", which basically states that a little dirt will never hurt, today we live in a "super-clean" world, especially in North America. We think that the more sterile our environment is, the better – correct? Well, it is not exactly so. Through the overuse of anti-bacterial and anti-viral soaps and cleansers, the filtering of our air and the sealing off of our homes from any outside influences which are thought to have an adverse effect on our health, we have effectively diminished our contact with the many antigens that formerly would have stimulated our immune systems in a healthy manner. The belief is that at present, our immune system may have drifted away from fighting infection and instead may have turned its attention to driving its allergic component. This is one of the reasons why there is such an overall increase in so many types of allergy.

This, obviously, is too far in the other direction from the norm. The hygiene pendulum has swung too far to the right.

What is optimal for us is to be somewhere close to the middle mark. For infants, total health care, including hygiene, is the responsibility of the caregiver. By the time your child reaches 4 to 5 years of age you should slowly let him take over this responsibility for personal hygiene under your supervision. At 8 years of age, your child should be totally responsible for his or her own hygiene.

There is no general rule as to how clean a person must be. Standards of cleanliness usually depend on family background as well as access to the basics such as clean water, soap, a toothbrush, toothpaste, nail clippers and a hairbrush. It also depends on where you live. In the 1960's (as I observed when working up north) people working in far northern climates bathed infrequently, due to the extreme weather conditions.

Your child's hygiene depends directly on the example you set. Remember, you are the model he learns from. His level of hygiene will mimic yours.

Hygiene involves total body care. This includes the hair, the nails, the whole body (including vagina and foreskin). It also includes the cleanliness and tidiness of one's clothes.

My father used to say you can tell the quality of a man by his fingernails, his handshake, the shine on his shoes and the crease in his pants. I think that this is not so far from the truth. I believe that good hygiene, academic achievement and self-esteem can all be considered parts of one package. So do not underestimate the positive effect of good hygiene on your child's life outside his home.

In over 40 years of practice, I have not infrequently come across young children and even teens who have poor hygiene – foul breath, vile body odor, filthy nails, grass growing between the toes and unkempt, dirty hair. I see it in those who can well afford healthcare products as well as those who can't. In this day and age this is inexcusable. I have seen children become social outcasts because of their poor hygiene – and it is a pity.

Underarm odor may begin as early as 6 to 7 years of age. If it occurs with no sweating, then use powder. If there is sweating, any underarm deodorant is fine to use.

Bad breath can occur at any age. The common causes of bad breath are dental and/or gum disease, chronically inflamed tonsils and/or adenoids, chronic sinusitis, gastroesophageal regurgitation, diet, and food lodged in tonsil creases. The hunt is on!!

By 3 years of age you should be able to retract the foreskin of uncircumsized boys to at least visualize the tip of the penis. Retract it (only as far as you can) and clean the head of the penis with every bath. Older boys should be taught to do this on their own. You may notice a white, cheesy material under the foreskin. This is called smegma, a collection of dead skin. It helps to free the foreskin from the head of the penis. It is not an infection or a result of poor hygiene. It does not require removal. If it comes to the surface, just gently wipe it away.

For girls, the outer vaginal area should be cleaned with every bath. Gently spread the labia and with a soft washcloth and warm water clean from front to back.

As far as hair is concerned, the style and length the child prefers really don't matter in the long run. Just make sure that it gets washed at least 2 to 3 times a week (more often is preferable).

As far as the orderliness of the child's bedroom is concerned, it is his problem, not yours. No one ever became ill or had a social problem (except with their parents) from a messy room. If you do not like what you see, just keep the door closed.

Remember, a little dirt will never hurt. But please do us all a huge favour: please make sure to empty your child's hockey bag and sanitize both it and its contents on a regular basis. The same goes for Dad's hockey bag!!!

Immunizations – Advisability (Yea or Nay?)

"To immunize or not to immunize?" – that is the question.

There is a growing number of caregivers who have joined the "anti-immunization" club. It is time to take off my kid gloves and try to make some sense of the value of routine childhood immunizations.

If you search long enough it is certain that you will find evidence to support whatever view you hold, no matter what the subject. If there is scarce information we question, "Why?" If there is good information (well researched) we question its validity. If it is information of questionable quality, not well researched or validated, we nevertheless gravitate toward it. Why? Because that is just human nature. We seem to be pulled toward the "cons" and to dismiss the "pros."

Caregivers who refuse to have their children immunized do so basically out of fear. They fear that routine childhood immunizations (either the vaccine itself or the components with which it is made) may do more harm than good. This fear, I believe, is the direct result of lack of proper education. I understand this reticence fully and do respect any parent with concerns about immunizations. Past truths have been known to become today's lies. That is, what we thought was safe before has sometimes been proven not to be now.

So then, where is the public to get its information? By far, most of the education comes via the Internet and media specials (TV, newspapers and magazines). All too often these reports tend to sensationalize the so-called potential negative effects of routine immunizations. Unfortunately, much of this information does not hold up to true scientific scrutiny. The Internet has thousands of sites available providing unsubstantiated information as to the ills of immunizations. Any layperson reading these articles certainly would have serious concerns about immunizing his child.

Many who practice alternative medicine believe that immunizations can do more harm than good. They strongly believe that immunity for any disease is best gained from contact with the offending virus or bacteria – that is the "natural" way. They maintain that vaccines only "pollute" the body with foreign substances that are harmful.

We still know very little about the immune system. Our knowledge is growing by leaps and bounds almost on a daily basis. We do know that young infants have an immature immune system. We also know that despite this fact, they are able to have an excellent immune response to many foreign substances, including routine inoculations. This immune response builds up memory and antibodies to help ward off illness resulting from future contact with these same foreign agents. From the time of birth an infant is challenged on a daily basis with thousands of new antigens (foreign substances), which stimulate their immune system.

If you were to ask parents when their child is older and is about to get his first skateboard, whether or not they were going to buy a helmet, wrist pads, elbow pads as well as knee pads, the answer would be a universal "yes". "Why?" I ask. The answer is obvious and always the same – in order to protect the child. You can see the helmet and you can feel the helmet. The protection is right there in front of you in a very tangible way. Unfortunately, you cannot see or feel the protection provided by routine childhood immunizations. If you could, I am positive that the anti-immunization faction of our community would soften its stance or, perhaps, no longer exist.

Yes, it is true; you can get natural immunity from direct contact with viruses and bacteria. Yes, the immunity is for the most part better than that given artificially from immunization – but at what cost? Remember, there were thousands of people who died of smallpox before developing natural immunity. Remember the thousands of people who died or became paralyzed by polio before developing natural immunity? What about the thousands of children who died from meningitis or overwhelming sepsis (infection) before they developed natural immunity? There were millions of children who survived their disease and, yes, developed immunity, but as a result of the disease, also developed serious complications such as hearing loss, seizures, mental retardation, spastic paralysis, learning disabilities and a host of other problems. In all the examples, the children were stricken by a virus or bacteria resulting in serious illness before the immune system could be primed to protect them. Those mentioned and many more diseases are now preventable with routine childhood immunization. Because of the lack of immunization in some underdeveloped countries measles is still a major killer – striking millions of children yearly.

As a doctor, parent, and grandparent, I am fully aware of parents' concern regarding the injection of foreign substances into our children's bodies. The argument is as follows: pollution is everywhere. We hear about it and read about it almost on a daily basis. Pollution is in the air, pollution is in the water, pollution is in our food, and so on. None of this news is good – it is well recognized that pollution is harmful to our health. Are we not just further polluting our children's bodies with vaccines and the other ingredients they contain for stabilization, the most feared of which are thimerosal and aluminum? To add to these concerns, recently there have been 3 new vaccines developed which are available for protection. More are on the way. Can this be good?

To adequately respond to the above questions so that a parent's mind can be put at ease, the answer cannot be a simple, "Yes, inoculations are beneficial." Caregivers want to know more. At present they seem to get much of their information, for reasons I cannot completely understand, from dubious sources. Whether in the news media, on the internet, from practitioners of alternative medicine or from books written by doctors, such information can be very convincing.

Nevertheless, I have been practicing pediatrics for over 40 years and I am constantly reading about immunizations. I attend at least 3 or 4 seminars yearly that deal with immunizations. I read the negative articles concerning immunizations so that I can better understand how to counsel my patients' caregivers. I am thoroughly convinced that routine immunizations are highly beneficial and are the best way we have, at present, to protect our children from serious illnesses. Short-term side effects may include a fever, as well as some soreness and swelling at the site of injection.

There is sufficient scientific data at present to reassure caregivers that there are no long-term negative side effects of any kind from any immunization. Thimerosal has not been used in any Canadian vaccines for a number of years (with the exception of the flu vaccine). In 2001, thimerosal was taken out of all routine vaccines in the USA. Since then, the incidence of autism has not diminished. Conclusions are that thimerosal, therefore, is not a trigger for the increased incidence of autism. Numerous reviews of data collected worldwide by reputable well-known scientists concerning the implication of the measles, mumps and rubella (MMR) vaccine as a trigger for autism again have shown no connection.

Aluminum, another suspected toxin is added to some vaccines to increase their effectiveness. In animal experiments it has been shown to be neurotoxic (adversely affect the brain) in large doses. However even though it is present in vaccines given early in infancy there has never been a direct connection made between aluminum and the potential toxic side effects. Additionally, about 70% of aluminum is excreted in the urine within 24 hours. Until there is actually scientific documentation of the adverse effect of aluminum in vaccines, all world agencies dealing with vaccinations and their potential danger recommend the universal use of every vaccine available. This includes those countries that routinely immunize infants with the hepatitis B vaccine (which may contain aluminum) in addition to the other routine infant immunizations Aluminum is not present in the MMR or chicken pox vaccines.

The main problem we are seeing at present is the limited duration of the time of protection from any one immunization. We are now realizing that lifelong protection does not necessarily result for each individual immunization. Examples of these at present would be the whooping cough vaccine, chicken pox vaccine and meningococcal C vaccine. I am sure others will follow. As well, some of the newer vaccines have only been administered for 7 years or less. An example of these are the human papilloma virus vaccine and the multi-strain meningococcal vaccine. Only time will tell us how long protection will last. Agencies around the world are following how long vaccine immunity persists. If or when immunity to any vaccine is found to reach a non-protective level, booster doses will be recommended.

Whom do you trust? Who is the voice of reason? Your doctor, the pharmaceutical company, the government, anti-vaccine groups, TV, the Internet, books or anecdotal stories? No one ever said that it would be easy for you to make the all-important health decisions for your child. I know how difficult it is for parents to come to the sensible conclusion. Hopefully, with time, the cloud of confusion concerning vaccines will be cleared 100%. My choice, at present, is that I am 100% for vaccinating all children with every appropriate vaccine now available.

I have 7 grandchildren. All have been fully immunized. What I do for my own I would recommend for yours.

The bottom line: to immunize or not to immunize your child is your decision – educate yourself.

In this pediatrician's eyes, "Be Wise, Have Your Child Immunized."

Immunization (Pain Prevention)

The discomfort from an immunization needle is obvious, but as much pain (or more) may be produced by its anticipation – "needle phobia". Trust me, this anticipation only increases from the time your child realizes that he is to receive a vaccination to the time he actually receives it. It may start as early as 15–18 months and is always present by 2 years of age. The word "needle" conjures up fear even in grown adults. The greatest reluctance a child has with a doctor's visit is the fear of the needle. The longer he knows before, the more horrible these imaginings become. They rapidly escalate as time passes. This for sure will lead to a "resistance struggle" of titanic proportion. The result is a very unhappy child, a very distraught parent and a doctor who is unable to examine a very uncooperative patient – your child. I would still have all my hair (or maybe just half) if I did not have the stress of this struggle at least 5 times daily.

Taking the Ouch Out of the Ouch

• If your child asks prior to the doctor's visit if an immunization is required and you know for sure that it is, I suggest you respond by saying, "I think so, but we will have to ask the doctor" or "We will see" or " I am not sure"– speak very calmly. Try everything to delay the answer "Yes".

• Instead of the word "pain" use the term "owie", "boo-boo", "mosquito bite" or "pinch". These are less harsh words associated more with only minor discomfort.

• Never threaten, even in a joking fashion, that if your child is not good the doctor will give him a needle. In fact I wouldn't use the word "needle" at all.

• A caregiver should never display any personal apprehension about receiving a needle when vaccinations are discussed – your child will see your expression or hear your tone of voice and respond negatively.

• Reassure your child that the doctor always gives a "gentle owie"– never tell your child that it will not hurt. You will instantly lose trust and credibility.

• For the apprehensive child, giving him acetaminophen or ibuprofen one hour prior to the doctor's visit, with reassurance that discomfort will be diminished, may be psychologically effective, although it really has only a placebo effect.

• There are patches and sprays available to be placed on the site of injection that are local anesthetics. They are applied at least one hour prior to the procedure. You may wish to talk to the doctor or his nurse to find out where this site will be for your child if you do not already know. As a rule, in children under one year of age, immunizations are given in the outer aspect, of the upper thigh(s). In children over one year of age it is the outer aspect of the upper arm(s) approximately 3 cm or 1-1/2 in. below the outer shoulder blade. Remember, your child may be receiving more than one immunization at that visit – 2 patches may be required.

When actually in the examining room and ready for immunizations here are some tips:

• If there is more than one child, who goes first? The answer really depends on your family's make-up. Your doctor will best advise you as to the order. There is an old saying, "Girls rule and boys drool." Therefore, girls first. Some prefer the oldest to youngest while others the reverse. Bravest first or last is your choice. Over the years, in my own personal experience, I prefer to give it to the most apprehensive first (less time to think). If you have an infant and an older child both requiring immunizations, if possible, have the older child leave the room. After the baby has been immunized and has settled down, do the older child (if very apprehensive do him first).

• Other children should not watch and it may be advisable that they leave the room.

• Do not allow the child to watch. Hold the hand of the arm not receiving the immunization with your hand and turn his head away with your other hand. Speak calmly. Talk about something pleasant, sing a song together, have him count either forward or backward to 5, or say the alphabet slowly.

• For the younger infant, get right down to the baby's face and distract him by giving noisy kisses – the louder the better. Pick him up as soon as possible after immunization and give him a good cuddle. Again, make lots of noise, give lots of loud kisses and jostle him. Better still, hold the baby and feed him (breast especially) during the injection. Also, a 25% solution of sugar-water (1 cube of sugar with 10 mL (2 teaspoons) of water) administered by medicine cup, syringe or by baby sucking on a sugar-water soaked piece of gauze (held by you), starting 1–2 minutes prior to injection, may help to diminish discomfort in the infant under 6 months.

• For the older child, rubbing the injection site briskly beforehand may be helpful in diminishing the discomfort. Chilling the site usually is ineffective but may help to achieve compliance.

• A smart doctor will never, ever let the child see the syringe and needle before, during or after the vaccination – that's just cruel.

• If more than one immunization is to be given, coordination of movement between mother and doctor from one side to the other side should be planned so that the least time is spent between needles.

• Have a reward sticker or sucker handy right away. This will, hopefully, not allow the child to linger in negative thoughts.

• The least amount of discussion between you and your child once he knows that an immunization is imminent is the best. Trust me, saying, "It is not going to hurt" never works. Occasionally, I have to leave the child and mother alone for a few minutes for her to settle him. It is worth the wait even though it may take a few attempts. Most doctors are willing to take as much time as is needed to settle a child down – the more pleasant the visit can be made, the better the compliance for the next one.

Older children will try stalling tactics to avoid the deed. "Just wait a second" or "I have to tell you something," etc. Trust me, any delay will be directly related to escalation of the anxiety. Unfortunately, you may need to take physical control of the child in order for the procedure to be done.

It is unfortunate that there is no easy solution to prevent discomfort. Perhaps in the near future all immunizations will be given painlessly.

In the end, there is a great variability in discomfort tolerance among children. Some 2-year-olds will "take it like a man"(or woman!). Some older children will have to be practically "wrestled down." At my flu vaccine clinics I wear hockey goalie equipment for my own protection!

Immunization (Routine Vaccines)

At present, during the first 2 years of life, a total of 11 bacterial and/or viral vaccines are recommended. Diphtheria, tetanus, whooping cough, polio and H. influenza immunizations are combined in one vaccine. Four are given during the first 18 months of life. The pneumococcal vaccine is routinely given 3 times by 12 months of age. For high-risk children who may have an immune problem, a 4th dose of pneumococcal vaccine is given at 15–18 months of age. Meningococcal C vaccine is given once at 1 year of age. Measles, mumps and rubella are combined in a single vaccine and recommended at 12-15 months. Chicken pox vaccine is given at 15 months of age. In Canada all of these vaccinations are covered free of charge by public health.

Additional vaccines are also recommended for added protection for your infant. These include meningococcal C vaccine at 3 and 5 months of age, rotavirus vaccine – 2 or 3 doses given between 8 and 32 weeks of age, and meningococcal ACYW135 at 2 years of age. At present these vaccines are not covered by public health, but may be covered by private drug plans.

The measles, mumps, and MMR, rubella, chicken pox and rotavirus are live vaccines. All other vaccines are killed (inactivated).

The rotavirus (live) vaccine is given by mouth. The MMR and chicken pox vaccines are given subcutaneously. All other vaccines are given intramuscularly. The immunizations are given in the thigh until one year of age and thereafter in the arm(s).

At 4 years of age a combined vaccine of MMR and chicken pox is given.

At 5 years of age a booster is given for diphtheria, tetanus, whooping cough and polio.

At 15 years of age a booster for diphtheria, tetanus and whooping cough is given.

Between grade 7 and grade 8 hepatitis B (2 doses), meningococcal ACYW135 (1 dose), and human papilloma virus (3 doses) immunizations will be provided free of charge to all students attending school. At present, only females will be offered the human papilloma virus vaccine at school. It is, however, recommended for boys as well.

There are also travel vaccines. The most common are hepatitis A and B (2 doses) and typhoid vaccines and Dukoral (2 doses – for cholera and traveller's diarrhea). Others may be required depending on where you are travelling. There are no travel vaccines for children less than one year of age other than hepatitis B. Depending on your destination you may be better off going to a travel vaccine clinic. Do not make the mistake of leaving it too late to get proper immunizations for protection during your travels. See your doctor at least 6 weeks before travel so that all the necessary vaccinations can be arranged and given in a timely fashion.

Malaria prophylaxis may be recommended depending on your travel destination. This is given by mouth. It is taken the week before you go, while you are away and for one week after your return.

Because of the increase in the incidence of whooping cough in infants, over the past years the whooping cough vaccine has been added to the 15-year-old booster. It is felt that the increase in whooping cough is due to the increase of this illness in older teenagers and adults whose immunity to the disease has waned. Many adults who have a cough lasting for more than 2 or 3 months, especially one that is worse at night and is spasmodic, probably have whooping cough. The illness could be passed to unprotected infants. Recommendations at this time are that all adults should receive a booster dose of diphtheria, tetanus and whooping cough every 10 years. Herpes zoster vaccine (for chicken pox) is recommended for all adults over 60 years of age. This is to prevent shingles. Pneumococcal vaccine is recommended for all adults over 65 years of age. The vaccine is to prevent pneumococcal pneumonia. However, at this time vaccine specialists are questioning the need for it. **Please note that the exact immunization schedule may vary depending on the area in which you reside.**

Side Effects of Vaccinations

VACCINE	FEVER	INJECTION SITE Soreness, Swelling Redness	RASH	BODY ACHES AND PAINS	MOST COMMON CONTRAINDICATIONS
Rotavirus (Live)	NO	NO	NO	NO	NONE
Pentacel	YES	YES	NO	NO	NONE
MMR (Live)	YES	YES	YES	NO	True Egg Allergy ** see below
QUAD	UNLIKELY	YES	NO	NO	NONE
Chicken Pox (Live)	YES	YES	Few Lesions * see below	NO	NONE
Pneumococcal	YES	**YES**	NO	NO	NONE
Meningococcal	YES	YES	NO	NO	NONE
Hepatitis (A, B or A/B)	UNLIKELY	YES	NO	NO	NONE
Flu	YES	YES	NO	YES	True Egg Allergy
Adacel	UNLIKELY	YES	NO	NO	NONE

* **Giving acetaminophen or ibuprofen prior to immunization is unnecessary.**
** **Recent evidence shows no contraindication with egg allergy.**

Treatment

FEVER

- Fever (if occurs) usually begins 1–2 hours after immunization and may last for 2 days.
- Acetaminophen or ibuprofen – dose according to weight, not age.
- Dress the child lightly – we want to keep the heat out, not in.
- Cool baths or alcohol rubs are not necessary.
- Encourage drinking.

INJECTION SITE (soreness, swelling, redness)

- May occur a few hours after immunizations. Lasts less than 3 days.
- Acetaminophen or ibuprofen for pain.
- Apply ice 10 minutes on and 10 minutes off – then repeat.
- A hard, non-tender lump may be felt for weeks thereafter.

RASH (MMR)

- 2% of children may have fever and a light red rash on face and trunk 7–10 days after injection.
- May last 2-4 days. Treat fever. Children are not contagious.

CHICKEN POX

- 2%–4 % may have a few pock marks usually at site of injection 7–10 days after vaccination.
- Cover with long-sleeved shirt. No activity limitations or isolation. It is not contagious.

NOTE: A CHILD WITH A MILD COLD WITHOUT FEVER MAY BE VACCINATED.

- IF FEVER IS PRESENT — NO VACCINATION.

COLDS, VOMITING AND DIARRHEA ARE SELDOM THE RESULT OF VACCINATION.

A child should be seen after vaccination if – inconsolable or weak cry, temperature persists over 40°C (104°F) for 2 readings 4 hours apart, marked lethargy (weakness), persistent irritability, persistent headache and/or vomiting, febrile seizure (convulsion).

- IF PREVIOUS SEVERE REACTION TO AN IMMUNIZATION HAS OCCURED – DISCUSS WITH YOUR DOCTOR.

Impetigo and Herpes Simplex (Cold Sores) Skin Infections

Impetigo is a superficial skin infection. It is most common in children with upper respiratory tract infections who tend to pick at their noses. It may be found anywhere on the body where the skin's integrity is broken. A child may scratch some mild irritated skin condition (commonly on the buttocks). With the breakdown of the skin's protective surface barrier, a bacteria, either streptococcus or staphylococcus (which are normally present on everyone's intact skin), invades the abrasion in the skin causing the area to become infected. The initial abrasion itself may not be visible to the naked eye.

When chicken pox was common, scratched lesions would frequently become infected by impetigo. Chicken pox pitting of the skin would result after healing.

Clinically, the lesion starts as a red and inflamed small area. It then turns into a blister-like lesion, which may weep (i.e., be moist). Thereafter, yellow crusting occurs. The most common sites are found around the nose and mouth, but they may occur anywhere on the body where the skin's integrity has been compromised. From the primary lesion other lesions may occur anywhere on the body.

Children who have eczema and develop chicken pox often have a more severe reaction to the pox, with resulting infection. These children need vigorous treatment and to be observed closely by the doctor during the acute phase.

Impetigo is **extremely contagious** and is spread by direct contact with the involved lesions.

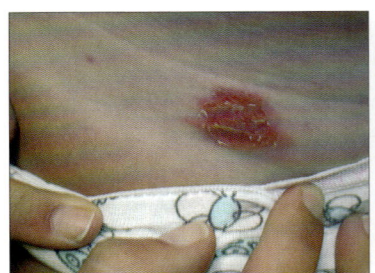
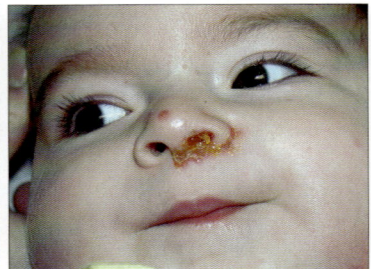
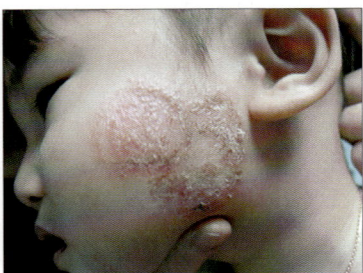

Impetigo　　　　　*Impetigo*　　　　　*Impetigo*

Treatment

If the lesions are localized, treatment consists of the application of an antibiotic cream for 7 to 10 days. If they are more widespread, an oral antibiotic, which covers both streptococcal and staphylococcal bacteria, is required to be taken for 10 days. The lesions should be left open and not covered with bandages. If they are moist, compresses with Buro-sol solution will help dry the lesions and hasten healing. Apply a compress 4-6 times daily for 5-10 minutes each time. Buro-sol powder or 1 tablespoon of bleach may be added to the bathwater to help dry lesions and "sterilize" the skin. Keep your child's fingernails cut short.

Because impetigo is so contagious, isolation of the patient should be implemented for at least one day after treatment is initiated

To prevent its spread to others, good handwashing technique is required. There should be no sharing of towels or washcloths. All bedding and clothing from the infected child should be washed separately at the highest washer temperature.

Complications of impetigo, although uncommon, can be serious. If the impetigo is due to a streptococcal infection, a post-streptococcal kidney inflammation called glomerulonephritis may occur.

Abscess formation is uncommon, but it still is a possibility. Flesh-eating disease is an extremely rare complication. Therefore, it is most important to manage the impetigo from the onset. Pitting of the skin is a cosmetic problem. If pitting results in an emotional difficulty for your child, then a referral to a dermatologist for possible dermabrasion should be considered.

Herpes Skin Infection

Herpes simplex 1 is a viral skin infection most commonly found on the lips or the skin around the lips. It does not occur inside the mouth.

It appears as a crop of blisters. They are itchy.

They are quite contagious and the child should be isolated until all the lesions have dried. Frequent handwashing is mandatory. The child should have his own eating utensils.

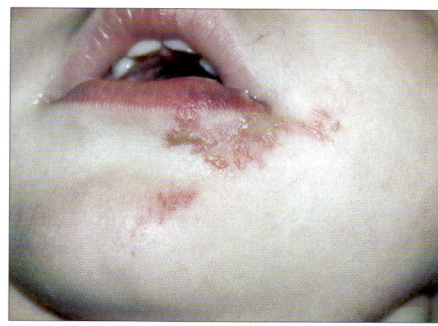
Herpes Simplex 1

The treatment varies depending on the stage in which the rash is diagnosed. If suspected early, as the first lesions are appearing, a topical antiviral agent may prevent its progression. Similarly, oral antiviral agents may be prescribed.

If the blisters are already present, then the above will not work. The treatment is to keep the lesions dry by frequent compressing with Buro-Sol solution or any other drying agent. If they become infected, then the treatment is the same as that for impetigo.

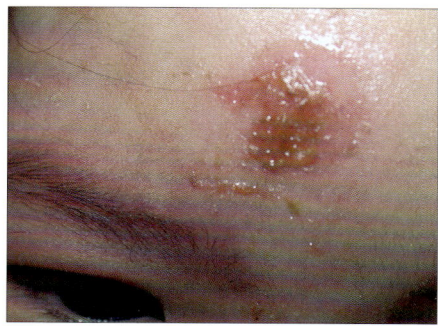
Herpes Simplex 1

Jaundice (Newborn)

Jaundice is a yellow discolouration of the skin and of the whites of the eye caused by elevated bilirubin levels in the blood. Bilirubin is a breakdown product of the red blood cells. The bilirubin produced is transferred to the liver as the blood circulates. It is extracted from the blood by the liver and transported to the intestinal system for subsequent excretion by way of the stool.

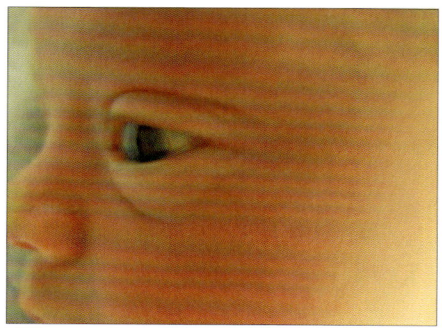
Jaundice

Day 1 Jaundice

The presence of jaundice in the first 24 hours of life is most likely to have an underlying cause, which will require identification and perhaps treatment.

Hemolytic Anemia

The most common cause of jaundice is a blood group incompatibility. The first suspected cause would be Rh incompatibility. In this case, the mother is Rh negative and the baby is Rh+. While the baby is in the mother's uterus, small amounts of the baby's blood are transferred over into the mother's circulation. Because it is considered "foreign" matter the mother makes antibodies against the Rh. These antibodies re-enter the fetal (baby's) circulation, causing a breakdown of the red blood cells. As a result, the bilirubin level is increased and jaundice appears. A similar process occurs with ABO blood incompatibility. Here the baby is either type A or B and the mother's blood group is O. Other minor variants of blood group incompatibility can also cause jaundice.

An ABO incompatibility is much more common than an Rh incompatibility.

Hereditary hemolytic anemias such as congenital spherocytosis and glucose 6 PD deficiency, as well as other defects in the red blood cell membrane, may also lead to an increased breakdown in the red blood cells – resulting in jaundice. With the hereditary condition, a positive family history is a clue to the problem.

There are drugs that mother may be taking that can cause hemolysis. (breakdown of the red cells.)

Infection

Infection should always be considered a possibility in a child who has become jaundiced starting from the first day of life. Suspicion of infection increases if there has been prolonged rupture of the membranes, maternal fever, discoloured amniotic fluid or low Apgar readings. The symptoms of sepsis (infection) are very elusive and variable. There may be a weak or high-pitched cry on baby's part, and there may be increased or decreased muscle tone, fever, vomiting or diarrhea, skin that appears to be an "off" colour, respiratory distress, or poor feeding along with the jaundice.

Day 2 Jaundice

The causes of jaundice on day 2 are the same as for day 1.

Days 3, 4, 5

Physiological jaundice – The lifespan of a newborn's red blood cells is shorter than that of a

6-month-old infant. Consequently, if the breakdown of these immature red blood cells occurs at a more rapid rate it results in jaundice. Physiological jaundice may last up to 2 weeks of age before slowly disappearing.

Breastfed jaundice: Infants may develop breastfed jaundice for 2 reasons. The first reason is an enzyme present in breast milk. This enzyme may cause the liver to slow down the excretion into the intestines of bilirubin from the blood. As a result of this slowdown the bilirubin builds up in the blood, resulting in jaundice. Normally, aside from the resulting jaundice, the infant is thriving without any other health problems. Breastfeeding-induced jaundice may last up to 2 months before disappearing. There is no need to stop breastfeeding. The second reason for breastfeeding-induced jaundice occurs with an infant who is receiving insufficient breast milk. Dehydration can occur and the jaundice is exaggerated. With rehydration the jaundice (bilirubin) level diminishes.

The above conditions account for over 98% of newborn jaundice. There are other, rare causes of jaundice such as galactosemia, among others. Remember, in the above instances I am referring only to healthy infants born at term and with normal birth weight. This particular section does not include a discussion of premature infants, infants with congenital infections such as rubella, or those having developmental or genetic problems.

Jaundice also may be prolonged in infants who have a large hemorrhage somewhere in their body. This hemorrhage is usually from a cephalhematoma, fracture of the femur or an intra-abdominal bleed. Prolonged jaundice may also be a symptom of an underactive thyroid gland. However, with newborn screening, a thyroid disorder would be ruled out.

Jaundice lasting for more than 3 months may be caused by hereditary problems with the transport system of bilirubin in the liver or by a blockage called biliary atresia.

Diagnosis of Neonatal Jaundice

As with many other illnesses this diagnosis is made by history, family history, physical examination and appropriate laboratory investigations.

If a hemolytic disease is considered, then blood grouping of both the mother and the infant will be done along with a CBC (complete blood count) and a blood film. The bilirubin level is measured for both the direct and indirect amounts of bilirubin. The blood film may be suggestive of a congenital hemolytic anemia. Blood levels for G6PD deficiency may be required.

If an infection is suspected, the infant will have a CBC, blood culture, lumbar puncture, urinalysis, urine culture and possibly a chest x-ray. He'll be started on antibiotics, and management thereafter will depend on the laboratory results and the clinical condition of the baby.

Treatment of Jaundice

The management of a newborn with jaundice depends on its underlying cause. Most often nothing is required except for closely monitoring the jaundice level.

For physiological or breast-milk jaundice no treatment is required. Breastfeeding should be continued. It is uncommon for either of these causes of jaundice to require phototherapy.

As stated above, if the jaundice is one of the symptoms of infection then antibiotics are the treatment.

Hemolytic diseases vary greatly in their severity. Some have very little hemolysis and others have a greater degree of it.

The management involves keeping the level of bilirubin below the level at which the bilirubin could cross the blood/brain barrier, resulting in damage to the central nervous system. Treatment, if required, is administered through single or double phototherapy. During phototherapy the baby's eyes are covered to prevent any eye damage and the skin is watched closely to ensure that there is no skin damage. While under phototherapy, the infant's jaundice level is monitored and when it returns to an acceptable level for the age, the phototherapy will be discontinued. It is rare that it subsequently arises for a second time, requiring the use of phototherapy again.

Exchange transfusions (whereby the infant's blood is exchanged with banked blood) are very uncommon now since the introduction of RhoGAM for Rh-negative mothers.

Putting a jaundiced baby by a window in order for him to get more sunshine will be ineffective for reducing his level of jaundice.

Labial Adhesions (Genital)

The labia are the skin folds at the opening of the vagina. These folds should be able to be opened easily to reveal the vaginal opening. If the inner labia (labia minora) stick together for a period of time they may become fused. The fusion appears as a thin membrane with a dark thin line down the centre. The vaginal opening will not be visible because of this adhesion.

Drops of urine can collect in the pocket created by the adhesion. This may lead to irritation and possibly a urinary tract infection.

The adhesion can be "melted" away with the use of an estrogen cream called Premarin.

The Premarin is applied with the finger directly onto the adhesion, twice a day, until the full vaginal opening is visible. This may take up to 4 to 6 weeks.

There are no side effects from the Premarin cream. If some of the cream when applied gets on the normal skin, this is harmless – no concern.

Once the vaginal opening has been re-established, with every subsequent bath the labia should be parted gently to prevent them from re-fusing. Coating the labia with a thin layer of diaper paste after bathing will also prevent the labia from adhering again.

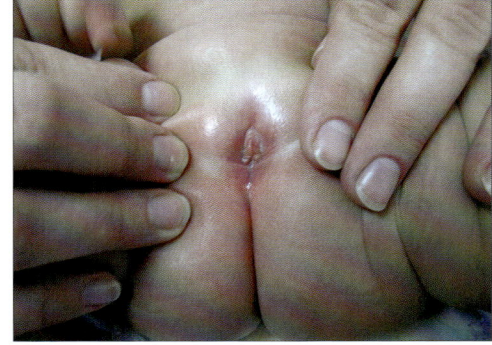

Labial Adhesion

Lactose Intolerance

Lactose is a sugar found in milk and dairy products. It is also present in breast milk.

Primary lactose intolerance may develop at any age. It is important, however, to note that the symptoms do not appear before 10–12 months of age. Why the onset symptoms of primary lactose intolerance may not occur until later in life is still a mystery.

Primary lactose intolerance is often found within families.

The symptoms of lactose intolerance vary from person to person. The common symptoms are abdominal bloating, passing of a lot of gas, abdominal discomfort and loose stools.

The degree of the individual's intolerance also varies. Some do not tolerate any lactose at all while others may tolerate varying amounts of it. If, however, the latter group exceeds these limits, symptoms of intolerance may occur.

As mentioned, primary lactose intolerance does not cause symptoms in infants who are less than 10 months of age. It is not the cause of colic, excessive gas, abdominal bloating or discomfort in that age group. Restricting lactose in the diet in either the mothers who are breast feeding or in a formula-fed infant itself will not decrease the symptoms. Even as I affirm this, there are always mothers who swear that their infant's symptoms were moderately reduced when lactose was restricted.

Secondary lactose intolerance can occur at any age. After a bout of diarrhea the stools may remain loose for 2–3 weeks or even longer. The diarrhea causes the lining of the small bowel to become thinned. With this thinning the small bowel is unable to produce lactase, which is the enzyme necessary to break down lactose into simple sugars, which in turn is required before absorption. The presence of lactose in the stool prolongs looseness of stools and thus the inability of the small bowel lining to heal itself. During the recovery phase, limiting the lactose content of the infant's or child's diet for 2 weeks will oftentimes speed up the recovery phase and help the stools return to normal more rapidly. After the bowel lining has healed, the infant or child can return to his routine formula or milk, and dairy products with no restrictions.

Lactose-free formulas and milk are readily available. Soy-based formulas are lactose-free and may be used for secondary lactose intolerance.

A probiotic may be helpful in returning the bowel flora (bacteria) to its normal state and have the effect of shortening the duration of the illness. Give for 5–10 days.

Lifestyle – Don't "Bug" Me!!

When I was a young kid, my mother was very diligent about keeping my two brothers and me spotless. We had a bath every night. To save on hot water mom used the same bathwater for each of us. Since I was the youngest, I was last, and got washed in my older brothers' grimy bathwater. Despite this I had a very healthy childhood – better than my brothers. Perhaps the dirty water contributed to building my immunity. I would like to emphasize that obsessive cleanliness is unnecessary whereas teaching the rules of simple proper hygiene is essential.

My feeling is that it is important to concentrate on giving your child a well-balanced diet and having him get lots of exercise rather than to overemphasize his general degree of cleanliness. "Dirt" does not cause disease. I am not referring to important personal hygiene of infants, toddlers and young children

"Bugs" (a.k.a. germs) are everywhere. There are good bugs and there are bad bugs. Bugs Bunny is a good bug. Bugs are everywhere – in the air and on your hair. They're on your skin, even your chin. They are throughout your gut, including your butt. They are in your mouth and on everything in the house. They reside in your nose and even between your toes. In other words, bugs cannot be avoided!

To complicate matters even further, individuals may carry "bad bugs" in their oral pharynx (mouth) but this does not cause them illness. Unfortunately, these bugs may be transmitted to another, otherwise healthy but susceptible individual, with resulting illness. An example of this is meningococcal disease. The carriers are completely undetectable unless appropriate laboratory investigations are done to show that they are in a carrying state.

Resistance to any viral or bacterial infection for which there is no active immunization develops only from exposure. In most cases the exposure leads to immunity without illness, the result being that future exposure does not lead to infection.

If "cleanliness is next to godliness", then there are a lot of sinners in everybody's neighbourhood. Personal hygiene is still very important. In tandem with good nutrition and lots of exercise illnesses can be minimized.

Remember this – children learn by example. You as a caregiver set the example which they learn from. I cannot overemphasize this point – caregivers are role models.

In early life you bathe your infant. Later you assist him. If taught properly, he is on his own by 3 to 4 years of age (under your supervision). Self-care is taught in stages. When one stage is accomplished, you move on to the next. All children move at different rates but will eventually get there.

Dental care starts with the eruption of the first teeth. They should be cleaned with a washcloth and, when the child has four teeth, a finger brush. When eight teeth are present, a child's toothbrush should be introduced with water in combination with (or without} a non-fluoride toothpaste. You must brush the teeth, because the child will only chew the toothbrush. At around two years of age toddlers can hold the toothbrush while you hold their hand and brush their teeth. At around three years of age most children should be able to brush their teeth on their own (under supervision).

Never leave a night bottle of milk or juice in an infant's crib for him to graze on throughout the night. This may help pacify the child but will also lead to dental decay, resulting in costly painful, dental care.

Nails should be cut on a regular basis. Cut the nails on the big toes straight across to prevent them from ingrowing.

Teach a little girl to wipe her external genitalia from front to back, thus avoiding bringing germs from the rectal area into the vagina. Avoid bubble baths – they may cause irritation and vaginitis. A urinary tract infection may result from either of the above.

Nothing smaller than your elbow should ever enter your child's ear. Cleaning the ear by inserting a cotton swab into the ear canal will only result in the packing of wax deeper into the ear. This may result in a minor hearing loss, as well as the child complaining of ear discomfort. The wax can be very difficult to remove.

To help prevent the spread of germs teach your child to sneeze and cough into his sleeve. Frequent handwashing helps. Don't forget to wash mittens, scarves and hats on a regular basis.

Eating snow (frozen acid rain) in small amounts will not cause illness. No self-respecting bug would reside out in the cold. Sticking his tongue onto an ice-cold railing will only happen once (every child will try it because that's the way it is and always has been).

Teaching your child the importance of regular changing of clothes is best done by example. How regular is up to you – daily, weekly, monthly – it is your choice! Living in Canada we have so many things to be thankful for. Don't get yourself overly "bugged" over a few bugs.

Lifestyle – Keeping Fit

Let's get down to basics. Good health depends on achieving and maintaining both a healthy mind and a healthy body. This depends on activity – mental activity for the mind and physical activity for the body. It is true that, "If you do not use it, you will lose it."

This section will concentrate on physical activity only.

Exercise is really just physical activity. The term "physical activity", however, sounds less demanding and onerous. It does not necessarily have to cost a lot to be valid or effective.

What are the benefits of keeping active and having a "sound body"? They are numerous, so let me just list them:

- A positive effect on self-esteem
- Better eating habits
- Better sleep hygiene
- Less prone to injuries and a more rapid recovery if one occurs
- Stimulation of the immune system, which improves coping with illness
- Lower blood pressure
- A stronger heart
- Better muscle tone
- Increased bone density

There are few negative effects for having a "sound body". The only one that I can think is that it might make other people jealous.

Unfortunately, in today's society, children do not have the freedom that we had in previous times. Children are limited as to where they are allowed to go and too often they require supervision. In the "old days" children as young as 6 and 7 were allowed the freedom to ride their bikes anywhere they wished. To swim in the creek. To climb trees. To explore. The only restriction was that they had to be home by suppertime. There was minimal concern for "street safety." Today we no longer have that luxury. Consequently, a great degree of independence, sense of adventure and just having active fun outdoors in the neighbourhood has to a large extent been taken away from our children – what a shame! When was the last time you saw a child on his own rolling down a hill, wading through a stream or riding a bike with his arms stretched out at his sides and the wind blowing in his face? All these activities helped to achieve and maintain an active and healthy body.

Now choices are limited to going to the park or enrolling our child in some organized physical activity (hockey, soccer, baseball, swimming or the martial arts, etc.). At least they are active.

What do some children do when they go to the park? Some sit and watch others. Some play in the sand. Others are pushed on a swing by a caregiver. These activities, while valid, are not nearly as physical as in yesteryear. Fortunately, there are children who are more active. They climb up and down the jungle gym and go up and down the slide.

For the inactive child the scene goes like this: "Oh yes, Doctor, Billy is very active. He is enrolled in hockey and soccer." But have you ever watched Billy and thousands of Billys like him? They stand in the middle of the soccer field or by the goal in hockey – watching. Others whiz by them and the only activity Billy really gets is moving his head back and forth as he watches. The same can be said for the passive child at recess. A large number of children, when you come right down to it, do very little physical activity on a regular basis. They need to be more engaged in the activity. Fortunately, many schools are actively trying to accomplish this.

Too many children are involved in sedentary activities – TV, video games, computer games, their iPod, exploring the Internet, text messaging, etc. Some of these activities may be good for the mind but certainly not for the body.

I cannot tell you how many times I have witnessed the following in my office. I ask a 7- or 8-year-old child to hop up onto my examining table, which is approximately 3-1/2 feet high. The first move is by a caregiver, who is going to lift the child onto the examining table. "Whoa," I quickly say and ask for the caregiver to sit down. I then ask the child to hop on my examining table. Some jump up without a problem while others might struggle and need a little coaching – but they all do it. How sad it is for me to watch a parent too willing to discourage the child from trying to accomplish such a small active manoeuvre. The smile on the child's face and the look of awe and slight embarrassment in the parent's eyes after it is accomplished are reward enough for me, and hopefully an example for the parent.

How do you help your child to be physically fit? First, you must set a good example and be active yourself – not just a sideline coach. Second, and most important, is to do physical activities as a family – now, that's fun!!!

Bring back hopscotch and skipping, family skate, biking together and "shooting hoops". So get moving and let's see some total family involvement in physical activity.

Lifestyle – Obesity (Unhealthy Weight)

Here we go again, another "evangelist" preaching on the sinful epidemic of childhood obesity – when is enough enough? – NEVER!!!

You are what you are for 4 reasons: your genetic background, which you have no control over; chronic illness, which may or may not be controllable; quantity and quality of input (diet), which is controllable; and, lastly caloric output (activity level), which is also controllable. Remember, you have a tremendous influence over your environment and that of your child. You must be a good role model. The old adage, "Don't do what I do, do what I tell you" just doesn't cut it in today's world. If you are obese as a parent that in itself at least doubles the chances of your having an obese child. In time, other factors not yet considered or discovered will be found to play a role in the development of obesity. It won't be one or the other, but a combination of many factors.

Genetics (besides diet) plays a major role in the amount of cholesterol and triglycerides in the bloodstream. Some families are blessed with "good genes" while others are burdened with "bad genes". Fortunately, those born with "good genes" are able to prevent excessive weight gain as well as elevated cholesterol and triglyceride levels regardless of their eating and lifestyle habits. Unfortunately, those born with "bad genes" will always have to struggle with weight and circulating lipid (cholesterol and triglyceride) problems. Even so, the struggle to control excessive weight gain and elevated lipids is worth it.

In the mid-20th century scientists were asked to picture what man would look like in the 22nd century. The description they gave us was of an extremely large head (to enclose a large brain) on a very small body. How wrong they may have been. The exact reverse proportions will likely be the norm – a small head on a large body.

In the past 20 years, with economic growth and expansion, it is unfortunate that our waistlines have done the same: grown and expanded. The increased rate of obesity in preschool children has tripled over the past 2 decades. We are all familiar with the reasons why, at present, there is such an explosion in the rate of obesity – diet combined with a lack of physical activity. Many of you have reached your saturation point, with information overload on the topic. Yet I would be remiss not to state that as parents we are enablers of obesity and we are killing our kids with kindness. We are setting young people up for a lifestyle that promotes poor health. It is easy to deflect the blame in any and as many directions as you wish, but the truth of it is that the parents are the determining factor. The responsibility belongs to the caregiver in charge. Through either lack of knowledge or stubbornness about adapting to better, healthier, lifestyle habits, obesity can be the result.

Did you know that the total number of fat cells in the body is determined within the first 2 years of life? After that time, there is little further increase in the number of fat cells, only an increase in how much they are filled. As a consequence, the foundation for a tendency toward obesity is laid down very early in life – fewer fat cells equal fewer to be filled. If we could prevent the tendency to be overweight as infants and toddlers we could probably prevent the development of a great deal of obesity in later childhood, as well as in adulthood. This can be accomplished by portion control to prevent overfeeding, and providing nutritious foods. In the end, it is the parent who should control what goes in the child's mouth and not the child!

Remember that sweet foods should not be used as a bribe in order to get your child to eat other, more wholesome foods. It would have been best if the word "dessert" had never been introduced. For every excess pound of fat carried by the body, the heart, with each beat, has to pump through an extra mile of blood vessels and lymphatics. Now that is a lot of work for your poor heart to perform beat after beat after beat.

Let us assume, for example, that a child's "ideal" weight is 100 pounds, but instead his weight is 115 pounds (15 pounds overweight). How significant is this? Carrying an extra 15 pounds daily is equal to carrying 105 extra pounds for one week. This means every week your child is doing the equivalent of hopping on his own back and carrying himself for 24 hours. To think of it in another way, each week for one whole day he has to strap 25-lb weights around each arm and each leg to carry for the full 24 hours. Difficult to picture, isn't it? By the way, Mom and Dad, how much extra weight would *you* have to carry?

Body mass index (BMI) charts are available for all ages. Following an infant's and child's height and weight with BMI charting is a good indicator of whether the child will be overweight and to what degree.

With our hurried pace of life it is so easy to take a quick way out. Fast foods have become an integral part of our diet. Oversized portions of food are common. Rich foods seem to have become the norm rather than a treat. How often are you having a proper homecooked meal? How often are you feeding your child unhealthy calories to fill a hungry tummy because the child will not eat the nutritious food that has been put in front of him?

Expert nutritionists continually emphasize that whole-grain cereals are better than those that are over-refined and laced with sugar; that lower-fat foods are healthier than those that are saturated with fats, especially trans fats; that water is far better for your child to drink than sugar-laden juices, pop or other sweetened drinks; that broiling is better than deep-frying; that the more basic the food, the healthier it is. With a little imagination and a good cookbook, food does not have to look and taste "blah". I am telling you that if you keep these guidelines to good dietary habits in mind and stick to them, both you and your children will learn to eat more healthily and be able to make better choices as to which foods and quantities are to be consumed.

Many infants and toddlers are overweight to varying degrees. Not all infants with "fullback-sized" thighs are going to end up being overweight or obese. There is, however, a significant number who will. There are still many unknown factors in the equation as to which chubby infant loses his baby fat and upon whom the fat will continue to accumulate. From our present knowledge, which of these children should we worry about? The answer will come from examining the family history. This includes a family history of obesity, of close family members with type 1 and/or type 2 diabetes or hypertension, of close relatives with early heart disease or cerebral vascular accidents and, lastly, a family history of a lipid problem. Children with this family history require lifelong monitoring. These children (especially if overweight) require screening by at least 3 years of age. They require a blood sugar and a total lipid screening initially. If these readings are normal, they should be repeated every 3 to 5 years. If an abnormality is found, action should be taken immediately to reverse the problem to prevent future possible complications. Their blood pressure should be measured yearly, and as well, their height and weight growth acceleration should be monitored along with recording of their BMI. Other investigations may be required on an individual basis.

We, as adults, realize how difficult it is to lose weight even when we are really motivated to do so. How many times have you tried to lose weight? How many diets have you tried? How many "weight-loss" pills have you popped? How many exercises classes have you joined and quit? How many nutritionists or other specialists have you gone to in an effort to lose weight? To make things worse, infants, toddlers, older children and early teens do not even have this motivation to lose weight. They have no idea as to the long-term health consequences of obesity. To put it bluntly, most children under 10 years of age and even older do not care about their weight. Without proper motivation, weight loss is next to impossible. There are, nevertheless, many things you the parent can do to prevent excessive weight gain in your child. These are seemingly easy to implement but actually require a lot of effort and motivation on your part to carry out.

First of all, childhood obesity should be viewed as a family affair. You cannot expect your child to adhere to one set of rules and the rest of the family to another. Foremost, as the parent you have to set the example. Fortunately, you have control over which foods enter the home. You should also have control as to what goes in the mouths of your children, from both a quality and quantity (portion size) perspective. Calorie-dense fast and junk foods should be minimized. They are overloaded with both fat and carbohydrates and their salt content is often very high. Outside the home, unfortunately, it may be a different story. It is difficult to control the consumption of undesirable foods when your children are out of your sight.

As an aside, do you know the amount of salt you and your children are ingesting each day? Less than 1500–2000 mg per day in adults is recommended. I would imagine that one-quarter of this is more than enough for children. Excess salt intake and hypertension are linked together.

One big problem encouraging childhood obesity stems from other caregivers, usually grandparents. Many equate weight with health. The heavier the baby, the healthier he or she is. This is a carryover from the "old country", where food was scarce. When your children are under their care, nothing gives a grandparent more pleasure than to fill them with food. They do this out of love and do not realize that their "love" is harmful for the grandchild's well-being. Difficult as it may be, you must do your best to explain to them the importance of proper nutrition. Getting the grandparents aboard, although it may be difficult, is worth trying and retrying.

When it comes to burning calories, I am not a fan of the word "exercise". This sounds like work. I prefer to use the term "activity". The amount of energy we expend on a daily basis is directly related to the intensity and duration of the physical activity we carry out. Physical activity should always be fun. No child is going to go to the gym for a high-energy "fat-burning" workout. You have to use your imagination to promote fitness. Each child responds differently and you have to find those activities that he/she enjoys. The more you participate as well, the greater will be the involvement, enjoyment and enthusiasm on the part of the child. It is really a win-win situation for both of you. By the way, playing soccer by standing in the middle of the field watching the ball going to either end of the field for a half-hour is not a "calorie burner"! The same applies to all sports – zooming up and down the field or hockey rink burns calories; being a "spectator athlete" burns zero. Sedentary activities such as TV, video games, computers, iPods, etc., should be limited in total to less than 2 hours each day.

Children should not be put on a restrictive diet until after finishing puberty. What you need to model early on is "smart eating" and practice portion control. You can reduce the child's caloric intake without his noticing it. A small plate with small portions has the same eye appeal as a greater amount of food on a bigger plate. Healthy snacks, including fruit and fresh vegetables (with lower-calorie dips) and plain popcorn, should be encouraged. Water should be exchanged for juice. For milk, 1% or skim milk is best. Make changes in consultation with your doctor. Research the vast amount of information available on nutrition, or ask for a referral to a nutritionist if you are stuck.

The general quality of your child's life is governed by what you allow in their mouths and their level of activity. This responsibility is in your hands.

So let's rumble! Make healthy lifestyle choices a family affair.

Lifestyle – Shape Up

Your ultimate height and weight are based on a simple formula. You are the sum of your genetic make-up plus your environment. You have very little control over your genetic make-up. What you inherit from your parents has a direct effect on your physical make-up, your personality, as well as susceptibility to certain diseases. You can do little to change your genetic make-up. However, you have a tremendous influence over your child's environment. I cannot over-emphasize that if you start early with good habits, these will be ingrained in your child forever. You must be a good role model. The old adage "Don't do what I do, do what I tell you" just doesn't cut it in today's world. Having obese parents at least doubles the chances of being an obese child.

Remember, you are the one who controls what enters your child's mouth – not the child. Here I am including all caregivers, especially grandparents, who just love to overindulge their grandchildren. Imprinting of good eating habits starts in the first year of life. Remember that sweet foods should not be used as a bribe in order to get your child to eat other more wholesome foods. I wish sometimes that the word "dessert" had never been introduced.

I hate to say it, Mom and Dad, but too many of us are killing our children with kindness. Poor eating habits nurtured by a caregiver set your child up for a life-long lifestyle that only promotes poor health. You may deflect the blame in many directions but the bottom line is that caregivers must take direct responsibility for permitting a child to become inactive and overeat.

The total number of fat cells in the body reaches its maximum at approximately 2 years of age. Few fat cells are added thereafter. If we could reduce the total number of fat cells in a child less than 2 years of age we could thereby help prevent obesity. A caregiver may think that chubby is cute – the chubbier the cuter. After 2 years of age, how fat you are is determined by how full each fat cell is. An obese infant has a greater chance of becoming an obese child, who has a greater chance of becoming an obese teenager, who has a greater chance of becoming an obese adult when compared to the infant who, at 2 years of age, is of normal weight and height (fewer fat cells).

Body mass index (BMI) charts are available for all ages. Following an infant's and child's height and weight with BMI charting is a good indicator of whether the child will be obese.

Let me put it more graphically. Every pound of fat is serviced by approximately 1 mile of blood vessels. If your child is 20 pounds overweight his heart has to pump through an extra 20 miles of blood vessels. Put another way, if he is 20 pounds overweight and his ideal weight is 100 lbs, this is equivalent to your child having to carry himself on his back for 24 hours every 5 days. This is a lot of stress on his heart over a number of years and will end up adversely affecting his quality of life, as well as shortening his lifespan.

With our fast pace of life it is tempting to take the quick and easy way out. Fast foods have become an integral part of our diet. Large portions are common. Rich desserts and junk food seem to have become an expectation rather than an occasional treat. How often does your family have a proper home-cooked meal? How often are you feeding your child empty calories to fill a hungry tummy because he won't eat what has been put in front of him?

It does not take an expert to know that whole-grain cereals are better than those that are laced with sugar; that low-fat foods are better than those saturated with fats, especially trans fats; that water is far better for your child to drink than juices, pop or other sweetened drinks; that broiling is better than frying. The plainer the food, the healthier it is. With a little imagination and a good cookbook, food does not have to taste "blah". I am telling you that if you make these changes in dietary habits and stick to them, both you and your children will learn to eat healthily and be able to make better choices as to which foods and quantities to consume.

I do not like the word "exercise". To me it has the connotation of work and effort. I would rather exchange it with the words "physical activity".

The amount of energy expended is directly related to the intensity of the activity and the length of time this activity is carried out.

I watched my grandson Jacob play a soccer game. During the half-hour game he was on the field only for approximately 10 to 12 minutes. During this time, however, he would zoom up and down the field chasing the ball. A number of other children did the same. However, there were at least two children just standing on the field watching where the ball was going. Now what did they get out of this as far as activity is concerned?

Let us be honest. There are some children who are active and those who tend to be sedentary. Both are products of their environment. Those who are active will benefit from anything that requires physical activity. This includes playing at recess, as well as after school activities. The inactive child, unfortunately, will probably benefit very little during these time periods.

I, therefore, throw the whole problem of lack of physical activity and poor dietary habits into the laps of the parents. This problem is a family affair – so turn off your TVs, computers, etc. Let's rumble!!

Lifestyle – Sound Body, Sound Mind

The 3 Rs– reading, 'riting and 'rithmetic have long been the acknowledged cornerstones for academic success. There are, however, some other important R's that are necessary to achieve this success. The first R is reason, also known as motivation. The child must have the desire to learn, a reason to do well. The reason is to be as successful academically as they can be in order to reap the rewards of higher academic achievement. A second R is that a child has to be *ready* to learn. If the child is not ready to learn he will not reach his potential. A large part of what is referred to as being ready is a child's physical and mental state while attending school. This depends on a number of factors. First, and foremost, is their nutrition. A child with an empty tummy will without doubt be behind his peers who have adequate nourishment during the day. This includes breakfast, morning snack, lunch, afternoon snack, supper and, lastly, a nighttime snack. Poor food choices may fill the tummy but do not provide optimal "fuel" to the brain for learning. A proper sleep habit is also very important for the brain to learn. Public-school children should be receiving up to 10 hours sleep at night and those in high school no less than 8-1/2 to 9 hours nightly. A well-rested mind when at school allows the child to concentrate fully on learning. For the emotionally troubled child, problems such as marital discord at home or problems at school such as being bullied, or emotional issues due to other causes, may also be factors in causing him to fail to reach his potential.

I suppose we can add another R – recess. Most public schools have two 15-minute recess periods a day. Unfortunately, there is no physical activity break in high school, only a spare. Recess, a time for physical activity, is as important to learning as time spent being taught in the classroom. There is a saying that goes "Your mind can absorb no more than your seat can endure." I have spoken to many children of all ages. I wondered what they were doing during recess. Were they just standing around doing nothing or were they engaging in physical activity? I am very pleased that I found out that the vast majority of them were active during recess. They may not be doing as much skipping or playing hopscotch as they did in my day, but they were running around playing tag, throwing a ball or Frisbee, or playing soccer. I cannot emphasize how important this playtime is not only for learning but, as well, for healthy physical development.

There are several studies that have been published that show a direct correlation between play or downtime and the child's improved performance in the classroom. Of interest, it has also been shown that if playtime occurs in a natural setting (the presence of trees, grass, plants and water – even fountains and a beautiful view), classroom learning is improved. In fact, it has been demonstrated that children with attention deficit hyperactivity disorder (ADHD) who spent time in nature during the school day scored better on concentration testing compared to those who did not. Likewise, physical activity as simple as having periodic walks outside for a child with ADHD has also been shown to improve scores for attention and concentration.

I cringe when parents inform me that their child was denied recess as punishment for some misdemeanour in the classroom. This should never occur. Other classes, such as science, math or language, are never denied as a punishment. Neither should they deny the child his recess.

Everyone's brain needs a time to rest – to "air out". It needs a time to reenergize its battery. It needs time to focus on areas other than academics. This is accomplished during recess. Because of recess, more is accomplished inside the classroom.

During recess, teachers on yard duty patrolling the playground have limited opportunities to really play with the children. They have to supervise and enforce proper rules of equipment use, break up potential fights and encourage kids to take turns, share, and play respectfully. It's called conflict resolution. I do applaud all teachers who recognize this important correlation between physical activity and learning, especially those who are able to get outside with their students and play with them. When teachers have the opportunity to play with their students, this can increase respect for the teacher and also create a greater willingness to learn by the pupil.

I am a great believer that you cannot separate a healthy mind from a healthy body. Physical activity before school, at recess time, after lunch and after school is of utmost importance for optimal learning. Five stars to all the schools that provide pre- and post-school activities.

Lymph Nodes (Glands)

You may not know that there are, in fact, 2 separate circulatory systems in the body. The system that everyone is familiar with is the circulatory system for the blood. There is another system called the lymphatic system. This system is responsible for draining tissue fluid and returning it to the circulatory system. Along the lymph channels are small "stopping depots" called lymph nodes. These act as filtering stations to keep the lymphatic system clean.

Lymph nodes are found throughout the body. Some are found very deep in the chest and abdominal cavity while others are superficial; that is, they are located just under the skin. Superficial lymph nodes are found in the neck, axillae (armpits) and groin.

Normally, they can be felt if carefully searched for. They are small, soft, round, the size of a pea, nontender and easily moved by your finger.

The most common cause of lymph gland enlargement is a secondary reaction caused by the flow of lymph from an area of inflammation or infection, usually one found in the skin. When the impurities are filtered through the lymph glands, the glands enlarge. The primary area of inflammation or infection may not even be visible to the naked eye. It may be the result of some minor irritation. Once the skin "insult" resolves, the lymph node returns to its normal size. If there is continual and repeated inflammation, then the lymph node may become fibrosed (filled with fibrous tissue) and remain palpable (able to be felt). This is called a "reactive gland". It may take months or longer for the gland to return to its normal state. Many times it remains enlarged.

Often the gland is first detected by the child and then brought to the attention of the caregiver. Other times the caregiver feels the bump when bathing the child, brushing his hair, changing him or just stroking him.

The gland is usually pea-sized, not tender to touch and mobile (moves freely). If you were to feel the area carefully you could probably feel many more nodes.

The first reaction in the minds of the alarmed parents is that the child has some dreadful disease.

I can reassure you that 40 years of experience has taught me that in 99.99% of cases these are benign reactive glands and pose no risk to the health of the child.

However, there are red flags to signal that you should seek medical attention:

- Glands seem to be enlarging, tender and, warm
- Associated fever
- A firm, nontender gland larger than a grape that is immobile (seems to be stuck to the underlying tissue)
- Loss of appetite, lethargy, and possible weight loss

The above red flags may indicate a potential problem occurring in the gland, one that requires further investigations and/or treatment.

The bottom line is, if you are concerned, see your doctor. It will often be an unnecessary visit but it will give you peace of mind, and that is what the art of good medicine should be about.

Masturbation

A parent reacts with alarm thinking, "Oh no, I am not ready for this" or "Don't tell me this is so."

It is masturbation, an act of self-pleasuring which toddlers may begin from 1-1/2 to 4 years of age. It is a means of self-comforting, physical pleasure that has little sexual connotation. The pleasure received should be considered no different than that received from thumb sucking, twirling of hair or using a comfort blanket.

Adults are the ones who have a problem with the child masturbating. It is a totally normal way in which a child is able to give himself physical pleasure. There is a tremendous misconception that masturbation by a child less than 4–5 years of age is inappropriate, abnormally sexual, and is a reflection of poor parenting skills. There is also the misconception that it will lead to some deviant sexual behaviour when the child is older. Nothing can be further from the truth.

Over the past 40 years I have met with parents concerned about their child's rubbing of his or her genitalia. Some children do it infrequently, others more often. Children can rub their genitalia against anything one can imagine; that includes *anything* (I leave you to complete the picture).

The problem is magnified in parents' minds when the child's tendency toward masturbation takes place outside the home. There is not a parent who does not feel the scrutiny of the eyes of others when their child is masturbating in public. They feel, "What must people be thinking?"

For children under 2-1/2 years of age, if you wish to lessen the behaviour, you basically cannot. All you can do is try to divert the child's attention to some other activity when you see it occurring. Nothing further should be done or said.

Children over 2-1/2 years of age can be gently reasoned with. They should be reassured that what they are doing, although it is not "bad", should, however, be done in privacy. They should be taught the proper names for their genitalia. They also should be taught that the genitalia are private and not to be shown to or touched by anyone other than a caregiver during bathing or a doctor during a physical examination.

Children are born to explore. Frequently, they will examine other children's genitalia, whether of the same or opposite sex. Under 5–6 years of age this should not be considered abnormal behaviour but more a showing of curiosity. Discreetly and gently redirect the children to some other activity. Reinforce to your child that his genitalia are private.

Parents must understand that masturbation is a normal behaviour and reflect this idea to the child. A child should never be reprimanded or told that he or she is naughty. Avoid any other negative reinforcements to curb something that is completely, perfectly natural and normal.

Measles (German) Rubella

I call this illness a mildly "sneaky" viral infection that is difficult to tell apart from many other viral illnesses. Only once or twice in the past 40 years have I actually made the correct clinical diagnosis of rubella. How many I have missed, I do not know.

The incubation period for rubella is between 2–3 weeks.

The contagious period is 2 days before the rash appears until 5 days after the rash's appearance.

Clinically, after the incubation period, there is first a mild upper respiratory tract infection consisting of a runny nose and a slight cough for 1 to 2 days. This is followed by mild enlargement of the glands at the back of the neck. A faint rash spreads from the face to the trunk and lasts for approximately 3–5 days. During the entire illness the child is only mildly ill.

Older children, especially females, may get aches and swelling of the joints. Again, this is usually only mild in nature. On rare occasions, German measles can be followed by chronic arthritis.

Treatment consists of the use of acetaminophen or ibuprofen for fever or discomfort.

Complications for the child who has rubella are rare.

Rubella infection when contracted by a woman during her first trimester, is very serious and may result in the birth of a baby that has significant congenital abnormalities. It is, therefore, extremely important that all women have their immune status for rubella clearly established before planning a family. If they are found to lack significant immunity, rubella vaccine will be given. It is advisable for women to keep from becoming pregnant for at least 3 months after the vaccination. Testing for the level of immunity one month after the vaccination is advisable to ensure that immunity has been increased and the vaccination has accomplished its purpose.

Although the vaccine has not been associated with causing fetal damage it is recommended that it not be given during pregnancy. If a mother who is pregnant is found to lack sufficient immunity, then the vaccine is recommended to be given after the birth of her baby.

Unfortunately, a baby born with congenital rubella will have many abnormalities. This is called the Rubella Syndrome. The rubella virus for such infants may be excreted in their oral/nasal secretions, urine and stool for up to one year. The virus may thus be spread inadvertently to other susceptible contacts. Any contact with a non-immune pregnant woman during the first trimester of pregnancy should therefore be avoided.

A live rubella vaccine is available in combination with mumps and measles vaccine. It is usually administered at 12-15 months of age with a booster at 1-1/2 to 4-1/2 years of age. Infants with a true egg allergy may safely receive the vaccine – discuss this with your doctor.

Measles (Red) Rubeola

With the institution of the measles vaccine the incidence of red measles has decreased dramatically. It is still, however, a major killer of children in Third-World countries where there are no vaccination programs.

The incubation period for red measles is 7–10 days from exposure to the onset of symptoms, and 14 days from exposure until the onset of the rash.

Before the appearance of a diagnostic rash, there is a period of 3–5 days when there is a fever, a very harsh, brassy cough, a profuse nasal discharge and red eyes. During this period, white spots on the gum line near the molar teeth will appear. These are called Koplik spots. Normally, these are only seen during a medical examination. The spots are diagnostic for measles, and with 100% certainty the rash will appear within 2 days.

The rash is very red. It usually starts on the head and spreads over the whole body in a descending fashion. The fever persists, usually with cough, runny nose and red eyes (sensitivity to light) for approximately 5 days after the onset of the rash.

The contagious period is during the time of incubation and lasts until the rash fades. Spread of measles is by contact with oral, eye or nasal secretions of an infected individual.

Treatment is supportive only, with use of acetaminophen or ibuprofen for the fever; it is important to maintain adequate hydration and treat any complications if they occur.

Complications can include middle-ear infections, pneumonia and encephalitis (inflammation of the brain). With intensive supportive treatment, death from measles infection is rare, but nevertheless may occur.

All infants born to mothers who have previously had red measles or the vaccine are protected for up to one year of age by the transfer of protective maternal antibodies that cross the placenta during pregnancy into the baby's circulation.

Immune serum gamma globulin given early after exposure may prevent or diminish the severity of the disease in children who have not been vaccinated with the measles vaccine. It is used, however, only for those known to have chronic debilitating illnesses, who are on immunosuppressive therapy or who are immunodeficient.

A live vaccine for measles, mumps and rubella (MMR) is recommended to be given at 12-15 months of age (not before) and a booster shot at 1-1/2 to 4-1/2 years of age.. Those infants who have a true egg allergy can often be given the vaccine safely – discuss with your doctor.

Some countries require measles immunization (if the person has not previously been vaccinated or had the clinical illness) to be given before allowing a person to enter that particular country. As a result, children under one year of age may require the vaccine. These children should also be revaccinated at 12 to15 months of age and then again at 1-1/2 to 4-1/2 years of age.

There are numerous scientific reviews on the vaccine that indicate there are no connections between the MMR vaccine and any chronic illness, including autism.

Medicine Administration – Method (By Mouth, Ear, Eye)

Oral (by mouth) medication

It has never ceased to amaze me that infants and toddlers will put almost anything in their mouths (dirt, toys, pencils, etc., etc., etc.,) and do so willingly, and with great glee. There are 3 things, however, that they will fight with all their might to resist opening their mouths for – these three are tooth brushing, eating nourishing food and taking medicine.

Some infants and toddlers seem to have a super-hero's sense of smell and taste. From 3 ft. away they are able to sense that something they really don't want is coming their way. Giving a child medicine often requires the patience of a teacher, the wisdom of a prophet, the skill of a magician, the attack plan of an army general and the strength of a fullback (and sometimes the whole team approach).

If the medicine is prescribed to be taken 4 times daily, the first dose is in the morning, the second dose is in the late morning, the third dose is mid-afternoon and a fourth dose is before bedtime. If prescribed 3 times daily then the first dose is given in the morning, the second dose in early afternoon, and the last dose at bedtime. If medicine is prescribed twice daily, the first dose is given in the morning and a second dose in the early evening. If prescribed for once daily, it does not matter the time of day you choose to administer it; however, be consistent on a daily basis. These schedules will allow you and the child to, hopefully, have an uninterrupted sleep.

Medicine may be administered by syringe, medicine cup, measuring spoon or dropper. Regular kitchen spoons vary in size. Using them to give you child medicine may result in the administration of an inaccurate amount of medication. If the child seems apprehensive and hesitant about taking medication, I advise you not to use a measuring spoon – administer either by syringe or dropper. Place small amounts between his gum and teeth, as far back as possible. There are fewer taste buds in this area so the taste will be somewhat hidden. When swallowed, repeat until all the medication has been taken. Avoid putting medicine on the back of the tongue or squirting it onto the palate. Both of these actions will induce gagging.

Parents always want to know, "Why won't they take the medicine?" The first reason is because of the taste and consistency – it's "yucky"! Although most medicines for children are flavoured, they still may have a somewhat bitter taste and/or a gritty texture, as well as a lasting aftertaste. Next reason: It is something that you usually do not give to your child: "What is with this stuff," they say? "Why are you being so overly nice to me? Something must be up." It is an unwanted, suspicious change in the daily routine. Even older children, who can swallow half a hot dog with one gulp, all of a sudden can't seem to swallow a tiny pill. Somehow, somewhere, one of the earliest things learned is that medicine is distasteful and is to be avoided at all costs.

Please note the following: If the instructions on the medication state that the meds should be given on an empty stomach, it does not mean that it cannot be disguised (see below). In order to have complete delivery of the medication some pills should not be crushed or chewed. Similarly, some capsules must be taken whole and not emptied to disguise their contents. Check with your pharmacist.

For my patients, I recommend the jam or "ram and slam" method. The 'jam method' is meant to disguise the medicine's taste. It is your choice whether you try jam, peanut butter, ice cream, maple syrup or a little of your child's favourite drink. I'm sure I could write a book on the thousands of methods used to hide the taste. Check with your pharmacist to ensure that whatever you are disguising the medicine in will not affect its potency. I would add that you should avoid using the word "medicine". You can call it anything else – just not medicine. Do not even tell the child that he is getting anything. Many pharmacies are able to change the flavour of the medicine to one that the child likes best. If the child refuses to take the medication from a spoon, you can try a syringe. Place the syringe between his cheek and his gums and slowly inject. The further back in his mouth you get, the greater the success getting him to swallow the medication. If, after all your efforts, you're unable to pry the child's lips apart, then you have to resort to the "ram and slam" method. This method may have to be accomplished with the help of 2 or more people. Hold the child's nose shut. This will force him to open his mouth to breathe. Once the mouth opens, then carefully "ram" the medicine in and quickly let go of the nose. Just as quickly, put one hand on the top of his head and the other under his chin and clamp his mouth closed. He will have no choice but to swallow the medicine. To prevent struggling, swaddling may be necessary. This method, although seemingly harsh and torturous to your child, is nevertheless effective. Believe me, you will not likely have to do this more than twice before your child realizes that it is not worth his effort to resist. To teach this lesson will be well worth the effort and save you hardship in the future when medication is again required.

If vomiting occurs within 15–20 minutes after taking the medication, it may be repeated. After that interval of time, enough medication will have been absorbed to do the job.

What about pills and capsules? Many children (and adults) have a pill phobia – even the most stoic of individuals. Most pills, when crushed, have a very bitter taste and, therefore, many children resist taking them. It is, however, worth a try to disguise as described above. Most of us have already tried placing a pill in a child's mouth and having them drink. Too often this leads to gagging and spitting out everything, including the pill. Try giving the child half a cracker or cookie to chew. Then give him the second half and the pill with it. Frequently, they will chew and then swallow the cracker or cookie and the pill will slip down whole.

Ultimately, it is rare to find anyone who likes taking medication. However, when it is needed the above are the only options. You just have to knuckle down, grit your teeth and pull up your sleeves to do it!!!

Ear medication

Lay the child on his side. Pull the ear up and back. This action straightens out the ear canal. Place the drops one at a time in the ear. Have the child remain still on his side for at least one minute so that the medication can reach all parts of the canal and not drip out as it will if he is allowed to sit upright immediately after administration.

Eyes–medication: See **Conjunctivitis (pink eye)**.

Meningococcal C Vaccine

There are 5 strains of the meningococcal bacteria that cause septicemia (blood infection) and/or meningitis. These diseases are very serious. For a child under 2 years, only meningococcal C vaccine is available. There is no vaccine for type B (one will be available late 2012). There is a vaccine available at 2 years of age that covers groups A, C, Y, W135.

The overall mortality rate for meningococcal disease is approximately 10%. Twenty percent of those who survive will have a permanent complication that can include brain damage, seizures, hearing loss, and loss of fingers or toes, or even arms and legs. Children who are spared from serious complications may still develop learning disabilities.

In the Canadian population, approximately 2 in 100,000 will develop this disease. The highest incidence is in the under-one-year-old age group.

In some Canadian provinces, government programs have been implemented for giving the meningococcal C vaccine free of charge. It is given at one year of age – but not before one year of age, according to their guidelines.

Unfortunately, these guidelines leave the child under one year of age unprotected.

I therefore recommend 2 doses of the vaccine, one to be given at 3 months and a second at 5 months of age. A booster dose should be given at one year of age.

Meningococcal Illness (A, B, C, Y, W135)

Meningococcal disease is caused by a bacterium called *Neisseria meningitides*. There are 5 serotypes of this bacterium – A, B, C, Y and W135. Of interest, this bacterium, which resides in the nasopharynx, can take genes from other bacteria and is capable of switching from A to B to C to Y or W135.

Three kinds of illness may result from infection. They are meningococcal pneumonia, meningococcal meningitis and meningococcal septicemia (infection in the blood). Meningococcal septicemia is the most serious of the three.

The meningococcal bacteria reside in the back of the throat and in the nasopharynx of "carriers." "Carriers" harbor the bacteria but do not get ill themselves. They can, however, spread the infection to others who are susceptible via oral droplets that are spread by coughing or sneezing, or by the sharing of straws, lipstick and lip balms, eating utensils or drinks (bottles and cans). The bacteria may also be spread from any inanimate object such as a desktop, pen, toys, electronic games or computer keyboards. In these cases, the bacteria have been deposited on a surface that a susceptible individual may touch and transfer the bacteria to their mouth and, thus, become infected.

The highest incidence for infection is in children under one year of age as well as those in their teenage years and young adults. The death rate for meningococcal disease is 10% to 15%

(higher if it is meningococcemia). Of those who survive the disease, at least 20% may have a severe permanent neurological deficit.

A vaccine for serotype B will be available in late 2012.

One vaccine is available for serotype C alone and another for serotypes A, C, Y, and W135. The vaccine for serotype C only can be started as early as 3 months of age and upward. The vaccine presently available for the combination of serotypes is only recommended for children over two years of age.

Serotype B, for which there is no vaccine at present, is the most common cause of meningococcal disease in children between the ages of 5 and 9 years – 80%. Over 10 years of age, serotypes Y and W135 become more common – 50%. Serotype C overall accounts for up to 30% to 40% of meningococcal infections. The vaccine for serotype C is the only vaccine available at present for children under two years of age (remember, children under one year of age are the most susceptible, followed by those from one to two years of age, to meningococcal disease).

I, therefore, highly recommend to all my caregivers that their infants receive the meningococcal C vaccine at 3 and 5 months of age, with a booster dose at one year. At two years of age they should receive the vaccine that covers all 4 serotypes. All children over 12 years of age, especially those in their mid-teens to early adulthood, should also be vaccinated with the 4-serotype vaccine. A vaccine for serotype group B is on its way. Be Wise – Immunize.

Molluscum Contagiosum

This is a viral infection of the skin that results in small raised bumps, often with a central dark spot. They may be single or multiple. They can occur anywhere on the body.

They are spread by direct contact with a lesion. They may also spread from one part of the body to another on an infected child.

The raised bumps are contagious as long as they are visible. The degree of transmissibility is extremely low.

If left untreated, the lesions usually remain 2–3 months. Unfortunately, they can also stay for up to 2 years.

By themselves they present no symptoms. They are mainly a cosmetic nuisance.

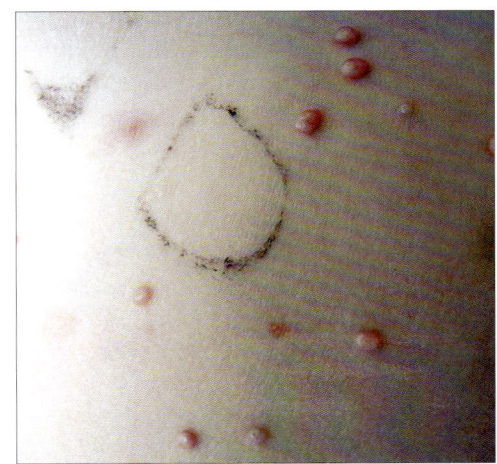

Molluscum

There are many different ways to manage these lesions: from doing nothing to using topical medication, cryotherapy with liquid nitrogen, or laser surgery. Therapy should be considered on an individual needs basis.

Mumps

Mumps is a mild viral illness that was very common before routine immunization with the mumps vaccine became available.

Symptoms include a low-grade fever, fatigue, headache and a tender swelling of the parotid gland on one or both sides. The parotid glands are usually unable to be felt unless they are enlarged. They are located in front of the lower half of each ear. When inflamed, they may be tender to the touch and cause pain on movement of the jaw. Discomfort may also occur with the drinking of citrus fruit juices.

The serum amylase in the blood is elevated.

The incubation period varies from 2–3 weeks after exposure. It is spread by oral droplets from an infected person. It is contagious for one day prior to swelling until the swelling subsides. Isolation is recommended during this time. The swelling diminishes 3–7 days after the onset of the illness.

Treatment

Prevention of mumps is accomplished by vaccination against this virus. The mumps vaccine is given in combination with the measles and rubella vaccines after one year of age and a booster dose follows between 18 months and 4-1/2 years of age. Vaccination results in over 95% protection. Those infants with a true egg allergy may still have the vaccine. This should be discussed with your doctor.

Pregnant women who have had mumps will give transient antibody protection to the newborn for approximately 6 months after birth.

For treatment, either acetaminophen or ibuprofen may be given to manage fever or discomfort.

The complications of mumps can often be worse than the disease. These include encephalitis (brain inflammation) – 1 in 200 children, pancreatitis, deafness and orchitis (inflammation of the testicles). Orchitis occurs rarely in the pre-adolescent age group. Twenty-five percent of adult males with mumps may have this complication. It may be one or both testicles that are affected. Resulting infertility is rare. Inflammation of one or both ovaries may occur in 5% of females. Again, infertility is rare.

There are other causes of inflammation of the parotid glands other than those due to the mumps virus. These most commonly result from other viruses. Rarely are they caused by a bacterial infection.There is a condition in childhood called recurrent parotid gland inflammation. This is a recurrent inflammation of the parotid gland. The etiology (cause) is uncertain. The prognosis is excellent. A stone in the parotid gland duct may also cause inflammation. Rarely, parotid gland inflammation may occur with certain autoimmune disorders.

To confirm a parotid gland inflammation, testing consists of measuring the serum amylase. An ultrasound or x-ray test, called a silogram, may also be required to rule out a parotid duct stone.

Neurodevelopment Assessment (18 Months of Age)

Does your child:	Yes	No
• Smile appropriately ("social" smile)?		
• Respond when called by name?		
• Look at you when talked to or played with (makes eye contact)?		
• Appear to be loving (likes to be cuddled) and show affection to people, pets and toys?		
• Socialize well – take interest in other children?		
• Play with toys appropriately (not just mouthing, fiddling or dropping them)?		
• Perform repetitive movements such as flapping of the hands, excessive finger movements in front of the face or constant rocking?		
• Like to spin the wheels of toys rather than play with them appropriately?		
• Spin excessively or run in circles for extended lengths of time?		
• Prefer to play alone rather than with others?		
• Enjoy playing peek-a-boo and hide-and-seek?		
• Engage in pretend play, for example, talking on the phone or taking care of a doll?		
• Point to what he wants?		
• Appear to be oversensitive to noise (covers ears)?		

Does your child:	Yes	No
• Walk?		
• Climb stairs?		
• Look at what you are pointing to?		
• Seem to understand what people say?		
• Sometimes stare at nothing or wander with no purpose?		
• Speak at least 10 understandable words? If less – how many?		
• Identify pictures in a book (example, when you say, "Show me the dog")?		
• Follow 1-step directions, e.g., "throw me the ball" or "bring me your shoes"?		
• Identify and point to at least 3 different body parts?		
• Hold a cup to drink?		
• Pick up and eat finger food?		
• Help with his own dressing by holding out his arms and legs?		
• Squat to pick up a toy without falling?		
• Push and pull toys while walking?		
• Stack 3 or more blocks?		
• Like to feel and stroke a piece of material or hair (for a long period of time)?		
• Display frequent severe temper tantrums (with minor triggers)?		

If you have any concerns, consult your doctor.

Adapted from the Modified Checklist for Autism in Toddlers (M-CHAT), Georgia State University, USA; the M-CHAT Screening Questionaire; and the Nipissing District Development Screen (NDDS). The above questionnaire is the one I use in my office. There are numerous others available to help the physician determine if the child is neurodevelopmentally on target for his age.

New Sibling Arrival (Management of the Older Sibling)

With the arrival of a newborn, in order to have a smooth transition, preparation for the event should also include the preparation of the sibling.

Remember, until now your first child has had 100% of your attention. When your new baby arrives, the focus of this attention will be dramatically shifted. How your child will react really depends on how you prepare him in advance for the arrival.

Never underestimate the traumatic effect that a new arrival can have on an older sibling

The preparation for helping a sibling to adjust should begin during your pregnancy. If possible, he should accompany you, the mother, to ultrasound appointments so that he starts to feel that he is part of the whole process. You should encourage him to feel your tummy as the baby grows and make special note when there is movement. Include him in the choosing of a name for the new baby, choosing the baby's clothes, decorating the room, and shopping for any of the items you need when the newborn arrives. The more he can take part in the whole process the better his adjustment will be.

Your child should also be prepared (appropriate to his age level) as to what will happen to both you and him when you go into labour and what he can expect during your hospital stay. The sooner after the birth he meets and sees his new sibling the better. Buy him a little toy baby doll so that he can have a new baby as well. Encourage him to treat his baby just as you do with the newborn. Encourage his participation (under your supervision) in the caring of the newborn.

Make sure that you set aside one-on-one time to spend with your older child. At this particular time he is in need of that special attention so that he does not feel left out. Rewarding him for good behaviour by saying "good job" or "you're a great helper" will help to ensure his acceptance of the new arrival.

If, for whatever reason (most likely jealousy), he does not "like" the baby and either bites or hits him, then all you need to do is hold his forearm firmly, make direct eye contact and say emphatically, "No hitting." Then go on with your daily routine and nothing further should be mentioned.

I do not recommend that you take your older child out of his crib and put him in a bed or change his room to make room for the newborn around the time of your labour and delivery. If you decide to switch your child to a big bed then do it a minimum of 2–3 months prior to the arrival of the newborn. I also recommend that if you plan to use your first child's crib store the crib until it is needed. Make as few changes as possible until you are certain your older child is completely comfortable with the idea of his new sibling. This may take 2 or 3 months or even longer. It is during this time that you should have few problems transferring him into a bed and even another room. Take your cues from him.

This is also not the time to begin potty training.

Some children regress when the newborn arrives. Toilet habits may temporarily reverse; baby talk may return; there may be a demand to reintroduce the pacifier. Feeding problems and sleep problems, temper tantrums, the child demanding to be fed, making unreasonable demands and physically trying to hurt the new arrival are just a few of the many occurrences that can surface. What your child is telling you is that he is not happy with his new lot in life – going from being "numero uno" to a position of merely second place. This child needs extra special attention and reassurance. Negative reinforcement should be avoided. You must listen to his needs and respond accordingly. He needs to be reassured of your love and that his place in the "pecking order" of your family has not changed.

Older children should be educated about safety precautions regarding the new baby. Their play may become a virtual safety hazard for your newborn – improperly carrying the baby, putting small objects in the baby's mouth, ears or nostrils, covering the baby with a blanket or moving the baby's limbs in a rough manner. All constitute a danger to the newborn which the older child must be made aware of.

The older child himself must be nurtured in order that he too loves the baby in a gentle fashion and handles him carefully, not like a toy or Fido the family pooch.

Newborn (Good News)

Things You Do Not Have to Worry About Concerning Your Newborn

You have finally arrived home with your newborn. Excited but exhausted – nothing could be greater. Nothing until you actually realize that you're going to have to make all the decisions concerning your baby, whose only way of communicating with you is to cry – an overwhelming responsibility suddenly presents itself.

You'll soon notice little things about your baby and wonder if there is a problem. Your self-appointed "advisory staff" often continues to fuel your anxiety.

Over the past 40 years of practice I have encountered approximately 40–50 "concerns" about their baby from new parents that are in fact "non-concerns". Here are some of the more common ones.

The skin

- Most babies are born with **dry, flaky skin** which they soon shed like a snake shedding its skin. No moisturizer is required.

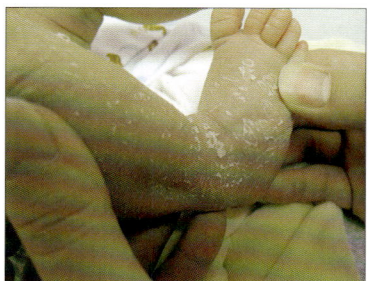 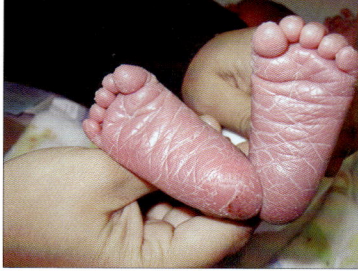 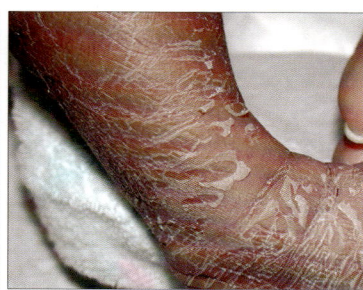

Dry Skin (Normal) *Dry Skin (Normal)* *Dry Skin (Normal)*

Varying sizes of **red blotches** with a white spot in the center and irregular edges are called **erythema toxicum neonatorum (ETN)**. They will disappear within 2 to 3 weeks of age.

- Pink blotches on the baby's upper eyelids are called "angel kisses" and the one at the back of the neck is called a "**stork bite**" – no problem.

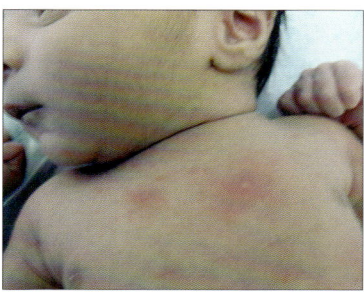 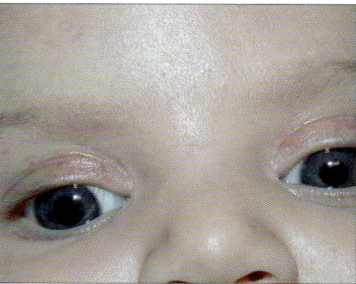 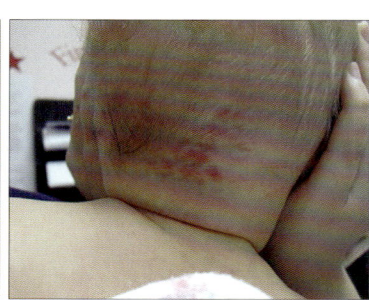

Erythema Toxicum Neonatorum *Angel Kisses* *Stork Bite*

- Varying sizes of **purple discolourations** that look like bruises may appear anywhere on the body. They are most common in the lower back region. These are called Mongolian spots and will disappear within two to three years.

- A **blue vein** crossing the bridge of the nose will disappear.

- Numerous little **white spots** on the baby's nose are called **milia**. They will slowly fade.

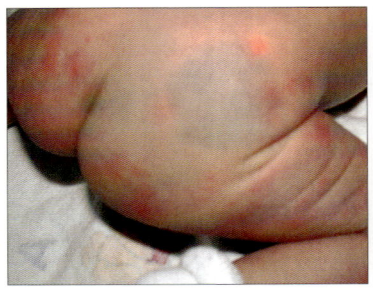
Mongolian Spots

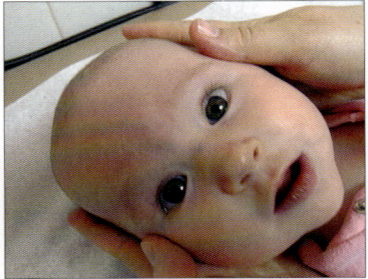
Nose – Blue Vein

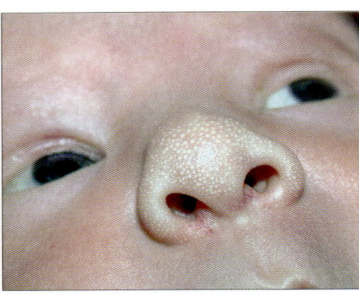
Milia

• At around two weeks of age numerous little "**pimples**" on the baby's cheeks are **baby acne** – no treatment required.

• Between the **eyebrows** may be a reddish discolouration that spreads up to the forehead – it may appear like an **Olympic torch flame**. This will slowly disappear by three years of age.

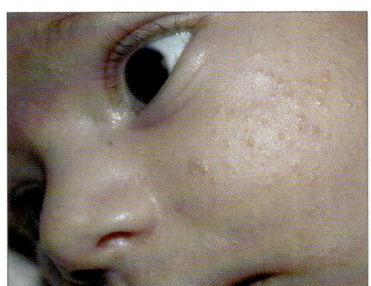
Baby Acne

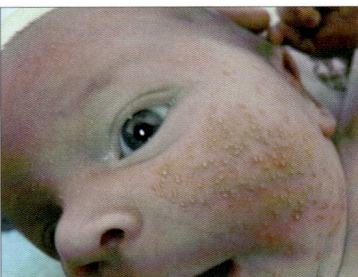
Severe Baby Acne

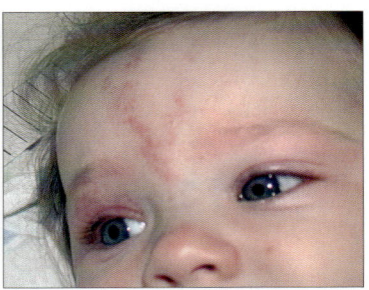
Olympic Torch Flame

Hair

• At a few weeks of age you may notice that the baby is losing hair. The amount varies and may result in total loss. Do not fret; it will grow back, although it may take several months or longer to do so.

Ear, nose and throat

• **Sneezing** (and **hiccupping**) is normal.

• Under the baby's **tongue** is a little band of tissue called the **frenulum**. As long as the baby is able to protrude (stick out) his tongue as far as the lower lip, there should be no interference with latching onto the breast, or with age, speech. A poor latch thought to be due to a tight frenulum is called a tongue

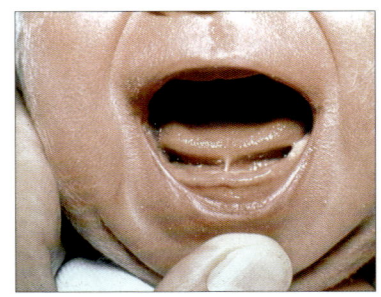
Tongue Tie

tie. It will be snipped by an ear, nose and throat (ENT) specialist.

• A mid-line alveolar cleft in the upper dental ridge will close in time, most often without any future dental problems.

• A **white-coated tongue** is just milk residue – clean it with a washcloth if you wish. A **sucking blister** may appear in the middle of the upper lip, especially with breastfed infants.

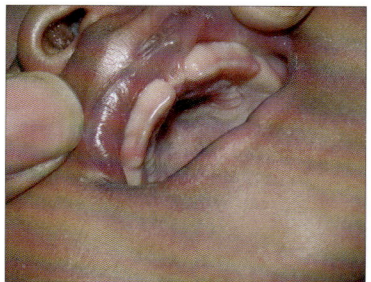
Alveolar Cleft

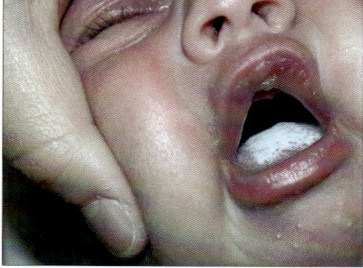
White-Coated Tongue

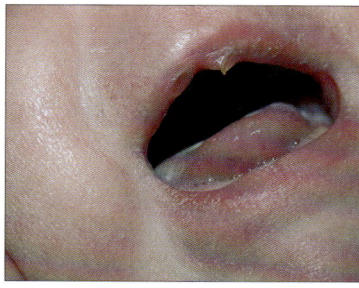
Sucking Blister

• **Stuffy nose**: if the baby can suck while feeding without having to stop to catch his breath, then the nasal stuffiness is bothering you and not the baby – no treatment required. You do not have to remove any mucus from the baby's nose.

• Do not remove any **wax** from the ears. Nothing smaller than your elbow should ever enter the ear canal.

Eyes

• **Eye colour** – brown eyes will stay brown, however, blue eyes may change colour by seven to eight months of age depending on the genetic background.

• A red crescent surrounding part of the iris (the coloured part) is a **sclera hemorrhage**. This occurred during passage through the birth canal – and it will disappear.

• **The whites of the eye may appear grey or blue** – no problem. They may also appear **yellow**. Most likely this is due to physiological newborn jaundice and will disappear within one to two weeks. Breastfeeding may also be the cause of jaundice. If this is the case it may last several weeks – again, no problem.

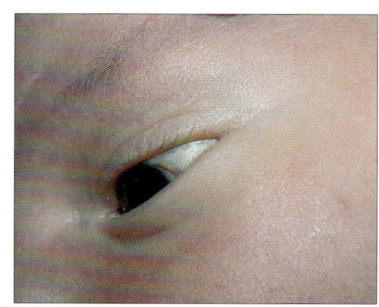
Scleral Hemorrhage

- Coordination of **eye movements** may not occur until 4–5 months of age.

- **Excessive tearing** in one or both eyes is due to blocked tear ducts. No treatment required. A little matter collecting in the corner of each eye, which is easily removed with a moist cotton ball, is also due to **blocked tear ducts**. The tear ducts may be intermittently blocked until 12 to 18 months of age.

Gastrointestinal system

- The **umbilical stump** may take two to three weeks before falling off. When it does, a few drops of blood may be noticed for 1-2 days – no problem.

- Sponge bathe the baby only until the stump has fallen off and dried. No treatment for the stump is required.

- The **belly button** may protrude and feel mushy to the touch. This is an **umbilical hernia**. Most disappear by a year and a half of age.

- A small piece of **fleshy skin** may protrude from the belly button area. This is called an **umbilical granuloma**. Most disappear on their own by six to eight months of age.

- After meconium stools, newborn stools are usually loose, yellow and seedy. Green stools are fine.

- An **anal skin** tag may protrude from the anus. This will regress within a few weeks.

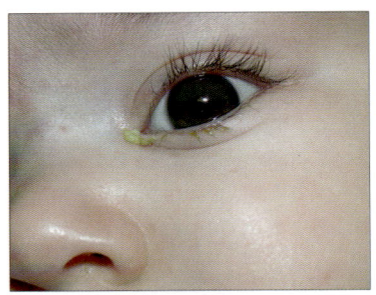
Blocked Tear Duct

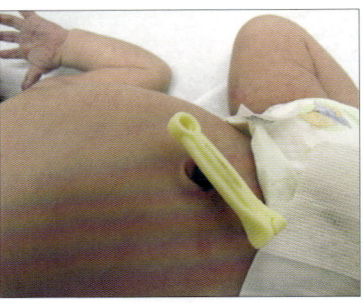
Umbilical Clamp

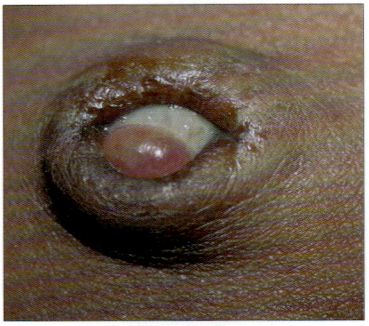
Umbilical Granuloma

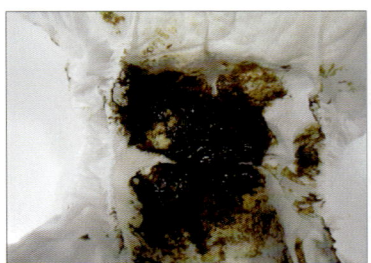
Meconium Newborn Stool

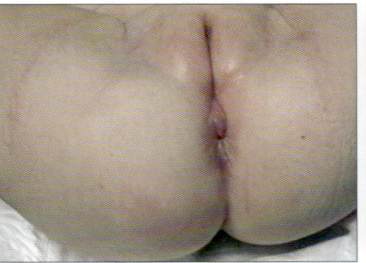
Anal Skin Tag

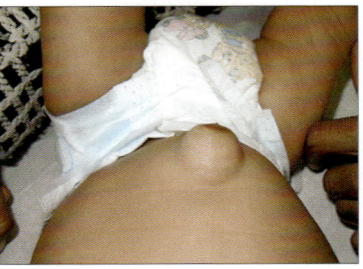
Umbilical Hernia

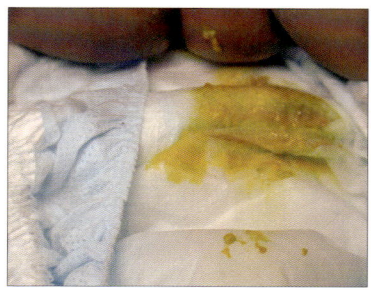
Normal Stool

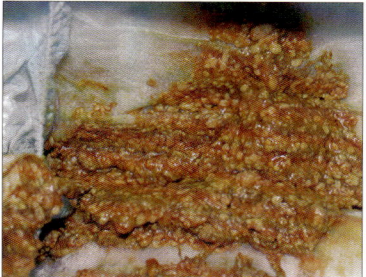
Normal Stool

Genital system

• **Swollen testicles** are due to water sacs around one or both testicles. They are called **hydroceles**. Most swellings disappear by one year of age.

• A small **skin tag** protruding from the baby's vagina will disappear.

• **Bleeding** from the **vagina** may occur. This is called pseudo menses – no concern.

• Pinkish discolouration on the diaper from urine is due to **urate crystals** and not blood. It may be a sign of underfeeding – check with your doctor.

• A mucusy, white **vaginal discharge** is normal and will disappear within a week or so.

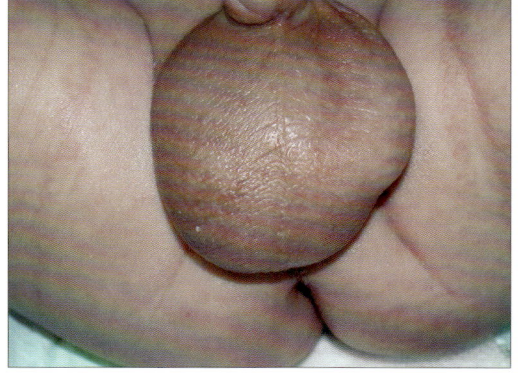
Right Hydrocele

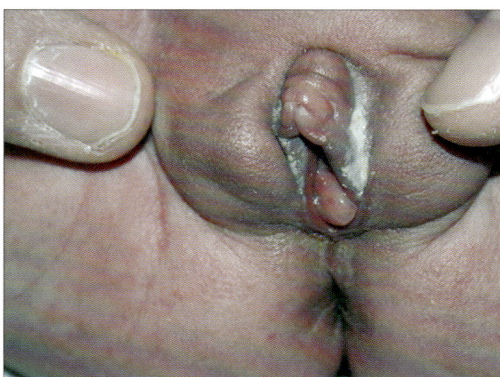
Vaginal Skin Tag

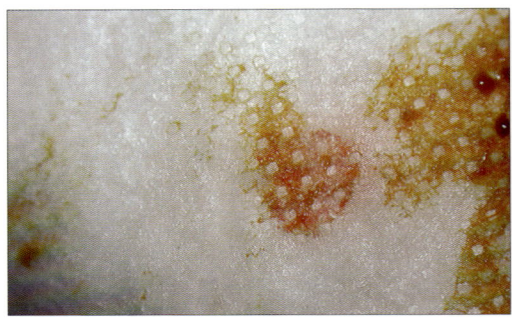
Urate Crystals

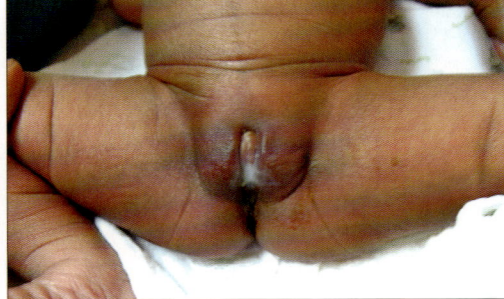
Vaginal Discharge

Respiratory system

• **"Mucusy" respirations** that sound loud and seem to vibrate through the chest are just the sound of the baby breathing through a web of mucus at the back of his throat. If the baby is feeding well, sleeping well, happy and does not appear distressed, there is no problem.

• At times the baby's respirations will seem to speed up for half a minute or so and then slow down – he may even pause for several seconds between breaths.

Central nervous system

• **Startling** – when the baby's arms and legs seem to shoot out, this is considered normal.

• **Quivering** of the limbs is also normal.

• A **soft, mushy swelling** at the back of the head on one or both sides is called a **cephalohematoma**. During the baby's passage through the birth canal, pressure has been put on the baby's head. This may cause some bleeding under the skin. It may vary in size. It will not harm the baby (during its reabsorption it may cause or add to mild jaundice). Over a period of months, it will be replaced by bone and the skull will remodel itself to leave the head normally shaped.

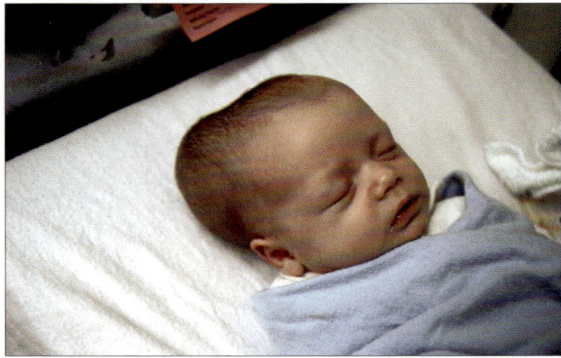
Cephalohematoma

Circulatory system

• The **hands** and **feet** appear **blue** and **cold**. This is due to the baby's high hemoglobin – no concern.

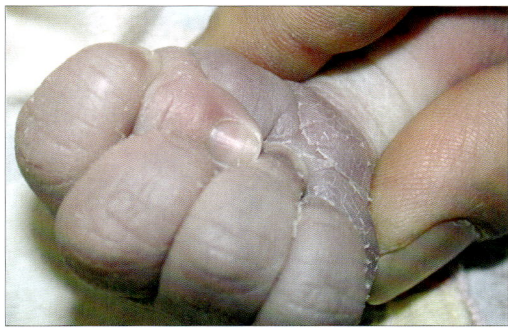
Normal Skin Colour

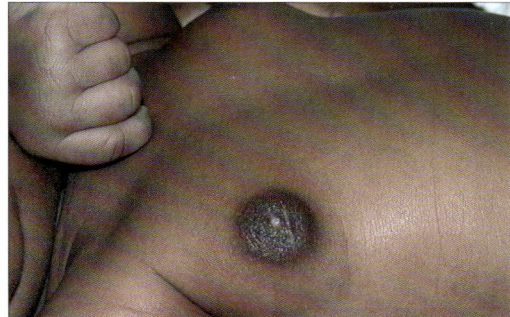
Breast Engorgement

Anatomical

• **Engorged, swollen breasts** in newborn boys and girls are normal. It is the excess of mother's hormones circulating in the baby's blood that causes the enlargement (occasionally milk may be expressed if the breast is pinched). After birth, the maternal hormones will diminish and within a few weeks the breast engorgement will as well.

• The **ribcage** may appear to be **concave** (caved in) in the middle of the chest – no concern.

• The bottom of the **ribcage** on either side seems to be flared outward – no problem.

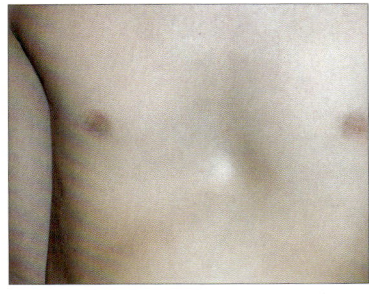
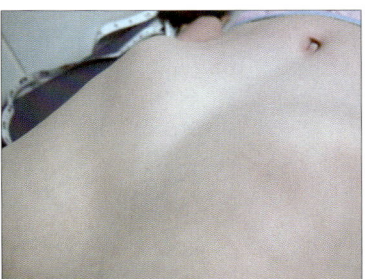
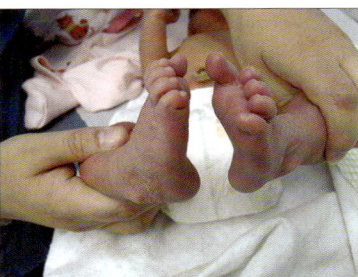

Pectus Excavatum (Sunken Chest)   *Rib Flaring*   *Normal Position of Feet*

• The **legs and feet** may seem **crooked, with bowing** – if you were cramped up for nine months yours would be too! They will straighten.

• At the bottom of the **chest cage,** in the middle, you may see and feel a bony prominence. This is the **xiphoid sternal process**. This is a normal bone at the end of the sternum. In time it will become less prominent.

• The **toenails** on one or both big toes may seem to be **ingrown**. The skin around the toe may be slightly reddened. This is normal and of no concern. If you were to pinch the toe, there would be no pain. Ingrown toenails are very tender to touch and often contain pus under the skin.

• In a straight line below a breast nipple, there may be one or more small brown pigmented indentations. These are **accessory nipples**. During the early development of the baby while in utero, there is a line of nipples on either side. These are not unlike the nipples on a cow. After further development only one pair of nipples remains and is present at birth. Occasionally, a remnant of other nipples may remain. They will not disappear and are a concern only for cosmetic reasons.

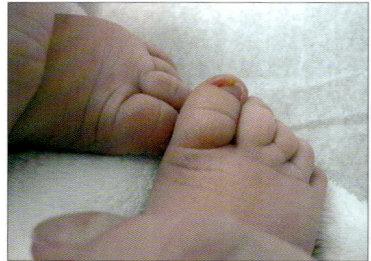
Normal Toes

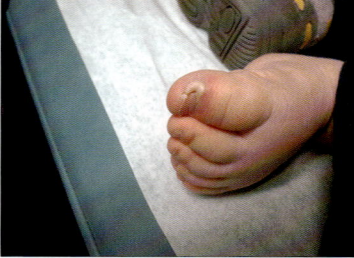
Ingrown Toenail (pus)

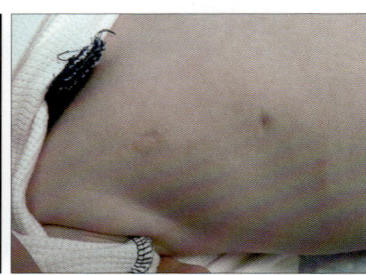
Accessory Nipple

• One or both **nipples** seem to be **white** as if containing a drop of milk. This "milk cyst" will disappear. One or both **nipples** may be **inverted** – no problem.

• At the lower end of the back, just above above the top of the buttocks, there may be a small indentation. The indentation is completely covered with normal skin. It is called a **pilonidal dimple**. Infrequently, its base is not covered with skin. A tract may be present leading into the spine. This is called a **pilonidal sinus**. It may leak fluid or become infected, and investigation as to its length will be required. Surgical removal may be indicated.

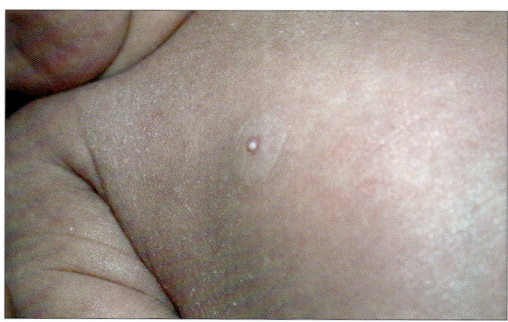
Milk Cyst

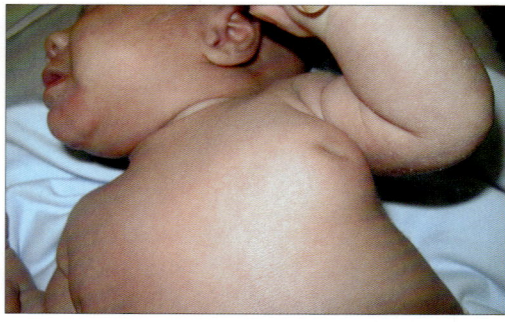
Inverted Nipples

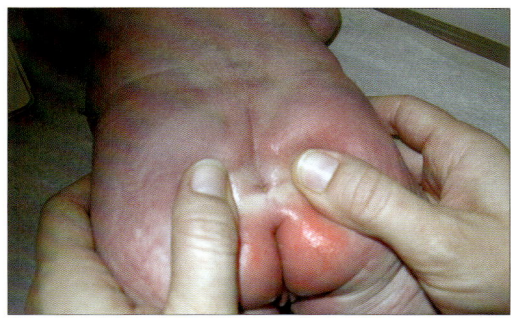
Pilonidal Dimple
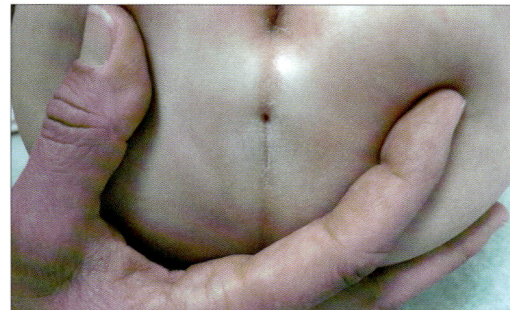
Pilonidal Sinus

I hope that by listing the above situations I have reduced some of your concerns so as to make life a little less stressful for you while you are adjusting to your most precious gift – your baby.

Night Sweating

Many infants' heads will sweat profusely during the night. In the morning the sheets where they were lying are soaked, as well as their hair.

They are otherwise entirely asymptomatic. No sweat is present on the rest of the body.

This is a very common phenomenon which concerns many parents. The cause of this is entirely unknown. It is not associated with any disease process in a child who otherwise is well.

All the parents need is reassurance that no problem exists.

Constant, excessive sweating of the whole body may be a symptom of other medical problems, such as an overactive thyroid gland or heart disease.

Night Terrors

When children experience night terrors it can be a very frightening experience for the parents as well. Night terrors usually begin between 2–3 years of age, but may not start to manifest until a few years later. Most children will outgrow them by 7–9 years of age. They usually happen infrequently, but for some children they may occur 3–4 times weekly. Approximately 15% of children may have the occasional night terror. Approximately 3% may have them on a more regular basis. They are more common in boys. Often, there is a family history. Night terrors are considered to be one of the sleep disorders.

The cause of night terrors is unknown. They occur during the deep sleep cycle.

The child usually falls asleep without a problem. One to three hours later, he may start to cry loudly, even to screech, to flail his limbs around, and become completely inconsolable. The child's eyes may be wide open and he may exhibit profuse sweating. He may speak out loud in his sleep, but his speech is often completely nonsensical. Wandering aimlessly may also occur. These episodes may last up to 10–30 minutes.

When the child wakes in the morning he/she does not remember the incident. Most times there is no known trigger. Night terrors are, however, more common when the child is overtired or over-excited before bed, or has had a recent stressful experience. There is no dietary trigger.

The only treatment that is required is to ensure that your child does not hurt himself. If there are frequent episodes which occur at specific times, then waking the child up just before those times may alter the sleep cycle and possibly prevent the incident. Do not try to wake the child up during a night terror. Investigations are not indicated. Medication is not indicated. The only treatment required is to be reassured that they are entirely benign in nature.

Nosebleeds (Epistaxis)

There is nothing like a good old-fashioned nosebleed in a child to raise the blood pressure of a parent rapidly. I sincerely doubt that there are very many people alive who have not had at least one nosebleed.

Nosebleeds often occur in individuals with a bleeding disorder or low platelets or from taking blood-thinning medication. The vast majority of them, however, thankfully do not result from any of these underlying problems.

Although nosebleeds may occur spontaneously, the vast majority are secondary to some type of trauma. Sometimes the trauma is obvious – a blow to the nose. Other times it is not obvious. The most common cause is a child who picks at his nose. This frequently occurs at night. The child partially wakes up and unwittingly scratches the inside of his nose with his finger. He wakes up in the morning and the pillow and sheets are blood-stained.

In the septum (middle partition of the nose) there is an area approximately 1–2 cm from the tip of the nose called Little's area. Little's area is just above the cartilage that protrudes from the septum at the entrance of the nose. In this area the overlying skin is very thin. This area also has numerous small blood vessels. It is from this area that the bleeding occurs when traumatized.

Treatment

If possible, have the child clear the nasal passages by blowing his nose. Have him lean forward. This is to prevent blood from being swallowed, which can aggravate the stomach and result in vomiting. Pinch the tip of the nose between your index finger and thumb for 5–10 minutes by the clock. An ice pack placed on the bridge of the nose may help. If the nosebleed does not stop, pinch again for 15 minutes. If it still persists, medical attention is required. I do not advise you to pack the nose yourself.

Prevention

- Keep fingernails cut short.
- Maintain the humidity between 45% and 50%.
- Apply nasal lubricants.

Recurrent nosebleeds – treatment

- Cover Little's area with petroleum jelly twice daily to act as a protective covering.
- Your doctor may prescribe an estrogen cream to be applied twice daily to Little's area for approximately one month. The cream will thicken the skin in this area.
- Cauterization of Little's area may be done if the above do not work.

Orthopedic (Lower Limb(s) Problems)

While the baby is growing in the uterus he is in a very confined space. After birth, most infants have bowing of the lower limbs and in-turning of the feet. With time these normal anatomical occurrences will straighten. The vast majority do so by 3-4 years of age. No intervention is required. Do not listen to your "advisory staff". They will only increase your anxiety. If you're concerned, discuss this with your doctor rather than with your mother-in-law.

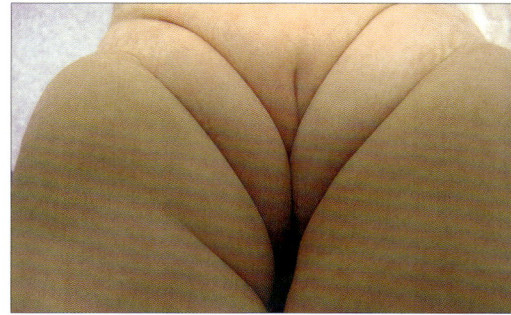
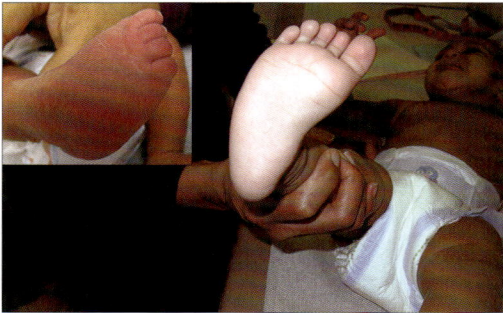

Dislocated Right Hip – Extra Skin Fold   *Club Foot / Metatarsal Varus*

Having been in practice for over 40 years, I have seen virtually every gait problem that concerns a parent. The orthopedic conditions that require intervention are: congenital dislocation of the hip, clubbed feet, and in-turning of the forefoot in an infant over one month of age – a condition that cannot be straightened by stretching exercises alone. All other orthopedic conditions in an otherwise normal child (with no underlying neurological or neuromuscular disease) do not require any intervention.

Some of the most commonly diagnosed and then subsequently treated conditions I see in my practice are foot or leg problems. These conditions for the most part never did and never will require any intervention. I am quite convinced if you were to take your child to a "specialist" who deals with feet, a chiropractor, a physiotherapist or a medical doctor who lacks sufficient knowledge about children's gait and bone development, your child would be treated. He would receive any one of the following "treatments"– an exercise program, special shoes, orthotics and/or various types of manipulation therapies. The practitioner would be more than happy to take your money for as long as you wish to pay. Can any of these therapies help? The practitioner would have you convinced so. You would be hoping for an improvement in your child's gait, so that you would convince yourself that it was happening. From wearing special shoes or orthotics, the condition being treated, to your eye, would be improved. However, the underlying cause being treated will not be corrected. The bottom line is that knowledgeable doctors (pediatric orthopedic specialists) feel there is a vast amount of over-treatment for normal physiological anatomical conditions: conditions that will either improve on their own in time or, if not, will not impede the child's participation in any physical activity.

Orthopedic conditions that do not have to be treated are as follows: flat-feet, toe walking, in-toeing, hypermobile foot, bowing of the legs and knocking of the knees. The most thorough way in which the doctor can examine a gait problem, is not only by physical examination of the child, in addition to watching him walk, but also by examining the bottom of the child's most-often worn pair of shoes. This helps him to determine if there is excessive pressure in any one particular area of the foot; so it is necessary to bring with you the shoes your child wears most.

The best way to strengthen your child's feet is to resist confing them in stiff shoes or boots. The support these provide prevents the muscles of the foot from strengthening on their own. Allow the child to walk without shoes whenever possible. Special high-priced shoes will not maintain or improve gait problems. All your child needs is footwear that protects the foot and is appropriate for the weather.

I would like to clear up a few misconceptions.

In-toeing

If you were to observe Olympic sprinters, you would notice that the very best of them have mild in-toeing. For this same condition in children corrective shoes are unnecessary even if the child trips

In-toeing

over his own feet. Often, tripping is worse when kids wear shoes, especially if those shoes are too large. Given time, the feet will straighten.

Flat-feet

All children are born with a fat pad under the sole of the foot. This fat pad may not disappear until they are 3 or 4 years of age. Therefore, the foot looks flat, but it is really only the fat. When the fat pad disappears an arch will appear. At 3–4 years of age, if the child curls the toes down while sitting and an arch appears, then he is not flat-footed. Even if the diagnosis of flat-feet is confirmed, it cannot be corrected. Orthotics will not correct or prevent the lower back pain due to flat-feet that some individuals will develop in later life.

Bowed Legs or Knock Knees

As you are walking down the street you will notice that people have differing gaits. Some have their knees touching while for others it would be possible to drive a tricycle through the gap. Could these "malformations" have been corrected had they been treated in early childhood? The answer, unfortunately, is "No." Orthotics or special boots are not the answer. The use of night splints is no longer in vogue. Correction can be done only with surgery. No self- respecting surgeon would operate on these conditions. The reasons are that most will self- correct on their own in time, a general anesthetic and a lengthy operative procedure would be required, with a very long recovery phase, and, lastly, the underlying conditions do not cause any health problems, for knees, hips or back.

Hypermobile Feet

When walking, if the child's foot or feet appear to be rolling inward so that he is walking mainly on his instep, this would indicate a loose ankle joint. The inside of the shoes take the brunt of the impact and shows most of the wear. For this condition, the ankle joint requires strengthening. This can be accomplished with the following exercise: have the child walk barefooted along a 2 m board that simply lies on the floor. Have half of his foot on the board and the other half hanging over the edge. Holding his hand for balance, allow him to take several steps. Then have him turn around and do the same with the other half of his foot. Then switch feet. Repeat each side 4–5 times a day for 2 or 3 minutes. Make it a game. This exercise will help strengthen his ankle and the problem should be resolved within 6–10 months if you do the exercise religiously. Wearing no shoes at all is preferable. Orthotics or special boots may appear to produce a normal gait but will not solve the underlying problem.

Toe Walking

Many toddlers prefer to walk on their tiptoes. If the feet can be easily bent back upwards so that there is a 90° angle or more with the lower leg, then there is no tightening of the Achilles tendon (the band at the back of the heel extending up to the lower leg). As well, if the child is able to stand with the whole foot (toe to heel) on the floor, this again is evidence that there is no tightening of the tendon. For the vast majority of toddlers who walk on their toes, this requires no treatment. If you look at the bottom of the shoes you will probably see some wear at the heel, which indicates that the child is able to put the heel down. Constantly reminding children to walk "properly" is unnecessary and will probably stress your child. By 3–4 years of age or earlier, the gait will be normal.

Concerns

All of the above conditions are those most commonly found in both legs or feet. It may be a concern if the condition occurs in only one leg or has not been present before and then just appears. A limp or hip, leg or foot pain which is not caused by trauma, are a concern as well.

Shoes

Remember, shoes are for protection and not correction. There is a lot less concern about feet and gait in areas of the world where shoes are not worn. Shoes should be fitted by someone who specializes in children shoes. Toe room in new shoes should be no more than 1.5 cm (this will allow for growth). New shoes will probably be required every 4–6 months. If the toes are close to the end of the shoe it is time for new shoes. Trying to economize is a good thing but when it comes to footwear, I do not recommend the use of secondhand shoes.

The Sitting Position

The best sitting position for the toddler is with his legs crossed in front of him or with his legs and feet out in front of him. Discourage him from sitting on his feet while they are turned in (feet used as a pillow) or with his legs spread out to each side in the M position.

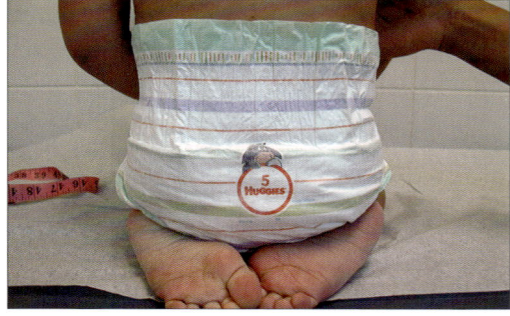   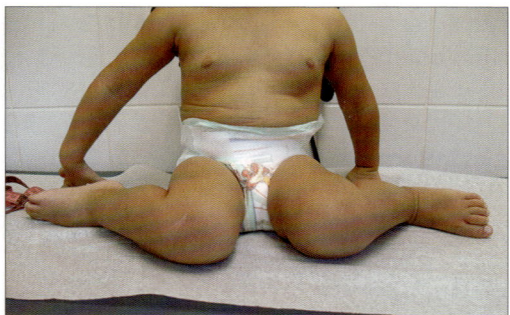

Improper Sitting Position   *Improper Sitting Position*

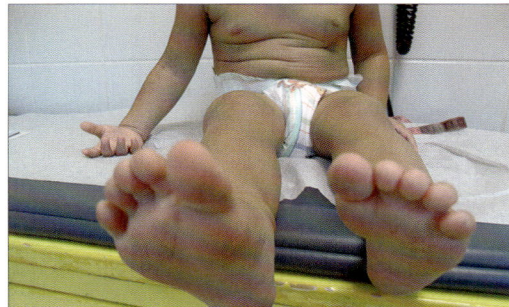
Proper Sitting Position

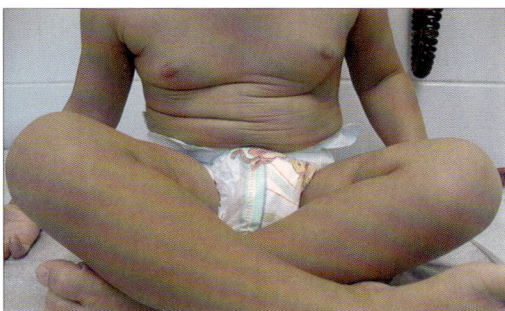
Proper Sitting Position

If you are not satisfied with your doctor's explanation of a foot or gait problem, request a consultation with a pediatric orthopedic surgeon.

Penis – Foreskin

The foreskin is the tissue that covers the glans (head) of the penis. It can vary in length from child to child. Basically, it is there to protect the glans from trauma, the elements, irritation and infection. Some believe that it also enhances sexual pleasure.

The care of the foreskin is quite simple. The penis should be washed the same as any other part of the body. It is not necessary to retract the foreskin. When the child is approximately 2 years of age his doctor will decide if there is a problem involving a tight foreskin, which may require gentle retraction. If your baby's foreskin can be retracted to reveal the tip of the penis then nothing further is required. When your son begins to have natural erections, the foreskin will be stretched sufficiently on its own.

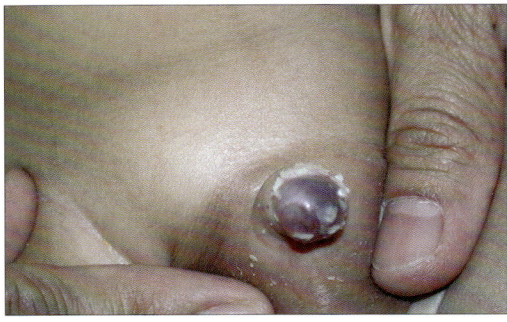
Smegma

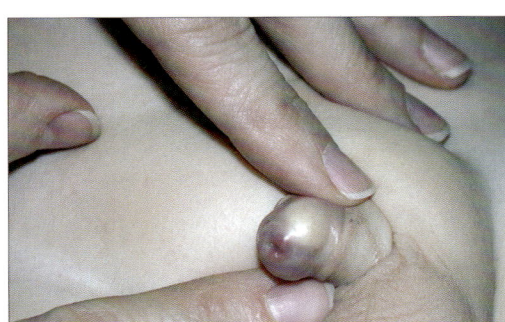
Smegma

Smegma

The secretions under the foreskin, which are creamy white in colour, are known as smegma (which is composed of dead skin cells). This secretion helps to break down the adhesions between the foreskin and the penis. This is important for future ease of retraction of the foreskin. It should be treated no differently than any other bodily secretion, such as wax in the ears. It has nothing to do with poor hygiene or infection. It can either be washed away or just left alone. Once the foreskin can be easily retracted, teach the child to pull it back and wash the head of the penis with each shower or bath.

Phimosis

Phimosis is a tightening of the foreskin whereby it cannot be retracted to visualize the tip of the penis. It is more common when the foreskin is long.

There are 2 types of phimosis:

1. Physiological infantile phimosis: This is the development of a nonretractable foreskin. This is more common in boys whose foreskins are very long.

2. Pathological phimosis: The foreskin, which previously could be partially retracted, is repeatedly and somewhat forcefully retracted by a caregiver trying to expose more of the glans. This continual irritation results in the foreskin adhering to the glans. Adherence can also occur if there are repeated foreskin infections.

The symptoms of phimosis may be negligible or there may be a weak urine stream, with or without ballooning of the foreskin during urination.

By 2-3 years of age, you should be able to retract the foreskin to visualize the tip of the urethra (penis). If this is the case nothing further is required. With time, as the child grows, the adherence of the foreskin to the glans of the penis will slowly loosen.

If, by 3–4 years of age the foreskin still can't be retracted to reveal the tip of the urethra, then cortisone cream will be prescribed by your doctor. It is to be applied to the mucous membrane at the end of the foreskin. This is done twice a day for 4–8 weeks. By that time, the foreskin should be easily retracted to see the tip of the urethra. This is the goal.

If the above procedures do not accomplish the desired results (the ability to see the tip of the urethra) I will suggest the following: If there are no recurrent infections of the foreskin or urinary tract, then one can wait as long as one wants. If, however, there is a single urinary tract infection or infections of the foreskin, then a surgical procedure is needed. This could involve either making a slit in the foreskin (dorsal slit) without circumcision, or a full circumcision. Both are outpatient surgical procedures done by a surgeon with the use of local anesthetic or, if necessary, a light general anesthetic.

If pathological phimosis is present, surgery is usually required.

Paraphimosis

Paraphimosis occurs if the foreskin is retracted behind the glans of the penis and subsequently cannot be brought forward to its normal resting position. If this occurs, the tightness created behind the head of the penis is similar to putting an elastic band tightly around the shaft of the penis. Blood flow returning from the head of the penis to the body is obstructed. Swelling of the head of the penis, as well as its turning dusky in appearance, will result. It usually is quite painful.

If paraphimosis has occurred, place ice on the penis for 5–10 minutes to help decrease the swelling. If still you cannot pull the foreskin over the glans then the child should be taken to the emergency department as quickly as possible. It may require surgical release.

Although this occurs primarily in uncircumcised males, if your child is circumcised and an insufficient amount of foreskin has been removed, then paraphimosis can still occur.

Balanitis

Balanitis is an inflammation of the foreskin. The foreskin becomes red in colour, swollen and tender to touch and pus may be present at the foreskin opening. There is often pain upon urination. The foreskin is tight and cannot be retracted.

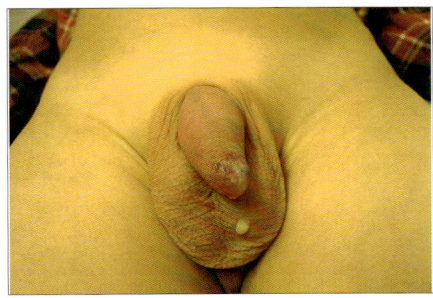
Balanitis

It occurs more often with boys who have a long foreskin and/or phimosis.

Inadequate hygiene or excessive irritation may be what triggers balanitis.

The treatment consists of warm baths, acetaminophen or ibuprofen to relieve the discomfort. A topical antibiotic cream, and often an oral antibiotic is necessary.

If there is recurrent balanitis, a surgical procedure such as a dorsal slit or circumcision may be required.

Penis (Structural Problems)

Hypospadias

In boys, the terminal urethra (where the urine comes out) is normally at the tip of the head of the penis and in the centre.

Hypospadias occurs when the urethral opening is located more toward the bottom of the head of the penis. With hypospadias your son's penis may look partially circumcised.

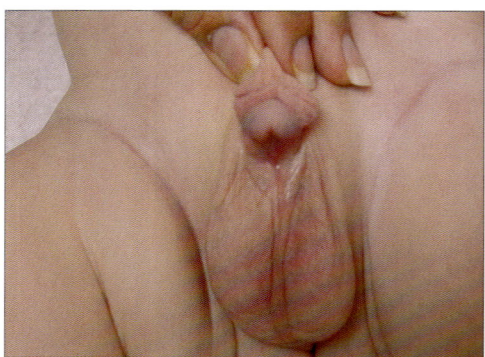
Hypospadias

There is normally only one opening where the urine comes out. However, with hypospadias more than one may be present. You should try to observe to determine which opening has the main stream of urine. If there is a weak urine stream (from birth on) with only dribbling of urine, your doctor should be informed immediately – that is, he should have a good urine stream from birth – "hit you in the eye at 5 paces."

The presence of hypospadias may also indicate an anatomical problem with one or both kidneys. Your doctor may order an ultrasound of the kidneys. Most often there is no problem at all. Sometimes, however, a minor abnormality that requires no treatment may be present.

Hypospadias requires surgical correction. No circumcision should be done on an infant who has hypospadias since the foreskin needs to be intact because it is used during surgical correction.

The surgery is usually done before 6 months of age. More than one surgical procedure may be necessary depending on the number of openings present and degree of severity of the hypospadias.

Chordee

A tight band of tissue, a chordee, may be present on the underside of the penis. This may cause the penis to be difficult to straighten. It may also be the cause of the urine stream going to oneside.

If the band of tissue is considered to be tight, surgical correction is advised and should be done some time during infancy. This is not a surgical emergency.

Posterior Urethral Valves

The urethra is a smooth tube which allows the urine to flow freely as the baby urinates. All boys should be observed as to having a strong urine stream as soon as possible after birth. This is accomplished by a caregiver's observation of the infant during urination (most often during a diaper change or sponge bath). By 3 days of age, if you're uncertain, then allow the baby to sleep with the diaper open. By checking where it is wet you will be able to determine whether he has a strong stream. If there is only a dribbling stream, the presence of posterior urethral valves is suspected.

When there is a problem, the valves present in the urethra narrow the urethra diameter to a point where urine outflow is blocked.

An ultrasound usually demonstrates a dilated bladder.

If this condition is present, it is considered a surgical emergency. If left uncorrected, the urine will back up and dilate the bladder, then the ureters, and finally the kidneys. Permanent damage to the urinary system may occur in time if the valves are not removed as soon after birth as possible.

Penis Hygiene

There are many myths and misconceptions concerning the cleaning of the uncircumcised penis, as well as retraction of the foreskin.

If your son has a good urine stream, then essentially very little has to be done as far as hygiene is concerned. Secretions under the foreskin called smegma are present to help break down adhesions between the foreskin and the head of the penis. This is not a sign of infection or poor hygiene. If there is smegma present on any part of the exposed head of the penis, gently clean it off.

Vigorous retraction of the foreskin is unnecessary. At around 2 years of age, during bathing, you may begin to gently retract the foreskin as far back as you can without any force and no further. Then clean the exposed tip of the penis if visible. If retraction is impossible yet he has a good urine stream, then nothing is required. When he gets older, he will start having natural erections, which will free the foreskin from the head of the penis – the way "Mother Nature" intended. Remember – never try to forcibly pull the foreskin back. There are basically two things a male infant or toddler will almost instinctively not do. The first is to open his mouth when you want him to. The second is to allow you to retract his foreskin.

Picky Eater (Prevention and Treatment)

Good habits started early and constantly reinforced will last a lifetime. This includes feeding habits. Food imprinting or taste preferences begin early in life. I believe you can make vegetables an infant's preference over sweets. Much depends on your presentation by way of facial expression and verbally when you introduce solids. Screwing up your face and using a tone of voice with negative inflections will be picked up by your infant. This may be the only reason why your child dislikes a particular food. I prefer introducing fruit last, after vegetables and meats. The reason for this is that you will never have a problem getting an infant or child to eat something with a sweet taste. At the same time, I do not recommend sweets as a reward at the end of eating a nutritious meal. The only reward for eating should be the satisfaction of having a satiated tummy. When you introduce a new food, it may take up to 10 tries before it is accepted. Also, try to provide the food in a texture that the child prefers and not in the consistency you think he should have.

Remember, you have control over what, where and when your child eats. Your child, however, has control over how much and how often he accepts it. Studies have shown that if a toddler is left on his own to choose from a smorgasbord of food he will end up consuming a balanced, nutritional diet over a period of time.

Eating can be a powerful tool a child can use against you, the parent, if you allow it to happen. Mealtime should never be wartime – a constant struggle. You will not win. Any good army general knows that if you keep losing battles over and over again a better strategy of attack is required. Periodical refusal to eat – a so-called hunger strike – is a baby's common tactic. Why this happens is uncertain. It may take a few weeks before the infant's appetite returns to its previous level. During this time you must be patient. Never force-feed the child. His hunger will eventually dictate the amount ingested.

By 8 to 10 months of age most infants are ready to self-feed – some a little later. Encourage this independence. Forget about the mess – the rewards that you and your child gain by his independence far outweigh the time it takes to clean him, the high chair and anywhere up to 10 feet of the space surrounding him! Whether he feeds himself with his fingers, a utensil, or both does not matter – what is important is that he is doing it on his own. While feeding the infant (after five to six months of age), you should not put the food directly into his mouth. Instead hold it just in front of his mouth and let him lean forward with his head toward you to eat. Do not make mealtime a game. Feeding is for feeding. Trying to entice your infant to eat with various games will eventually have a negative affect on his ability to eat on his own. For an infant or child who refuses to eat or just dilly-dallies at the table, select a time limit for eating – say 15 minutes. When the time is up, take the food away and mealtime is over. Do not offer alternatives. Do not fill him with empty calories. Do not offer him milk or juice. Mealtime is at the table. Do not fall into the trap of running around after him to feed him. A small nutritious snack may be offered between meals. However, he must wait for the next meal to satisfy his hunger. Believe it, when he is hungry enough, food will be consumed. He may have to miss two or three meals until he knows the routine. Stay the course; he will not starve himself. It is going to be a lot harder on you than on him. Trust me – it works, but you must not give in. If you do you will only be giving him control. Is that the way it is supposed to be? Again, dig down deep and resist feeding him. I know how difficult this will be for you. However, within a few days baby will have learned a lesson about mealtime that will make your life a lot simpler. Mealtime should be a pleasure for you both – and not a war zone.

All of baby's caregivers need to be united and aware of the guidelines you have set. Consistency is extremely important in the management of the picky eater. Unfortunately, grandparents have a much different idea as to what and how to feed your child. They tend to undermine even your best wishes as to how the child should be fed – there is often a lack of cooperation. They will attack your parenting skills with a myriad of questions concerning how and what you feed the baby. This will not only be frustrating to you but also raises questions in your own mind that suggests you are doing the wrong thing. This will only result in failure in your attempts to reverse your child's poor eating habits, and more, if there is a lot of contact between the child and non-complying grandparents. The grandparents must be made to understand that what you are trying to do is in the best interest of your child even though it appears to go against their "grand-parental instincts". They need to follow your feeding guidelines and not theirs.

Remember that no child has ever voluntarily starved himself. The best and only appetite stimulant in the world is hunger itself. Vitamins do not stimulate the appetite, nor are there any medicines or magic potions that do. What I commonly see in practice is a parent who tries to satisfy the child's hunger and empty tummy by filling it with lots of milk, water and juice. Up to 30 or 40 oz of milk and juice are ingested daily. Filling his tummy with fluids will certainly suppress his appetite for solids (for the child over one year of age 18 to 20 oz daily of milk is all that is nutritionally necessary). Little or no solids, such as eggs, meats, and cereals containing much-needed iron, will be ingested when appetite is suppressed. This for sure will result in a moderate to severe nutritional anemia (low hemoglobin) within a few months.

When plotting a picky eater on the growth grid, if there is a tailing off in the weight as compared to the height, then there is more at play than just being a picky eater. The same is true if the weight decelerates, falling more than 2 percentiles from the previous rate of growth. This child may have a some disorder which requires further investigation.

What to do?

Remember the previous protocol:

If your child refuses to sit at the table and eat, do not chase him around the room trying to force even a minimal amount of nutrition into him. During mealtime, he either sits in his high chair or a regular chair – nowhere else. Set a time limit for the meal to be finished. Once that time is up mealtime is over and away he goes. Nutritional snacks only may be given between meals (fruit or vegetables).

If sweets and other non-nutritional foods are absent from the home, then empty tummies will not be filled with empty calories.

You must withhold all liquids until small quantities of solids are ingested. Only after that is accomplished can fluids be given. For a child over 1 year of age, 18–20 ounces of milk is sufficient daily.

Make sure that you provide a texture of food that your child will accept (not what you or others think he should accept).

Involve the child in the shopping, preparation of the food, and setting of the table. Make it an adventure. This will instill in him a sense of power over what he eats and will have a positive effect on his eating habits. Add lots of colour and design to the food on his plate. It is amazing how creative you and your child can get to make food visually appealing and attractive. Place small quantities on a large plate (it gives the appearance that there is only a very small quantity of food on the plate). Try cutting or making interesting shapes. Use colourful plates, glasses and cutlery. Soups can be healthfully chock full of vegetables and meats (either puréed or not). Whole wheat pasta with meat, cheese and tomato sauce is also nutritious. Encourage him just to taste and that is all. Set a good example. If he sees you eating it, he will eventually join in. There are many cookbooks available that will provide you with nutritious recipes for children of all ages.

Encourage the use of finger foods from as early as six to eight months of age. As stated, this will encourage independence. Even if no teeth are present, many soft foods can be gummed and swallowed without choking. When serving hot dogs, cut them into thin, long slices (less chance to aspirate). Again, by a year of age, most children should be feeding themselves (with minimal assistance).

You must set a good example. Meals should not be consumed in front of the TV but at the kitchen table. Do not turn your nose up at any particular food. Eating properly with good table manners will be a learning experience for your child.

Ultimately, what and how your child eats depends on you and you alone. As the caregiver, you must and should be the teacher and take the lead – not the child. If you have lost control, you must take the time and put in the effort to regain it. Once this is accomplished, both you and your child will be winners. Bon appétit!

Pinworms (Bowel)

Pinworms are a very common cause of infection of the intestinal tract. Pinworms can occur in all socio-economic groups. They are not the result of poor hygiene. Pinworms are spread from person to person by the fecal-oral route (hand to anus or feces, and then hand to mouth). Crowded living conditions encourage the spread of pinworms.

Symptoms range from hardly any at all to a mild or constant scratching of the anal or vaginal areas.

Any infant female with recurrent inflammation of the vagina or recurrent urinary tract infections should be treated for pinworm. During the night, pinworms crawl out of the anus into the vagina. They carry with them fecal material containing bacteria, which in turn results in infection.

The diagnosis is most often made by clinical symptoms alone. Sometimes a Scotch tape test consisting of a piece of sticky tape touched to the anus in the middle of the night and subsequently examined for pinworms by the laboratory, is done. This will confirm the diagnosis. I seldom do a Scotch tape test and usually treat patients for pinworm if I am suspicious of a pinworm infection.

Treatment is simple and effective (a single dose of medication). If one member of the family has pinworms then all family members should be treated.

Proper handwashing techniques, especially after changing a diaper after a bowel movement, help to prevent the spread of pinworms.

Note: The presence of itchiness in the anal area along with a bright red circular rash around the anus may indicate a streptococcus infection. A culture of the area should be done, and if a strep infection is present, oral antibiotics are required.

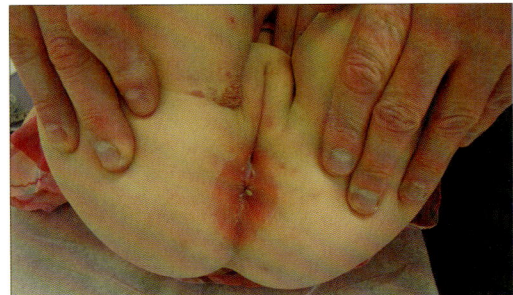
Perianal Strep Infection

Pneumonia

Pneumonia is a serious viral or bacterial infection in the small airways of the lungs. The younger and smaller the infant, the more serious is the concern.

It begins with a mild upper respiratory tract infection (runny nose and cough). Within 2–3 days a fever and cough develops.

The infant becomes progressively more ill:

• With more persistent and severe cough
• With persistence and worsening of the fever
• Displays diminishing appetite
• Has increasing lethargy (becomes less playful)
• Starts breathing using his tummy muscles
• Increases the use of his chest muscles to breathe and visibly shows indrawing of the tissue between the ribs as he breathes
• Experiences an increase in the respiratory rate

These symptoms usually evolve over a period of a few days.

On examination of the child's chest, the physician will hear rales (like the crackling of plastic wrap).

It is very important that the physician listen to the child's chest when the child is quiet no matter how long it takes. This is because it is impossible to assess a child's chest if he is crying.

A chest x-ray should be done to confirm the diagnosis of pneumonia.

Children with viral pneumonia are not as ill as those with bacterial pneumonia. Many children with viral pneumonia have what is called "walking pneumonia". Here the chest x-ray looks a lot worse than the actual clinical condition of the child.

Once the pneumonia has been confirmed by chest x-ray most doctors will treat the child with what they consider the most appropriate antibiotic.

Acetaminophen or ibuprofen is given for fever. Any other medication, such as a cough suppressant, decongestant or expectorant, is not indicated and, in fact, is even contraindicated. If the child is hospitalized, supportive care may be required to maintain hydration.

Pneumonia is frequently overdiagnosed both clinically and by x-ray findings. Remember, the radiologist does not have the patient in front of him, only the x-ray. All too often, increased lung markings are diagnosed by the radiologist as pneumonia.

If there is any confirmed patch of pneumonia on the x-ray, it is advisable that 4–6 weeks later a repeat chest x-ray be done to ensure the process has completely cleared. If this is not done and the child unfortunately gets another bout of pneumonia involving the same area, without this repeat x-ray, the physician will not know if this is a new infection or a flare-up of the previous one.

A child who has recurrent pneumonia should have further investigations to rule out cystic fibrosis, absent IgA, recurrent aspiration or any other underlying cause.

Pyelectasis (Newborn Kidney Obstruction)

Pyelectasis is a condition of the kidneys that is sometimes diagnosed in the fetus during a routine prenatal ultrasound of mother's abdomen; this check is done during the later stages of pregnancy for determining the status of the unborn fetus.

The kidney basically has two parts – the outer part, which consists of the filtration system, and an inner part, the collection system. The collection system is called the renal pelvis. It collects the urine from the filtration system and connects to the ureters, where the urine is passed down into the bladder and from there out of the body into the diaper. The vast majority of infants with the diagnosis of pyelectasis have no underlying reason for the pyelectasis. However, there are basically 2 causes that should be examined in order to be ruled out. The first is urine reflux from the bladder backwards up one or both ureters to the renal pelvis (normally there should be no reflux at all). The second is obstruction at the ureteropelvic junction (the site where the renal pelvis joins the upper end of the ureter).

Pylectasis is a dilation of one or both of the renal pelvi. On an ultrasound a normal renal pelvis measures less than 5 mm in diameter. Those renal pelvi measuring between 5–10 mm are diagnosed as having pyelectasis. Those whose size is greater than 10 mm are usually diagnosed as having hydronephrosis (enlarged kidney), which is a more serious condition.

If this is present after birth, the infant will be put on an antibiotic called trimethoprim to prevent a urinary tract infection.

An ultrasound of the kidneys is usually done within the first week or two of life to determine if the problem has corrected on its own. If so, the medication is stopped and the problem is considered to have been resolved.

If pyelectasis is still present, the infant is usually continued on the preventative antibiotic and the ultrasound is repeated at approximately 1 month of age. If improvement is noted an ultrasound will be done in another 1–2 months' time to ensure that resolution is continuing to occur. If this is the progression, the prophylactic antibiotic will be discontinued.

If, however, the ultrasound (at one month) shows no resolution, or perhaps a worsening of the condition, a voiding cystourethrogram (VCUG) will be done to rule out reflux. During this procedure, a catheter is inserted into the bladder. Dye is injected into the bladder to determine if there is any reflux (backward flow of urine towards the kidney) up one or both of the ureters. If there is significant reflux, the infant will be more susceptible to a kidney infection. The preventative antibiotics will be continued. Ultrasounds will be done every 3 to 4 months to monitor the pyelectasis. At one year of age the VCUG will be repeated. If reflux persists, the child will most likely be referred to a pediatric urologist for an opinion concerning future management of the problem.

In the absence of reflux, if the pyelectasis still persists without showing improvement, or is in fact worsening, then a procedure will be done to rule out an obstruction (at the location where the renal pelvis connects to the upper ureter). This is done by a diuretic lasix renal scan. If obstruction is present a pediatric urologist referral is made and surgery may be required to relieve the obstruction.

In the absence of either obstruction or reflux an ultrasound will be done every 3 to 4 months. Once the process starts to improve, further ultrasounds will be done every 6 months until complete resolution occurs. The prophylactic antibiotic will be discontinued once an improvement is noted.

There are studies in progress to determine the value of the use of prophylactic antibiotics in treating pyelectasis, as well as for recurrent urinary tract infections, with or without reflux. At present this is still a disputed issue within the medical community.

It is my experience that the vast majority of children with pyelectasis clear on their own with no resulting urinary tract infections and without requiring any type of surgical intervention.

Rash (Diaper)

General

The skin is not only the largest "organ" of the body but also the one that is the most exposed to public scrutiny. Any blemish is thought to be undesirable, even diaper rash, which is concealed from everyone except the caregiver. A blemish is a blemish no matter where on the body – not to be tolerated. Caregivers often become upset when any kind of rash appears in any place on the infant's body, no matter how minor, and not uncommonly, even if it is visible only to the parent.

The Common Diaper Rash

Why some babies never seem to have diaper rashes while others do, having a diaper rash almost every time you expose their behinds, is a mystery. Perhaps it is for the same reason that some people figuratively speaking, are thick-skinned and others are thin-skinned!

The intact superficial layer of skin acts as a barrier to prevent the development of a diaper rash. Any break in the barrier, whether it is visible or a "micro-abrasion" (one that cannot be seen), can lead to a diaper rash.

A diaper rash is an inflammatory eruption in the skin of the diaper area. Occasionally, it can become secondarily infected either by a bacteria, or more commonly, yeast.

There are basically 4 predisposing factors that may lead to a breakdown in the skin barrier. These include warmth, moisture, friction (from diaper chafing), contact with urine and fecal material. These irritants promote skin irritation and disruption of the superficial skin barrier. External elements are now able to "invade" the underlying skin – a diaper rash can be the result.

Most commonly, the rash appears on the skin next to the genital area and may include the genitals. The creases may be spared. A diaper rash can vary in intensity from only mild redness in the diaper area to severe excoriation (breakdown) of the skin. When it is excoriated, the baby may cry when urinating or when feces come in contact with the rash. At other times he may be just irritable. Excoriation is most often caused by the ammonia in the urine ("ammoniacal diaper rash").

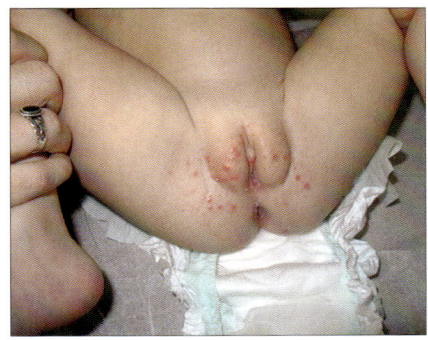

Common Diaper Rash

Treatment

The cornerstone for most treatments is to create a barrier between the rash and the environment when the baby is diapered. This can be accomplished by applying a thick layer of diaper paste or ointment – the thicker the layer the better – like icing on a cake. Cover the barrier with petroleum jelly so as to prevent it from sticking to the diaper.

Disposable diapers are superior to cotton when treating a diaper rash. Change the diaper frequently and use one that is one size larger than you normally use, to prevent irritation by friction. This will lessen any contact of the skin with the urine and feces.

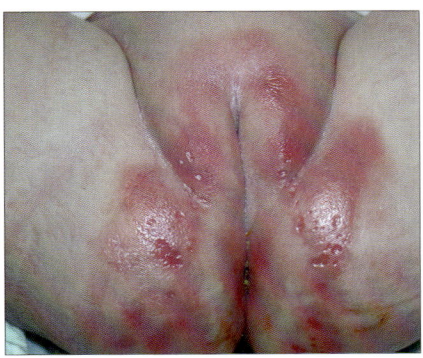

Ammoniacal Diaper Rash

Exposure of the area to the air for as long as possible will help greatly in the healing process. During exposure (no diaper) do not apply any barrier cream, because direct exposure of the skin to the air is important. Living without a diaper is a lot less messy with infant girls than boys (as boys can urinate a much longer distance than their female counterparts), but it is very important for healing.

To avoid further irritation, use mineral oil rather than water to remove any residual barrier cream. Excessive wiping may only irritate the skin and slow the healing process.

The baby may be bathed in lukewarm water, once or twice daily. Use a mild soap that is fragrance free. A fragrance-free bath oil may be added to the bathwater to help soothe the irritated skin. Pat rather than rub the baby dry, using a soft towel. This will avoid further friction.

An alcohol-free unscented diaper wipe or a warm, soft, damp washcloth is the best choice to cleanse the baby's skin between diaper changes.

A mild topical steroid cream or ointment may be necessary to use if there is no response to the above recommendations. This will require a doctor's prescription. The steroid cream should be used sparingly no more than 3 times a day. The barrier paste or ointment is applied on top of the steroid cream. Steroid ointments should not be used for more than 10 to 14 days at any one time. If possible, avoid their use on the scrotum. If there is little or no response after 1 week, another visit to the doctor is advised.

A diaper rash that does not respond to the above conservative management protocol may be caused by a superimposed yeast or bacterial infection. Appropriate topical medications will be prescribed by your doctor.

All common diaper rashes will resolve in time with no lasting scarring. Occasionally, there may be a temporary loss of pigmentation in the skin that is involved. In time a normal colour will return.

Streptococcal anal rash

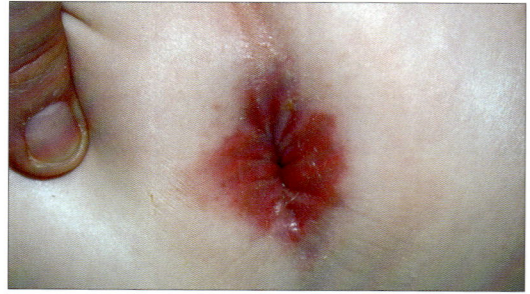

Streptococcal Anal Rash

A fiery-red rash with a well-demarcated edge which surrounds the anus is most likely caused by a streptococcal bacteria infection. Topical antibiotics alone may not work. An oral antibiotic is oftentimes required.

The most serious long-term side effects of having diaper rash are negligible for the infant but can cause great and long-lasting anxiety for the caregiver.

Staphylococcal diaper rash

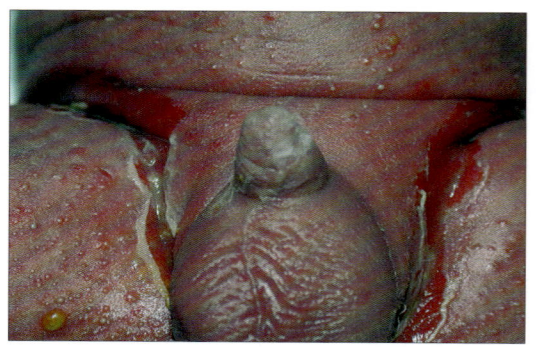

Staphylococcal Diaper Rash

Although uncommon, a staphylococcal diaper rash requires early diagnosis and treatment to prevent further spread.

The rash is very inflamed and "angry" in appearance. There are varying sizes of blister-like lesions that are filled with pus.

A culture of one of the fluid-filled lesions should be done.

The treatment requires the use of both topical and oral antibiotics.

Primarily, all in all, diaper rashes just happen. They are not, for the most part, due to poor hygiene or inattentive care, as your advisory staff will suggest.

Head and Neck Moisture Rashes

From constantly licking the lips, the wet-dry effect may cause irritation. Protect the skin with petroleum jelly or a lip balm.

A frequent rash that may go unnoticed is one that occurs under the chin. Here, moisture from drooling, as well as milk or food spit out of the baby's mouth, may gather. The result is an excoriated rash under his many chins.

Always keep the area under his chin dry. If a rash occurs it is often improved quickly with the use of a cortisone cream prescribed by the doctor. Once the area has improved, lightly powder the area after cleaning and drying carefully.

Ringworm Rash (Tinea Corpus)

Ringworm is a fungal infection of the skin.

It is not caused by poor hygiene, and although contracted by direct contact, it is not very contagious.

It can appear on any site of the body. Commonly, it is found in the groin area.

It appears as a well-demarcated, round skin lesion. If looked at closely the outer red ring may be seen to be composed of numerous tiny blister-like lesions. Inside the circle, the skin is rough, with a pale to light red colour.

It is only mildly itchy.

The treatment is by use of antifungal medication, usually applied twice a day for approximately 3 weeks.

A tinea infection (as ringworm is also called) may commonly be found between the toes of the feet. Its location is strictly between the toes

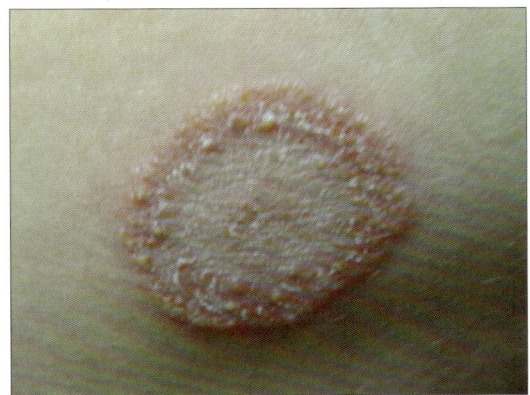

Ringworm Rash

at the base, where the skin of one toe connects to the next. Dry, cracked skin on the toes or the underside of the toes is not ringworm infection; it is just dry skin.

These tinea lesions are usually very itchy.

Treatment for tinea between the toes is the same as for tinea on other areas of the body. Make sure that the child dries between his toes after bathing or swimming as residual moisture encourages fungal infection.

Roseola (Fever and Rash)

This viral illness occurs in infants between 6 months and 20 months of age. It is spread from infant to infant through oral secretions. Its level of contagiousness is very low. The virus does not affect the fetus of pregnant women.

Clinically, it is characterized by a fever lasting for 3–4 days. Very few other symptoms are present other than those associated with the fever, such as fussiness, diminished appetite and lethargy. The fever disappears, and as it does, a fine red rash begins to appear, mainly on the trunk, and spreads to the arms, legs and occasionally the face. The rash then fades in 1–2 days.

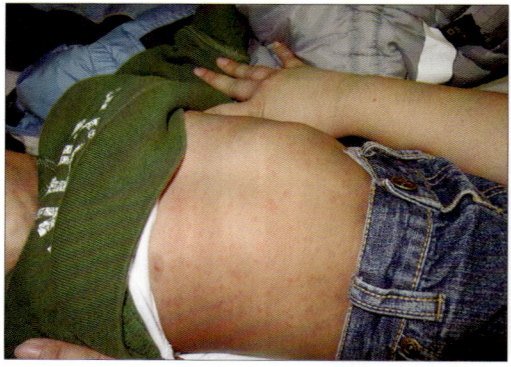 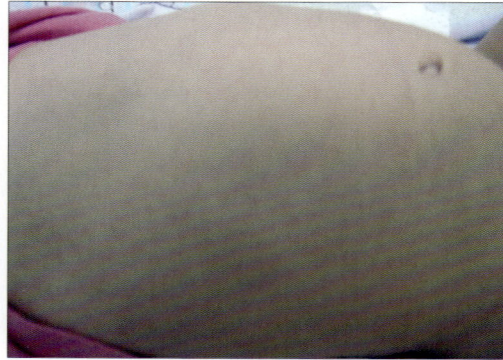

Roseola

Roseola differs from all other viral illnesses by the sequence of events. These events are quite precise. Roseola never presents with fever and rash together. When the fever fades, the rash appears.

Supportive care with the use of acetaminophen or ibuprofen for fever is the only treatment.

The one complication to roseola can be a febrile seizure.

Roseola is contagious during the febrile phase only.

One of the clinical problems in identifying this illness occurs when an antibiotic is prescribed during the fever stage. When the subsequent rash appears, a mistaken diagnosis of drug allergy could be made. Most physicians who deal with children should be able to differentiate between the rash of roseola and that of an allergic reaction. No child should be labelled as having an antibiotic allergy for the rest of his life unless the doctor involved is 100% sure that the child's rash is due to allergy and is not viral in nature. Unfortunately, all too often, this certainty is not the case. The scenario that results is that years later the child may have need of that very antibiotic as the one of choice; however, the parent states that the child has an allergy to it. A roseola rash is not a drug allergy rash. If there is any doubt between the two, allergy skin testing for the antibiotic should be done.

Rotavirus (Gastroenteritis)

Acute gastroenteritis is an illness with symptoms such as vomiting and/or diarrhea and is most often associated with a fever. It can vary in severity from a very mild case to one that leads to severe dehydration, a shock-like state and even death. The younger the infant, the more susceptible he is to becoming dehydrated. A small infant can lose enough fluid and electrolytes with one large single bowel movement to cause moderate to severe dehydration.

Gastroenteritis in infants and toddlers is most often the result of a viral infection. The most common virus is called rotavirus. Over 95% of all children are infected by rotavirus at least once by 5 years of age. In Canada, rotavirus is responsible for at least 60,000 doctor visits, 30,000 emergency room visits and 7000 hospitalizations each year. It affects mainly infants between 6 months of age and 3 years of age. The peak incidence is in the spring. However, it can also occur at any other time during the year.

There is a high likelihood that other members of the family will also develop gastroenteritis because of the contagiousness of the rotavirus infection. Therefore, for a parent, there is not only the illness to deal with but also interruption of work and possible wage loss.

The virus is easily transmitted, most commonly by the fecal-oral route. It may also be airborne. Outbreaks have occurred as a result of contaminated water and food. Unfortunately, rotavirus is very hardy. It can survive on familiar objects such as toys, books and tabletops for extended periods of time (even up to months). It is quite resistant to most common cleansing agents. Medicated soaps are no more effective than tap water alone for hand washing. All this results in rotavirus being easily spread and very difficult to control.

The incubation period for gastroenteritis is 2 to 4 days. It most often begins with vomiting and fever lasting for 2 or 3 days, followed by profuse watery diarrhea for another 4 to 5 days. Transmission to other children may occur from within two days before and up to two weeks after the onset of clinical symptoms. Some degree of dehydration occurs in 80% of patients.

There is a vaccine available to protect your child from a rotavirus infection. It is a live oral vaccine. It offers 98% protection against severe rotavirus gastroenteritis. Two to three doses are required (depending on the vaccine used). They are given 2 months apart. It is best started between 6 and 12 weeks of age and completed by 32 weeks of age.

It is a very safe vaccine with negligible side effects. It offers excellent protection against a potentially serious bout of gastroenteritis due to rotavirus.

With the vaccines now being used, there is no connection between the administration of rotavirus vaccine and a bowel obstruction called intussusception.

Safety (Home)

We all take it for granted that as caregivers we would never intentionally or unintentionally do harm to our children. Unfortunately, on a daily basis, there are thousands of accidents that involve children, many of which could have been avoided if preventative measures had been taken.

When it comes to safety, think of 4 things – liquids, heights, size and reachables. Always remember that even the smallest of infants can move like lightning. Accidents happen in "the blink of an eye".

The best way you can "safety-proof" your home, in my opinion, is to get down on your hands and knees and crawl around. This is what the baby sees and you'll get a better understanding of what he can reach and where danger lurks. Never underestimate the skill, determination and reach of your infant or toddler when he wants something.

Infants have an inherent curiosity. This instinct starts as early as 3 months of age. They see, hear, touch and taste everything (except food!) As they become more mobile and better coordinated, their explorations expand. Nothing is sacred – anything that is graspable is grasped. It is then thoroughly examined by touch, sight and smell – then finally, the test taste.

To digress for a moment – this exploration should be interfered with only when it is necessary to keep your child out of harm's way. Their little minds are taking in and processing huge quantities of knowledge on a daily basis. This process is called learning by experience. What is learned will more than make up for the little bit of harmless dirt that finds its way into your infant's mouth.

Liquids

Always check the temperature of bathwater before immersing the baby in it. Never run tap water while the baby is in the bath. An infant, before gaining head control, can drown in as little water as would fill a saucer. Never leave your infant or toddler alone for even a second while he is in the bathtub.

All liquids that potentially can be ingested, such as cleaning fluids, soaps, paint thinners, etc. must be kept out of the child's reach. They are best kept locked in a cupboard.

Heights

Heights include the distance the baby may fall from a bed, change table or couch, as well as down stairs. Be sure to monitor your child's proximity and interaction with these hazards.

Size

Size refers to anything small enough that could go into the baby's mouth or ears or nose and potentially be swallowed or aspirated, or placed in one of the body's openings.

Reachables

Reachables are anything your child can reach, pull or grab onto. Never underestimate the agility of your child. These reachables include anything on tabletops, kitchen and bathroom counters, on stovetops or in cupboards, tablecloths that can be pulled and electrical outlets. Televisions on tables are especially dangerous.

It is up to you to do your homework and make your home as child-friendly and safe as possible. As your child's mobility increases new safety measures must be put in place.

Childproofing in any other environment that your child will spend time in is also of extreme importance – grandparents' home or home daycare are two examples.

Having a first-aid kit available is advised. It is also recommended that all caregivers take a cardiopulmonary resuscitation (CPR) course with refreshers every few years.

Have your local poison control centre phone number handy.

There are many books devoted entirely to making your home safe. There are also many companies that will inspect your home and safety-proof it accordingly.

Safety – Summer Ouchies

Ah, summertime, fun at last. But with summer lurks hidden danger ready to spoil your child's day: a hidden root to trip over, a friendly-looking weed to "rash upon you", a bug set on bugging you and so on. Many of these nasties cannot be avoided. The use of sunscreen, insect repellent and allergy medication will help minimize 3 summer woes.

Remember, children will explore everything. They will venture where you and I would fear to tread. They have few inhibitions. Therefore, they need to be under your constant vigilant supervision. Remember my old adage – "If in doubt don't let them do it!"

The following is a list of some common hazards. To be on the safe side, if you are not sure, always seek medical attention to prevent possible further complications.

Foreign Bodies

Splinters – If part of the splinter is sticking out of the skin remove it with tweezers. Pull it out in the same direction as it entered the skin. If it is embedded under the skin surface, first clean the skin, and then, using a sterilized sewing needle, lift off the skin above the splinter (it will be easier if the child is looking the other way). Once the splinter is exposed, extract it with tweezers. If you feel that it is embedded too deeply and would be difficult to remove, leave it alone. Eventually it will work its way out on its own.

Foreign bodies in the eyes – Stand behind the child, tilt the head back, open the eyelid (you may need help) and rinse with a glass of warm water. If the child feels that the object is still present, have him look in all directions. Look for a small speck in the white of the eye. Dab the speck with the corner of a piece of tissue. If this is unsuccessful, seek medical help. If you are unable to see a foreign body or if it is visible in the pupil (dark part of the eye), seek medical attention.

Insect stingers – Do not break the fluid sac if it is still intact. Remove with tweezers. If an insect has entered the nose, have the child blow his nose as hard as possible. If it is still present and can be seen, remove it with tweezers. If it is in the ear and you can see it, then remove it with tweezers. When in doubt, seek medical attention.

Burns

First-degree burns shows as redness in the skin alone. Reduce the pain by using cold water compresses, acetaminophen or ibuprofen and any over-the-counter topical burn pain reliever if necessary.

Second-degree burns involve the whole outer epidermis, resulting in blistering. Do not break the blister. It acts as a bandage. Cold compresses, as well as acetaminophen or ibuprofen, will help reduce the discomfort. If it is dirty, cover it with a sterile gauze after gently cleaning with warm, soapy water. Change the gauze daily. If it is difficult to remove the gauze, soak the area in warm water. This will help loosen the gauze, making it easier to remove. It will take approximately 5 days for new skin to form. At that time any remaining blisters may be safely broken and the dead skin removed with sterile scissors. The area involved will be quite sensitive for 1 to 2 weeks. Leave it uncovered after 5 days. If at any time it appears to be infected (presence of pus, bad odor or spreading of the redness around the burn area) then seek medical attention.

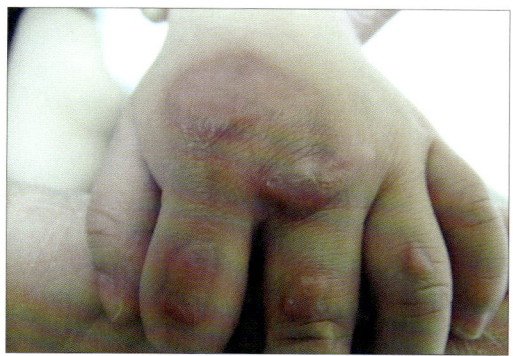

Fireplace Burn

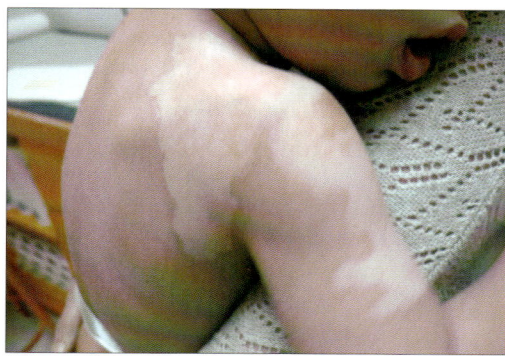

Liquid Burn (3 Months)

Third-degree burns involve the deeper areas of the skin. They occur more often with dry burns (from barbecue tops, hot coals or ovens, for example). They are often deeper than you may think from their appearance. Cool them down with cold water. Cover the area with a cold cloth. If the hand or foot is affected, cover the involved limb with a plastic bag. Seek medical attention at once.

Insect Bites

For the most part these require little or no care. Ice packs applied to the area will minimize swelling. Over-the-counter anti-itch medication may be applied (saliva works as well) to prevent scratching. Cut the child's fingernails short to prevent scratching and possible secondary infection. Remember, the area around the eye is like a dry sponge. A reaction to a small insect bite here can lead to major swelling around the eye. The eye itself may be closed. Do not panic. Although it looks terrible it is most often nontender and it appears many times worse than it actually is. Apply ice if possible for 10 minutes at a time. In a few days, the swelling will disappear. An

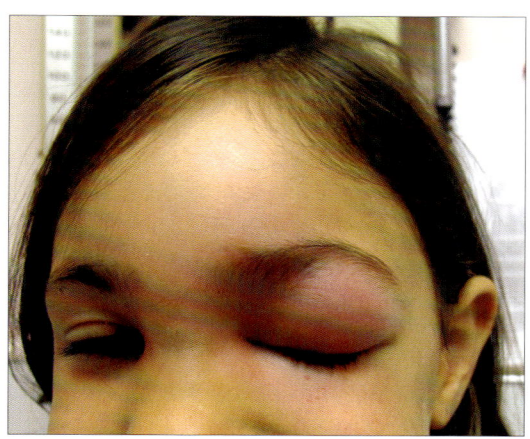

Insect Bite

antihistamine given orally will help to diminish swelling, as well as itchiness.

Trauma

Head – The skull is very thick and difficult to crack (especially the front and back of the skull). The sides of the skull, over the ears, however, have thin bone plates (especially in infants and toddlers). Seek medical attention if there is soft-tissue swelling after trauma in these areas. Other symptoms that require medical attention are loss of consciousness, loss of memory of the event (if the child is old enough to talk), vomiting 2 or 3 times, persistent drowsiness, clear fluid or blood leaking from the nose or ear, behavioural changes, persistent headache or visual disturbance.

If none of the above is present, apply ice if necessary. Acetaminophen or ibuprofen can be used for pain control. Maintain a normal diet. Light activity only is recommended for the child for one day after the incident. The usual naps during the day are allowed. If the child seems to be okay at bedtime you do not have to wake him up at all. (See also Head Injury)

Twists

Oftentimes it is difficult to tell whether a twist has resulted in a strain or a fracture. It takes a lot of force to break a bone. Most finger, toe, ankle and wrist injuries are only sprains. They can only truly be assessed once the child has stopped crying and allows you to investigate the injury. Unfortunately, with children (as well as with many adults) the dramatics of an injury often outweigh its severity. Injuries are most likely only sprains if there is no obvious deformity. Swelling over the ankle bone after a twisting injury is most commonly a sprain and not a fracture. If the child allows you to put pressure on the injured area and move it, the likelihood of a fracture is minimal. An acronym for the treatment of a sprain is R.I.C.E. – Rest, Ice, Compression (if swollen) and Elevation above the level of the heart.

If the child is reluctant to move the limb, look for any bony deformity or pain on deep pressure. If this is present, immobilize the area with a splint (a piece of wood, for example, or part of a hockey stick or a magazine) and seek medical assistance. With the upper limbs, if there is no obvious trauma to the arm and the child is still reluctant to lift it, a fracture of the collarbone may be present. It will be tender to light pressure. Soreness in the elbow area can result after a pull (such as being swung while being held below the elbows). This action can result in dislocation in the elbow joint. It is called a "pulled elbow". A sudden pull forward while being held by a hand or wrist can cause the same. Put the arm in a sling and seek medical assistance.

At the beach your child should wear beach shoes. These will help prevent cuts, twists and stubbed toes.

Nosebleeds

Nosebleeds can occur spontaneously or from minor trauma (picking, or a blow to the nose). Often they occur while the child is sleeping. In this instance the child partially wakes up and unknowingly puts his finger in his nose and that results in a nosebleed. Many times, the child does not wake up and in the morning blood is noticed on the pillowcase.

To minimize the swallowing of blood, have the child lean forward with his head between his legs. Swallowing blood can lead to vomiting and restart the nosebleed. If possible, have him blow his nose to remove any blood clots from his nose. Pinch the nose at the tip for 5–10 minutes by the clock. Ice placed over the bridge of the nose will help.

If you are unable to stop the blood flow, seek medical assistance.

Tooth Trauma

If the tooth is not loose nothing has to be done. If it is loose (5 mm or more) or driven into the gums, a dentist should be consulted.

If a primary tooth is lost, this is not a problem – let the tooth fairy handle it. If a secondary tooth is lost, clean it with warm water and if possible put it back into the socket. If you are unable to do this, transport it in milk or saliva. The quicker a dentist is seen, the better the chance of successful reimplantation.

If, following tooth trauma, approximately 1–3 weeks later there is tenderness or swelling in the area around the tooth, then an infection may be present or the tooth may be cracked beneath the surface of the gums. Consult a dentist. If the colour of the tooth slowly (over weeks) turns grey the tooth has most likely died. Your dentist may extract it or leave it in as a "spacer".

Lacerations of the tongue, gums or inner lips will self-heal. Suturing is not required.

Wound Bleeding

Clean the area with warm, soapy water and apply direct pressure until the bleeding stops. If suturing is thought to be required, then medical assistance is necessary. If no assistance is needed, clean and cover the wound for 3 or 4 days.

Sore Ear

A child may complain of a sore ear after swimming. Gently pull on the ear upward or push on the soft tissue just in front of the ear canal opening. If it is tender, then the child has swimmer's ear (infection of the ear canal). Ear drops are required for 5-7 days. The swimming can be resumed when the child feels better.

Rashes

During the summertime I am confronted with a "gazillion" different rashes. Most of these are difficult to diagnose. If the rash is very itchy and the child has been playing in a wooded area, poison oak or ivy is likely the culprit (especially if the rash presents on the exposed parts of the body). Clean the area with soapy water and use cool compresses and topical anti-itch preparations; oral antihistamines may also be used. Baking soda in tepid water baths is comforting (half a box in the bathwater). Keep the child's fingernails cut short.

If the rash worsens, spreads or seems infected (with pus or a bad odor) seek help. Topical or oral antibiotics, as well as topical cortisone, may be required.

Food Poisoning

Use safe drinking water and wash all fruits and vegetables well. Cook meat until 66°C–82°C (150°F–180°F). Hamburger meat, as well as chicken, should not be pink inside. Discard any food left unrefrigerated for more than 2 hours (one hour if the temperature is over 32°C (90°F) outside). Any cream, other dairy products or mayonnaise should be eaten or discarded after 1 hour.

In conclusion, it is impossible to cover every potential mishap in such a limited space. My advice to you is "If in doubt, don't do it" or "Throw it out." Have a good first-aid kit available along with a first-aid book. Take a CPR course (or refresher course if more than 3 years has elapsed since the last one).

During any mishap someone must keep calm and use common sense; always err on the side of safety.

P.S.: Keep those shoelaces tied – with a double (maybe triple) knot and have a great and safe summer.

Safety (Top-10 Summer Tips)

We take our children to the beach. We sit and watch in wonderment as the child fills his mouth with sand when we cannot even pry his mouth open to nibble on a carrot or taste a teaspoon of peas. Small insects are picked up, squashed between the fingers and then popped into the mouth – unbelievable! Pebbles and twigs are put into every imaginable opening in his body with great delight. How he is able to get enough dirt under his fingernails or in between his toes to plant a garden is mind-boggling.

1. **Sun protection** – For all children over 4 months of age, apply a sunscreen with a 30 sun protection factor (SPF) or more, 15 minutes before going out into the sun, and reapply frequently.

2. **Water safety** – You cannot take your eyes off your child while he is swimming or playing in or near water. An infant can drown in as little water as would fill a soup bowl. Swimming lessons can be started at 6 months of age. However, no child, no matter how proficient a swimmer he is, should be left unattended. Be careful with the use of flotation devices. Ensure that they are government approved, the proper size for the weight of your child, and well secured when in the water.

3. **Playground safety** – Ensure that your child uses age-appropriate playground equipment and has been instructed on how to use it safely. Protective helmets may be a nuisance but may prevent serious head injuries.

Age-appropriate "streetproofing" with regard to interacting with other people is essential and should be frequently reviewed.

4. **Burns** – Nothing is yummier than a barbecued hotdog or hamburger. An accidental burn, however, can be very painful and may lead to permanent scarring.

5. **Food poisoning** – Summertime is picnic time. Remember that many foods spoil if left out in the heat or even at room temperature too long or if not adequately cooked on the barbecue. Unconsumed food should be discarded after 3 hours at room temperature and after 1-1/2 hours if outside (sooner the higher the temperature is).

6. It is the caregiver's responsibility to ensure that the child is wearing the proper protective gear recommended for the activity.

7. Always have your child carry identification – first name and phone number.

8. While at the beach, I suggest your child wear water shoes to protect his feet.

9. For children over 6 months of age, DEET should be used if insects are a problem (sunscreen first, with DEET on top).

10. Take a first-aid kit with you for any outdoor adventures.

Sinusitis

Sinusitis in children is uncommon and far too often it is an overdiagnosed infection.

There are basically 4 sinuses in the skull. The maxillary sinuses are behind the cheekbone area. The frontal sinuses are behind the skull of the forehead. The ethmoid sinuses are between the eyes behind the upper nasal area. The sphenoid sinuses are behind the ethmoid sinuses.

The sinuses are not fully formed at birth. They become enlarged to their normal adult size over a period of several years. The maxillary sinuses are the sinuses that most commonly become infected. Up until 2-3 years of age the maxillary sinuses are very small. Because they are not as yet fully developed, sinusitis in a child under 3–4 years of age is very uncommon.

The clinical symptoms of sinusitis can vary from very mild to severe. There remains no 100% consensus on how to diagnose sinusitis in children.

A persistent yellow-green nasal discharge lasting for more than 2 weeks is the most common symptom for the clinical diagnosis of sinusitis. X-rays of the sinuses are difficult to interpret. A cloudy-looking sinus on an x-ray may just be tears and not infected fluid. The only diagnostic tool to confirm sinusitis would be a CT scan of the sinuses. This, of course, is completely impractical. The end result is that the child usually gets treated with a course of antibiotics. The child usually improves; however, it may be just the natural course of the illness and not the result of using an antibiotic. In my opinion, it is preferable that these children be treated with a saline nasal rinse 3 times daily for at least a week. If, after this approach, the discharge persists, then perhaps a course of antibiotics should be considered.

The clinical diagnosis of sinusitis is easier to make if the following symptoms are present:

- Pain over the sinus area
- Fever
- Headache in the infected sinus area
- Persistent green nasal discharge
- Tenderness with pressure over the sinus area
- Symptoms are usually on one side only but can be on both
- Soft-tissue swelling under the eye

With these symptoms the diagnosis of sinusitis is probable. The child should be treated with a course of antibiotics along with the use of nasal rinses. Acetaminophen and/or ibuprofen are used for fever and pain control.

To reemphasize, help clear the nasal passages and even the sinuses with the use of a nasal saltwater rinse. Three or more times a day is usually all that is needed.

Remember, a yellow-green nasal discharge does not necessarily mean that there is a bacterial infection. Viral infections can cause the same.

Sleep

Many "experts" have written on the subject of sleep and your baby. Each may have his own way to help your baby have a long, uninterrupted sleep at night. Unfortunately, what works for one may not work for another. That is why there are many different techniques which try to help you manage any sleep issues that may occur. All that has been written on sleep has one common denominator – starting early after the first months of life with consistent, structured sleep routines will result in fewer sleep concerns later on. The following is the way I see it.

Despite what you may have read, heard, or thought, no otherwise healthy infant has ever come to harm by not sleeping. Unfortunately, I cannot say the same for the caregivers. They are the ones who truly suffer.

The question most frequently asked by new parents is, "When is my baby going to sleep through the night?" Parents long for the time when they can just climb into bed at the day's end and have a full night's sleep. A grand thought indeed! When? Ultimately it depends on you, so read on.

Here is my non-scientific formula for how much sleep your baby needs: the amount needed equals the amount you think he needs. Interestingly enough, this also calculates to be exactly the amount you need. Unfortunately, the infant may not agree with this tabulation. After all, his total workload all day and all night is to eat, sleep, and cry. With no job, no responsibilities, life is great! Great for him, but not so great for mom and dad!!!

Infants are self-centred. They are not aware of your needs. Day or night – it makes no difference to them. They want what they want when they want it. It is your job to provide what they need when they need it.

There are many articles written that tell you how much sleep the baby requires depending on his or her age. How this is calculated is beyond me. Each baby is an individual and, as such, has individual needs and accordingly seeks the amount of sleep he requires. You can never force a baby to sleep more. Then how much sleep does an infant require? I will answer this question with another question: "How much wood could a woodchuck chuck if a woodchuck could chuck wood?" It makes just as much sense as the above question. Who really knows?

I am a firm believer that you cannot spoil your baby during the first few months of life. Your job then, is to meet your baby's needs. This is a most important time for bonding. However, many of the baby's needs after 4 months become wants. Between 4 to 7 months of age you must pay close attention to separating the needs from the wants. If you cater to the wants, they then become habits. Bad habits started early and reinforced over a period of time become difficult to break. The longer you wait, the more difficult it becomes to break an ingrained behavioural pattern. A sleep problem is by far the most common need that becomes a want and then a habit. Once an infant has taken control over his sleep pattern, the result is the "gotcha" syndrome. That is, the baby has "got" you. You have inadvertently given the power that is yours to your baby. You soon become sleep deprived. There is confusion as to what you should do, especially with all the unsolicited advice offered by your "advisory staff." Common sense becomes harder to use. Your coping skills become further eroded. In time, you yourself could require professional help – or at least something to calm your nerves.

Let's rewind the tape and go back to the beginning to see what we can possibly do to prevent all of this. First, ask how much sleep your baby needs? The answer – there is no answer. He basically needs what he gets, whether it is 6 or 16 hours a day. Remember that every infant is different, so never compare one with the other.

Routines should be started early. Infants thrive on routines and structure. It is very important that all caregivers maintain the same routine. I cannot over-stress the importance of routines and structure in all aspects of your infant's life. Routines started early in life and continually reinforced will last a life-time. Therefore, getting off to a good start is important for your infant and for your sanity. It's inevitable that you will not be happy if you allow your infant to take the control of sleep routines from you.

Remember your baby should be encouraged to sleep on his back until at least 8 months of age to reduce the possibility of SIDS.

I feel very strongly that the actual falling asleep should occur in the crib and not in your arms.

Because of concerns over their newborn baby, many anxious parents will allow the baby to sleep in a bassinet alongside their bed. This is also very convenient if you are breastfeeding, and is fine. The only problem is that every time the baby moves you will be woken up, so it is not such a good idea, especially if you become sleep deprived. Although it may be inconvenient to place the child elsewhere, I personally prefer that the baby sleep in his own room. Using a baby monitor will help you to keep in contact with him when he cries. The final choice is yours. The bottom line is that if you prefer the baby to share your room in a bassinet, that is an option. However, sharing your bed is a no-no. (Also see Bed Sharing)

As with adults, during sleep the baby will alternate between light and deep sleep. This cycle repeats itself throughout the night. When he's in a deep sleep, you could fire off a cannon and the baby would probably not wake up. When the infant is in the light sleep stage, he has two options of behaviour. He can "self-soothe" himself and go back into a deep sleep or wake up. He will only wake up if he has something to gain by it. This gain is usually to receive your attention by being picked up, cuddled or perhaps fed. Remove this reward and he will most likely put himself back to sleep or not wake up at all. This, however, can be a very difficult task for parents to carry out. There is a maternal need to "rescue" the baby. It is interesting that fathers do not have this same drive and are more prepared to allow the baby to cry (even when the mom is the one to go to the baby). This can become a source of contention between parents.

If a sleep problem develops, it is very important that both parents be of the same mindset about handling the problem, and carry out the same plan of action. If a caregiver cannot tolerate listening to her child cry, and continually "saves" him, then she is not ready to initiate a preventative plan. Read on.

Sleep issues are more common in infants who are breastfed as compared to those who are formula fed. By 4 months of age, once fed, a baby should be able to sleep 5–8 hours at night before waking for his next feed. With breastfed infants, there may be some doubt as to how much milk was delivered at the last feed. As a result, when the baby wakes up it is your maternal instinct to put him to the breast. The baby soon settles and falls asleep (usually in mother's arms). This scenario is repeated numerous times during the night. Is the baby truly hungry? The answer, most often, is that these "feeding times" are not for his nourishment but are baby's attempts to use you as a "human pacifier". From his point of view, this is great. However, it is not so good from yours. You have just created the "gotcha" syndrome – that is, the baby has got you. If this is the case, I suggest that at the last evening feed, you "top him up" with a supplement of either expressed breast milk or formula – as much as he wants. This may not help the problem of the frequent waking up; however, at least you will know that the baby's tummy is full and he is not crying from hunger. If hunger is a reason for waking, a supplement may be started at one month of age. Most infants who upon awakening, begin to cry and then stop as soon as they are picked up, do so for attention. The hungry infant usually will not stop crying until fed. I must admit, however, that it is sometimes difficult to distinguish between a cry for attention and one of hunger – so if in doubt – feed. Your guilty conscience about your baby being hungry will override everything else. Convincing a mom that she is just being used as a pacifier is a difficult idea to promote.

Between 4 to 6 months of age the baby should be getting up no more than once or at the most twice a night. When he wakes up, allow him to cry for 5 to 10 minutes. Try not to pick him up.

Often, an infant, at about 8 months of age, will wake at 6 a.m. ready to go. You, however, wish to sleep another hour or so. You may have a hard time convincing him to go back to sleep. Putting toys in his bed for him to play with may encourage quiet play while you get a little more shut-eye. Change the toys on a regular basis so he is not bored. A quick feed and a diaper change may also help. If not, your day has begun.

The above is a rough guideline for what normally happens. Any sleep time lasting longer is a bonus.

Here are some suggestions that may help if an infant continues to cry and will not settle on his own:

• If the baby is using your breast as a pacifier, instead of the breast offer him a few ounces of sugar water: 1 teaspoon of sugar in 90 cc (3 ounces) of water. After a few nights, switch to plain water. Then slowly reduce the amount offered. He will soon realize that this is not what he really wants and will put himself back to sleep. Your partner can play a very active role in changing this frequent-waking-habit.
• Swaddle (wrap) the baby tightly (for infants under 4 months of age).
• Play soft music or white noise (e.g., the hum of a fan; a CD with the sound of rain, rushing water or waves hitting the beach).
• Rock the crib gently (stay out of sight).
• Rub his tummy and sing to him (works best if infant is under 3 months of age). With older infants, if they see you, they want you.
• Lie down on the floor beside the crib so he is unable to see you and keep repeating the sound that he became used to hearing while in your tummy – shhhh-shhhhh.
• Try Dr. Harvey Karp's 5 S's – Swaddle tightly, hold him with his back against your Stomach, Stick your finger or pacifier in his mouth, Sway gently from side to side and keep repeating the shhhh- shhhh-shhhh sound.
• Leave your scent in his crib. This can be accomplished in a number of ways. You can rub one of your worn T-shirts on his sheets. Another method is, when drying his sheets and pajamas, to put one of your worn (not washed) T-shirts in the dryer. With an infant over 8 months of age, leave one of your T-shirts to snuggle.
• Try a pacifier – remember, however, that you are the one who has to keep getting up to pop it back into his mouth each time it pops out. In the short term it's fine; however, in the long term it's not a very good strategy.
• Stand by the door, out of sight. Keep repeating the shhhh-shhhh sound loudly. Intermittently throw in key phrases such as "you are okay, you're fine, everything is okay" and "go to sleep". Do this until the baby falls asleep. Do not allow the baby to see you. It may take up to an hour or longer before the baby goes back to sleep. If the baby wakes up, repeat the process each time. On the second night do the same with the shhhh-shhhh sound. Keep the key phrases to a minimum. Repeat throughout the night as necessary. By the third night you probably will only have to say the shhhh-shhhh sound once or twice before he goes back to sleep. By the fourth night he should be sleeping throughout the night.

The biggest mistake that you could make, in my opinion, is to bring the baby into your own bed. You will certainly not be happy with the results. You may get a good night's sleep but you're going to have a tremendous struggle later when you are ready to return baby to his crib. You may be ready to transfer him to his own crib or bed, but, believe me, his views will be quite different. The only proven advantage of having the baby in bed with you is that it is an excellent method for birth control – all intimacy between spouses disappears.

Again, the actual falling asleep should occur in the crib. It really does not depend on the state of wakefulness that the baby is in when you put him down into the crib (that is, drowsy, fully alert or crying).

By 7 to 8 months of age the baby should be sleeping through the night. By this age the training of the baby to learn to put himself back to sleep should have been accomplished. Unfortunately, it is often during this period of time that the opposite occurs. It is the baby who trains the parent. How often I have heard a parent complaining that the infant does not sleep! The caregiver cannot stand to hear the baby cry. The baby is quickly picked up with the first peep and after a period of time cannot be left alone even for a short stretch. As a result, the infant is up several times during the night and it is quite difficult for the parent to settle him. No sooner is he put down than the whole cycle starts again. The only way the baby falls asleep is if he is being fed, walked or cuddled, is allowed to lie on the living room couch or sits on dad's lap watching TV. He is everywhere and anywhere except where he should be – learning to sleep – in the crib. Parents soon become exhausted and spend the whole night and day walking around like zombies (usually it's mom). Finally, out of desperation to get some sleep, they commit the ultimate no-no by bringing the baby into bed with them. Not too long after that one parent (usually dad) moves out into another room. Please do not fall into this trap. Eventually, at some later time, your child is going to have to learn to sleep on his own. The longer you wait to teach the baby this important lesson of putting himself back to sleep, the more difficult it will become. If the infant is crying and stops as soon as he is picked up, then you have the "gotcha syndrome". As mentioned before, the baby has learned that from a light sleep pattern, he can wake up, cry, and get the attention he demands rather than go back to sleep. What do you think he is likely to do? Out of habit he will wake up – it's you-know-who that has conditioned him to do so.

Some parents just cannot let their infant cry. This is true even though their doctor has advised them that no baby has ever harmed himself by crying. The only long-term adverse psychological effects of infant's prolonged crying will be on the caregiver – not the infant. For the parent who is not ready to take the power back from the baby, all I can do to reassure you is to say that at some time, between now and the child's honeymoon, things will improve – believe me, mothers out there, you will definitely not be accompanying them – I guarantee it.

If all other methods have failed and you are ready (both physically and emotionally) to teach the child to sleep through the night without waking, then I recommend "Ferberization". Again, if you are not physically and emotionally ready to do it then do not attempt at this time. Do not start this technique before 7 months of age. The following is the plan: If the baby is crying when he is put in the crib, or wakes up crying after falling asleep, wait 15 minutes. At that time go to the door of his room to have a brief look at him. Try not to let him see you. If all is well, even if he is standing up, leave. If he has vomited, clean up and change him with no additional communication and do it as quickly as possible, then put him back in the crib and leave. Repeat this process, adding 10 minutes – that is, wait 25 minutes before checking on the baby. Keep adding 10 minutes to the routine each time. Carry out this routine nightly. Remember, try not to let the baby see you. In 3 nights or sooner the baby will have learned that he will not be picked up. Then he will go back from a light sleep to a deep one on his own because he has nothing to gain by waking up. Remember that if you end up picking him up after waiting for 2 or 3 hours of crying, you might as well have done so after 5 minutes – you are not ready for "Ferberization" yet.

A note to the parents who decide to bed share (sleep with the baby in their bed) to promote nurturing and bonding and to make it more convenient to breastfeed: a number of studies have shown that whether you co-sleep or not makes little difference for any behavioural outcome as the child grows older. Remember, with co-sleeping there is a 40-fold increase in infant mortality by strangulation or suffocation when compared to those infants who are left to sleep in the crib. The highest incidence occurs in infants who are less than 3 months of age. Here are some safety tips for co-sleeping: Never co-sleep in a waterbed. The bottom sheet should be tight. There should be no space between the headboard or bedside tables and the bed. The side of the bed should not be against a wall. There should be no fluffy cushions and duvets, and be aware that cords from blinds can become easily become wrapped around your infant's neck. Do not smoke in bed or have alcohol before going to sleep. If you are a deep sleeper and are heavy-breasted, co-sleeping is definitely not advised. It is better to share the room than to share the bed – the baby sleeps in a crib beside your bed.

Do not leave a night bottle of milk, juice or any sweetened drink for the baby to graze on during the night. Similarly, never allow baby to suck on a pacifier sweetened with corn syrup or honey. These will surely lead to gum and dental disease – if necessary, leave unsweetened water only. A bad habit once initiated will be difficult to break, so don't start it!

Do not hang a pacifier around the baby's neck– strangulation is a potential.

To prevent flattening of the back of the head, change the baby's sleep position, with his head at one end of the crib one night and at the other end the next night. During waking hours allow the baby to have lots of "tummy time". This will keep the weight from continually being put on the back of his head.

For the older child who continues to get out of his bed and run to you in order to be settled, I suggest the following:

• Place a light chair beside his bed and sit there until he falls asleep. Keep any conversation and touching to a minimum. Do not lie in the child's bed with him. Repeat this for 3 nights.

- Do the same for the next 3 nights, but without any conversation, physical contact or looking at the child.
- For the next 4–5 days move the chair 1 or 2 m from the bed. Sit there quietly with as little eye contact or conversation as possible. When he falls asleep, leave the room. If he wakes up and calls you, then return.
- Next, move the chair to the doorway and repeat as above.
- Lastly, leave the chair in the doorway and inform your child that you will not be sitting in the chair, but that you will remain close by if he needs you. If he does need you, then sit in the chair, but do not enter his room.

With this method you should be able to "wean" your child slowly from the need of having you by his bedside to comfort him in order that he falls asleep. The process may take a short time for some and longer for others. Do not become frustrated. Patience is required.

If you have fallen into the trap of allowing your child to leave his room and sleep with you, I recommend the following (only when you, the parents, are fully ready to break the habit):

- Have the child sleep next to you in a sleeping bag or portable light bed. Do not allow him to sleep in your bed.
- Once this has been accomplished, move his bed halfway to your door.
- Again, once accomplished and when there is compliance, move his bed to the doorway.
- Every few days move his bed slowly down the hall and into his room until the final destination of the "trip" is reached – his own bed.

The most drastic solution if all else fails is to put him directly into his own bed: every time he comes out, without conversation take him back. If it continues, you tell him that if he leaves his room you will have to shut the door, but if he does not get up you will leave it open. If this does not work then you must shut the door and either hold it closed or lock it. This is, perhaps, the most difficult thing a parent can do. For a few nights you may find him sleeping at the foot of the door in the morning. Eventually he will learn that you mean business and that there is no point in getting out of bed – he will gradually learn this lesson. Believe me, it is going to be as hard on you as it is on him – but stay the course and don't back down.

If, despite your best efforts, you are not succeeding and are completely frustrated but still wish to do something concerning your child's sleep patterns and routines, I suggest you hire a sleep doula.

In the end, try your best. It could always be worse – you could have quadruplets!

Snoring (Adenoids and Sleep Apnea)

During sleep, all the tissues surrounding the upper airway relax. As a result the upper airway becomes narrowed. If the narrowing increases to the extent that air flow is obstructed during respirations, then snoring occurs. The sound of snoring is due to the passage of air through the narrowed upper airway during sleep.

One of the main causes of this narrowing of the upper airway that results in snoring is due to enlarged adenoids. Adenoids are a mass of tissue (mainly lymphatic) located at the back of the oral cavity, tucked up high where the nasal passages enter the oral pharynx (back of the mouth).

Their function, along with that of the tonsils, is to help keep bacteria from entering the lower respiratory tract. Unlike the tonsils, the adenoids are hidden within the oral cavity because of their upper, posterior location. The exact size can be determined only by an x-ray (or ultrasound) of the neck. This is usually not necessary, because if the child is snoring, it most likely indicates that the adenoids are enlarged.

Like the tonsils, adenoids vary in size.

Snoring on its own has no negative health implications, except for those people who are kept awake as the result of someone else's snoring and thus become sleep deprived.

If the adenoids are enlarged they may obstruct drainage of the nasal passages into the oral pharynx. This often results in a persistent nasal stuffiness and a clear nasal discharge as well as snoring. These symptoms are often mistaken for nasal allergies, resulting in inappropriate treatment. Oral or nasal medication will not shrink the adenoids. The symptoms are the result of a mechanical problem – enlarged adenoids. During the day the child may tend to breathe through the mouth only.

No matter how loud the snoring, if the child's sleep is uninterrupted, the adenoids do not require removal.

Symptoms of sleep apnea in children (which is often associated with enlarged adenoids) are:

- Restless sleeping
- Excessive fatigue during the day – this may result in poor school performance and behavioural issues
- Waking up during sleep because of difficulty in breathing along with gasping for air or snorting

Children who are overweight usually have a higher incidence of snoring and resulting sleep apnea. This is due to the presence of excessive fat in the tissue of the posterior oropharynx (causing further obstruction).

Reasons for consideration of removal of the adenoids other than sleep apnea are:

- Recurrent ear infections where tubes are required
- Recurrent sinusitis (very uncommon)
- Persistent mouth breathing that affects speech or dentition
- Difficulty co-ordinating breathing and swallowing while eating (tonsils often involved)
- Persistent bad breath assumed, at least in part, to be due to chronic infection of the adenoids
- Poor school performance thought to be related to being overtired

Removal of the tonsils and/or adenoids will not stimulate appetite unless they are so enlarged that swallowing is made difficult while eating. If the adenoids are subsequently removed the child will be able to swallow better and could become more willing to eat. This might perhaps lead to an increase of food intake with a resulting weight gain.

Unfortunately, the adenoids can grow back and may cause the same symptoms again.

Speech and Language Development

Warner Bros. Mel Blanc was on to something and showed real magic when he developed his cartoon characters. Elmer Fudd, Tweety and Sylvester, Yosemite Sam and others endeared themselves to the world in part, because of their speech impediments.

The ability to connect with other people and share our thoughts and feelings by speaking is uniquely human and sets us apart from other species.

Strong communication skills are important to every aspect of your child's development. Communication skills affect the way he interacts socially with peers and impact his behaviour, both at home and in group activities.

Once at school strong oral skills (speaking and understanding) are important to ensure that your child is able to follow classroom instructions and participate fully in the classroom program. Oral language skills are also crucial for the development of reading and writing.

The terms *speech* and *language* are often used interchangeably but they are not the same. Speech is *how* we say something whereas language is *what* we say. Put simply, if a child says 'tair' for chair he has a *speech* problem. However if he calls the chair a 'table' he has a *language* problem.

Speech

Speech is the way we communicate vocally. This is in contrast to sign language, pictures or symbols, and facial expressions, which are non-verbal ways of communicating.

The most common speech difficulties include the following:

Articulation

Articulation refers to the production of speech sounds. Some sounds (e.g. /s/,/r/ and /th/) develop later than others (e.g. /p/,/m/ and /t/). Following is a chart with developmental norms.

Sound produced	Age 50% of children produce sound	Age 90% of children produce sound
p, m. b, n, w	1 year	3 years
h	1 year	4 years
k, g, d	2 years	4 years
t, ng	2 years	6 years
f, y	2.5 years	4 years
r, l	3 years	6 years
s	3 years	8 years
ch, sh	3.5 years	7 years
z	3.5 years	8 years
j	4 years	7 years
v	4 years	8 years
th	4.5 years	7 years
zh	6 years	8 years

Adapted from: http://www.norris160.org/resource/elementary/petsched/Speech%20Info/iowa-nebraska_articulation_norms.htm

When should I be concerned about my child's articulation?

- If at any point your child seems to be frustrated or upset when you cannot understand him.
- If by 2 years of age you can't understand approximately half of what your child says.
- If by 3 years of age you can't understand almost everything your child says.

What should I do if I'm concerned?

- Ask your doctor for a referral to a speech-language pathologist.
- Ask your doctor for a referral to a clinical audiologist for a hearing assessment.

Voice

What is it?

In order to produce most speech sounds, air from the lungs passes through the vocal cords causing them to vibrate. Voice difficulties can result from misuse or overuse of the vocal cords.

When should I be concerned?

- If your child's voice seems to always be hoarse or if he loses his voice often.
- If his pitch is too high.
- If his speech sounds too nasal (air coming out of the nose) or if he sounds stuffed up (nasal passages blocked).

What should I do?

- Ask your doctor for a referral to an ear, nose and throat specialist (otolaryngologist).
- If medical causes are ruled out you may then be referred to a speech-language pathologist.

Stuttering

What is it?

Some children between 2-1/2 and 4 years of age (and sometimes as late as 7 years of age) go through a period of "normal nonfluency" in which they repeat sounds, syllables or words and there are *ahs* and *ums* or pauses in their speech. Repetitions appear easy and effortless. The child seems unaware of any difficulty and does not show signs of tension when talking. Usually this period of nonfluency lasts no more than 6 months. However, there may be occasional recurrences.

What should I do if my child is experiencing a period of normal nonfluency?

- Pay attention to *what* your child is saying rather than how he is saying it.
- Let him feel that he has your undivided attention and that you will wait as long as necessary for him to complete his message.
- If he appears to be stuck, don't say the word for him. Maintain eye-contact and wait patiently for him to say the word. You may then repeat what he said so he has no doubt that you have heard him. Try to ensure that others respond in the same way.
- Reduce your own rate of speech to provide your child with a model of slow, relaxed speech. Since your child isn't aware of a speech problem telling him to slow down or think about what he wants to say will only make him self-conscious about his speech.

When should I be concerned?
- If at any point your child's speech seems to be getting worse rather than better over time
- If he shows any signs of struggle or vocal tension when talking
- If he expresses frustration or self-consciousness about his speech

What should I do?
Ask your doctor for a referral to a speech-language pathologist.

If in doubt, it is always best to err on the side of caution.

Language

Children are said to have a *language* difficulty when they have trouble:
- understanding what is said to them and/or
- putting words together to express themselves and interact with others

Language Development (See Table 2 on pages 313–315)
By around one year of age your child should have one or two "words" that are used meaningfully. Even if the pronunciation is not correct the child uses the word consistently to refer to the same thing, such as "mama" for mother or "baba" for bottle. By this time your child should also be able to follow very simple instructions such as "Give Mommy the book" or "Show me your nose."

My rule of thumb is that by 20 months of age your child should be saying 20 words (this rule holds true even if it seems as though older siblings are talking for him). By the time your child is between two and three years of age he should be putting words together in short, simple sentences such as "Look, Mommy, doggie." Or "I eat cookie." He will also be able to follow simple 2-step directions such as "Get your book and bring it to mommy."

Over the next year your child's vocabulary should increase dramatically. Sentences should become longer and more complex and similarly the complexity of the language that he understands will continue to increase.

As well, your child should demonstrate an interest in using his oral language skills to interact and engage with adults and peers.

What can I do to support my child's language development?
Children develop language by interacting with the people around them and with their environment.

- Provide your child with a stimulating environment in which he is exposed to many new experiences.

• Talk about what you are doing as you are doing it. For example, when giving your child a bath, talk about what you are washing on your child's body (e.g., "Mommy is washing your hands. Now Mommy is washing your arms.").

• Talk about what the child is doing to provide the vocabulary that he needs (e.g., "You are driving the *fast* car.")

• Read to your child often and provide many opportunities for him to interact with books by turning the pages and pointing to pictures. As he gets older, discuss the content of the book with him.

• If your child comes to talk to you about something, use this as an opportunity to extend the conversation by asking questions, using new vocabulary and clarifying and expanding upon what your child has said. Balance questions with comments.

When should I be concerned about my child's language development?

• If you are not seeing a steady progression in your child's use and understanding of language
• If your child appears frustrated because of an inability to communicate his wants or needs
• If your child is having difficulty interacting with other children and is not "using his words" as expected for his age

What should I do?

• Ask your doctor for a referral to a speech-language pathologist.
• Ask for a referral to a clinical audiologist to rule out hearing problems.

English as a Second Language

What if English is not my first language?

As a rule, parents should speak to their child in the language they are most comfortable using. This allows the child to build a solid foundation in that language, which will help, not hinder, his later development of English.

What if more than one language is used in the home?

Children being exposed to more than one language at home generally follow the same pattern of development as single-language learners (i.e., single words, then two-word combinations, etc.). (See Table 2).

If two languages are used in the home and parents want their child to learn both, it is best for one parent to speak in one language and the other parent in the second language.

You might also want to do activities that combine both languages. For example, both parents can read the same book to the child but in their chosen language.

If there is a delay in your child's language development in both languages there may be an underlying language difficulty.

When should I be concerned?

• If you feel that your child's language skills are not developing steadily from month to month
• If by 20 months your child does not use 20 words understandable to you, in both languages combined (for example, 12 words in the first language and 8 words in the second language).

What should I do?

• Ask your doctor for a referral to a speech-language pathologist.
• Ask your doctor for a referral to a clinical audiologist to assess his hearing.

Selective Mutism (the reluctant speaker)

What is it?

Selective mutism is the refusal of the child to speak in specific social situations (e.g., school) despite speaking freely in other situations.

Children with selective mutism are often described as being extremely shy. However if a child is still not speaking after several months of school the possibility of an underlying anxiety condition should be considered.

When considering whether or not a child is selectively mute, be sure to determine whether the child's difficulty results from lack of knowledge or comfort with the language being spoken in the particular situation.

What should I do if the selective mutism continues?

• Ask your doctor if there is a pediatric anxiety clinic in your area to which your child can be referred.
• Consult with the speech-language pathologist, psychologist or social worker at your child's school - or with the preschool speech-language pathology services in your area.

Hearing

Most hospitals have an infant screening program to assess infants' hearing in order to identify a hearing loss. Early identification is very important, as hearing properly is critical to your child's speech and language development. If you have any concerns about your child's hearing, ask your doctor for a referral to a clinical audiologist.

To Sum Up

You should see continuous development of your child's speech and language skills over time in keeping with the guidelines provided. If you have any concerns about your child's speech and/or language development, it is always best to err on the side of caution and ask your doctor for a referral to a speech-language pathologist. It is also important to rule out hearing loss through a hearing assessment by a clinical audiologist.

If you have concerns about your child's speech or language, make sure you refrain from talking about your concerns in front of him. Making your child self-conscious about communication can make the problem worse and it certainly will not help his self-esteem. Communicating should be a pleasure for both you and your child, never a painful confrontation.

Below are general guidelines for your child's speech and language development. Some children will reach these milestones a little earlier and some a little later. What is important is that your child isn't too far off these times and that you are seeing steady progress in his development of speech and language.

Table 2*

3 months of age

– Responds to your voice by turning his head or becoming quiet
– Has different cried that mean 'I'm hungry' or 'I'm tired' or 'I'm in pain'
– Repeats the same sound (known as cooing)

4 to 6 months of age

– Shows interest in sounds around him.
– Starts to "babble", repeating sounds such as "pa," "ba" or "ma".
– Is starting to use sounds to get your attention and to get you to meet his wants or needs.

7 months to 1 year of age

– Turns and looks at your face when spoken to.

– Is interested in songs, games and nursery rhymes, such as "pat-a-cake".
– Understands some words such as "milk", "juice", or "daddy".
– Is producing more and more sounds and uses "speech sounds" to hold your attention.
– Somewhere around this time your child will say his "first words" such as "mama", "dada", or "bye-bye".

12 to 18 months of age

– Follows a simple one-step direction such as "come here".
– Uses three to five words meaningfully.
– Combines strings of sounds together as though he is speaking in sentences.
– Use gestures such as shaking his head for "no" or waving "bye bye".
– Shows an interest in picture books.
– Brings toys or books to show to someone.

18 to 24 months of age

– Uses at least 20 words by 20 months of age and is acquiring new words quickly.
– Combines words.
– Uses more speech sounds such as /n/, /d/, /g/, /w/.
– Points to parts of his body if asked.
– Engages in pretend play with toys.
– Follows simple commands such as "Bring Mommy your shoes."
– Responds to simple questions such as, "Where is your dolly?" or commands such as "Push the car" by using a word or gesture.
– Enjoys being read to and sharing simple books with an adult.
– Enjoys hearing the same stories or rhymes over and over again.

24 to 30 months of age

– Uses 100 to 150 words.
– Is beginning to use pronouns such as "me" and "mine".
– Combines words to form phrases ("Daddy go bye-bye", "where car", "more push").
– Words sound clearer.
– Interacts with another child by offering a toy.
– Can hold a book and turn the pages.
– Can scribble with a crayon.

2-1/2 to 3 years of age

– Is becoming easier to understand.

– Has a word for most things.
– Asks for items by naming them.
– Uses some longer words.
– Combines words into short sentences.
– Uses more grammatical markers such as plural /s/ and correct verb tense .
– Understands the concepts such as "more", "big", "little", "in", "hot", "cold".
– Is aware of sounds such as the telephone or doorbell and will respond to them.
– Understands two-step commands such as "Get your book and put it on the table."
– Takes turns when playing with other children.
– Seems concerned if another child is upset.
– Plays with toys using a sequence of actions, for example, fills his truck with sand, "drives" truck to another location and empties sand from truck.
– Remembers and understands familiar stories.
– Recognizes some signs such as a stop sign.

3 to 4 years of age

– Understands who, what, and where questions.
– Uses sentences with 5 to 8 words.
– Can tell a simple story; can talk about past events that have happened away from home.
– Is affectionate toward a favourite friend.
– Engages in pretend play with toys.
– Speech can be understood by others most of the time.

4 to 5 years

– Can follow longer directions involving three or more steps ("Get the crayons, bring them to Mommy and then sit down on the chair.")
– Forms long and detailed sentences using adult grammar.
– Hears and understands almost everything you say to him.
– Enjoys listening to stories and can answer simple questions about the story.
– Can tell a story with a beginning, middle, and end.
– Can generate simple rhymes (cat-bat).
– Matches some letters with their sounds (letter /b/ says "buh; letter /t/, says "tuh").
– Speaks clearly and fluently and is understood by strangers almost all the time.
– Can say most sounds correctly but may still have difficulty saying the /s/, /r/, /th/ and /v/ sounds.

* Adapted from the Ontario Preschool Speech-Language Services pamphlet and The American Speech-Language-Hearing Association (ASHA) website.

Spider Nevi – Veins (Telangiectasias)

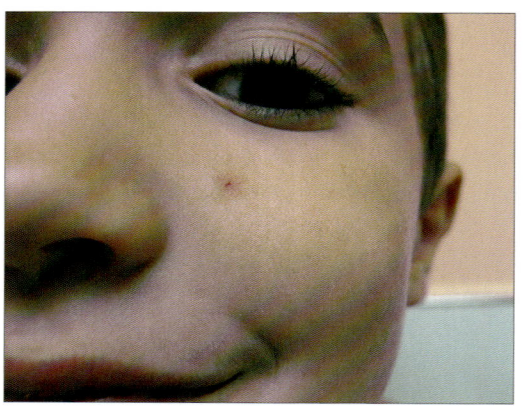
Spider Nevus

Telangiectasias are little veins that come to the surface of the skin and spread out appearing not unlike a spider's legs. If you were to touch the very centre of them with the tip of a pencil they would temporarily disappear.

Spider nevi in adults occur during pregnancy or with various other conditions. In children, however, they most commonly occur spontaneously without any underlying cause.

Although they can fade away with age, most often they remain.

If their appearance is bothersome to the child, then for cosmetic reasons they may be removed with laser therapy.

There is a hereditary form of multiple telangiectasia where they are present on the skin and also on internal body organs.

Spitting Up (Regurgitation)

Spitting up is a very common occurrence in infants. It starts soon after birth, at a few days of age. It may continue until the infant is 8 to 12 months of age.

It can occur during feeds, during burping or even between feeds.

The amount of the spit-up ranges from less than a teaspoon to what appears to be the whole feed.

It occurs equally in breastfed babies and formula-fed babies.

The spitting up may come out of the nose as well as the mouth. If this happens, there usually are no concerns.

What is the cause? When formula or breast milk is swallowed it passes down the esophagus (swallowing tube) into the stomach. The stomach then contracts to push the milk into the intestine. When this occurs, the opening where the esophagus enters the stomach normally closes, thus preventing any regurgitation. Unfortunately, in many infants, this closure is not fully formed and when the stomach contracts the result is regurgitation or spitting up. It may take up to one year for the closure to form and to function completely, at which time the regurgitation will cease.

There is little concern about persistent spitting up if the child meets the following criteria:

1. It is painless.
2. It is not projectile (shooting out like a fire hose).
3. It does not contain blood or bile.
4. Weight gain is occurring at an acceptable rate.

If the infant meets the above criteria then the spitting up is of no concern. It will stop by the time the child is 8 to 12 months of age. The one problem posed by the infant's spitting up is for the mom; she will probably continually carry the scent of "eau de regurgitation" during this time period.

Essentially, no treatment is required. A simple change in formula is not the answer. One of the pre-thickened formulas, however, may be helpful. Alternatively, you can thicken the formula you are using with cereal (one tablespoon per ounce of formula). The size of the opening of the bottle's nipple may have to be increased with a heated small-gauge metal knitting needle. Heat the point end and push it in and out of the nipple opening to enlarge its size. If you are breast-feeding obviously this doesn't help!

Feeding with less bending of the baby at the waist may help with the passage of milk from the stomach into the intestine and thus lessen regurgitation. Smaller, more frequent feeds can also be tried.

After feeding you may allow the baby to lie on his tummy for a half-hour. Fifty percent of the milk in the baby's tummy will empty into the small bowel within the first half-hour after feeding. Tummy time, therefore, may diminish any regurgitation. Do not allow the baby to sleep on his tummy during this time unless he is under your watchful eye.

If pain (fussiness) is present during or immediately after feeding or the child seems to refuse feeding, inflammation of the esophagus may be present. This inflammation is due to acid (present in the milk that is regurgitated from the stomach) irritating the esophagus. An antacid will be prescribed by your doctor. This condition is called reflux esophagitis. Improvement should be noted within a few days of starting the medication.

Pyloric Stenosis

If the reflux becomes persistently projectile (shoots out like a firehose), an ultrasound of the abdomen is necessary to rule out pyloric stenosis. Pyloric stenosis is more common in boys than girls – 4:1. It is also more common if another sibling has had pyloric stenosis. It begins with simple regurgitation which progressively increases to a point where it becomes projectile.

It occurs most frequently during the second and third week of life. Pyloric stenosis is the result of a tightening of the muscle at the beginning of the small bowel where the stomach enters it. Because the opening is now much more narrow, when the stomach contracts, the milk is forcibly pushed back up the esophagus and out the mouth. This condition is painless. The diagnosis is confirmed by an ultrasound of the tummy which shows a thickened pyloric muscle. It will require surgical correction.

If the infant has had excessive regurgitation and is not gaining weight, there are two considerations. First, the infant may not be receiving sufficient calories to maintain weight (especially if the vomiting is in large amounts). Thickened formula as described above may help. Medications are available that may help ease stomach emptying, resulting in a decrease in the degree of spitting up. The infant's weight should be followed closely. A second possibility, although uncommon, is a milk protein intolerance or allergy. This may present with only symptoms of vomiting and poor weight gain. Commonly, with cow's-milk protein allergy other symptoms, such as loose stools and fussiness, are also present. A family history of milk intolerance may be present. If this is diagnosed, a formula change, to a formula that is completely hydrolyzed (broken down) may be required. Breastfeeding mothers should eliminate all milk protein products and soy from their diet.

If the spitting up persists after one year of age, an upper GI series may be required to ensure that everything is in its proper place anatomically. The esophageal/gastric junction (where the swallowing tube enters the stomach) will be examined to rule out a hiatus hernia (failure of closure at the junction of the esophagus and stomach). If a hiatus hernia is present, as long as the infant is gaining weight without evidence of reflux esophagitis, no treatment is required. If, however, there is persistent esophagitis and/or inadequate weight gain, surgical correction of the hernia may be necessary. Surgical correction is a rare occurrence. In my over 40 years of experience, none has been required in my practice.

Fresh blood may be present in the spit-up of breastfed babies. This is most commonly the result of swallowing blood from the mother's irritated nipple during feeding. Express a little breast milk to see if this is the problem. If so, breast cream, with or without a breast shield, will be required for mom until healing occurs. Continue breastfeeding.

The sudden onset of severe abdominal pain (and I mean severe – with a reaction as if he has been hit with a cannonball) along with vomiting (often green bile-stained) indicates a bowel obstruction until proven otherwise. This requires immediate attention.

Coughing during feeding is uncommon. It may be caused by some "silent reflux". Silent reflux is suspected when there is regurgitation but not always to the degree that it comes out of the mouth. A small amount of milk may enter the windpipe, causing the cough. The reflux may be prevented by thickening the formula as described earlier.

To conclude, nearly all infants will spit up to varying degrees. Fortunately, for most, it is entirely benign in nature and is a nuisance only to the caregiver and not the infant.

Streetproofing

The year was 1967.

Jack says goodbye to his mother. "Have fun and don't forget to be home for supper!" she calls after him. Off he goes on his bike with his friends to the park. They ride their bikes up and down the hills, through puddles and along a ledge where there is a 5-foot drop. Then, whizzing down the side streets without a care in the world, they head for the beach. There they run in and out of the water with their shoes on and skip stones to see who can get the most skips. They grab an ice cream cone at the local vendor and off they go again – this time to see Mr. Moody, an old man living in a very old house. He has three cats and two dogs. He also has a fish pond filled with all sorts of coloured fish. Visiting Mr. Moody is like going to the zoo. After they play with the animals and trying to catch the fish with their hands, Mr. Moody usually tells them a story. By this time it's suppertime. Jack waves goodbye to Mr. Moody and his friends, and rides his bike as quickly as he can home for supper. "Did you have fun?" Mom asks. "It was great," Jack replies. "Wash your hands – dinner is on the table"

Fast forward to 2011 - the above scenario is a figment of my imagination and would never happen today. Mr. Moody would probably be suspected of being a pedophile.

In the past two to three decades our concerns about the safety of our children while they are outside the confines of home and backyard have escalated many-fold. Why? The answer is clear. We have great concerns over the presence of predators, pedophiles and abusers in our neighbourhoods who may harm our children. Unfortunately, in many cases these people are well-known and trusted by the family. This makes your child more easy prey.

One of the most important things that you can do to protect your child is to streetproof him. Age-appropriate instruction with demonstration and role playing is crucial when it comes to safety. Much material is available for you to accomplish this very necessary task.

I regret that, because of our paranoia, perhaps we are doing our children a disservice by putting so many restrictions on them. They are seldom left alone, out of our sight, unless they have a cell phone and report in hourly. I am quite sure that many parents would love to have a tracking device implanted under the skin of their child so that they could monitor their every movement. But this is a necessary reality of the 21st century.

Perhaps we could spend less time worrying and more time joining in our children's play and then maybe a little bit of the child in us would emerge – not such a bad thing. New wrinkle lines from worrying are really not necessary.

Stridor – Noisy-Breathing (Windpipe Narrowing)

As we breathe, we take air into our lungs (inhale – inspiration) and then let the air out (exhale – expiration). Any narrowing of the windpipe will lead, initially, to difficulty with inspiration. The symptoms noticed are a "barky" cough, indrawing between the ribs, a hoarse voice or cry and a squeaky noise called stridor when breathing in. The greater the narrowing the more severe are the symptoms.

Stridor occurs only when one inhales (when breathing in but not when breathing out).

In the newborn, a stridor may be one of the symptoms of a low calcium level in the blood.

Laryngomalacia

In the newborn and young infant the windpipe is soft. The force of inspiration can cause enough collapse of the windpipe to result in indrawing (chest wall draws in) with inspiration, accompanied by a stridor. The degree of stridor varies depending on the amount of narrowing of the windpipe during inspiration (breathing in).

The windpipe is surrounded by rings of cartilage. As the infant ages these cartilaginous rings stiffen to the point that they prevent the trachea (windpipe) from collapsing. This process may take up to several months or longer. During that time, symptoms of airway narrowing gradually disappear.

Laryngomalacia is the most common cause of windpipe narrowing. It may be mild, causing inspiratory stridor only when the child cries, or it may be continuous, with stridor occurring with each breath taken, along with indrawing of the chest wall.

Laryngomalacia is a clinical diagnosis made by the doctor. Often the diagnosis is confirmed by a simple maneouvre by the physician. When the infant's head is hyper-extended backward and his jaw is pulled forward, the stridor disappears. This maneouvre mechanically opens the airway. The stridor may also worsen if the neck is flexed. An ultrasound of the neck is only required if the diagnosis is unclear. With laryngomalacia the ultrasound is normal.

Most infants outgrow this condition without any intervention before one year of age.

Vocal Cords

A newborn, as well as an infant or child, with a vocal cord weakness or paralysis usually has stridor and a hoarse voice. Investigations will include an ultrasound of the neck as well as direct inspection of the vocal cords under a light anesthetic. Other investigations may be required depending on the findings.

A child who cries or screams a lot may develop inflammation of the vocal cords due to vocal abuse. With this condition, the hoarseness gets progressively worse during the day. Occasionally there may be stridor (usually when the child is excited, running or crying).

The treatment is to rest the vocal cords – with no yelling or screaming allowed.

Tracheal Narrowing

Pressure from an artery that crosses over the windpipe may cause the windpipe to narrow. This is diagnosed by laryngoscope examination under a light anesthetic. The diagnosis is confirmed by observation of the tracheal wall narrowing and pulsating at the same rate as the heart. Depending on the severity of the narrowing, surgery may be required to lift the artery off the tracheal wall.

Foreign Body

The sudden onset of stridor in an infant or child, especially during the day, should be considered an indication that there is a foreign body in the windpipe until proven otherwise. This can occur if the child (or older sibling) has put a small object into his mouth and it has been aspirated down the trachea. The symptoms vary depending on the degree of obstruction. They may be as mild as a stridor or, if there is complete obstruction, may be as serious as leading to respiratory arrest.

The Heimlich maneouvre will not dislodge a foreign body in the windpipe.

The diagnosis is confirmed by x-ray of the neck and/or chest. Only radio-opaque objects (those with some metal) will be seen on routine x-ray. Non-radio-opaque objects, such as plastic beads, wood or pieces of food, will not be seen on x-ray.

Treatment consists of removing the foreign body.

Epiglottitis

Epiglottitis is an infection of the glottis. The glottis is a small piece of tissue at the back of the throat which helps prevent food that has been swallowed from entering the windpipe during eating.

The infection is usually bacterial in origin and due to *Haemophilus influenzae*.

The child usually presents with a sore throat and difficulty in swallowing, as well as breathing. Stridor and indrawing are usually present. A fever may be present. The child appears very apprehensive and does not like to be moved. All his thoughts and efforts are focused on breathing.

If epiglottitis is suspected there should be no further ingestion of fluids or solids. The act of swallowing may result in the epiglottis completely obstructing the windpipe.

This condition is a surgical emergency. A tracheotomy or a breathing tube is usually required to allow the child to breathe while the infection is being treated with antibiotics.

Since the introduction of the haemophilus influenza vaccine, epiglottitis has become quite rare and occurs, for the most part, in children who have not been vaccinated.

Tracheitis (croup)

This is discussed on page 122.

Psychogenic causes

Persistent **daily** inspiratory stridor which may be accompanied by a croup-like cough, occurring in children over 4 years of age, may be a habit tic. This diagnosis is made after ruling out all other causes and by taking a good history from the caregiver. The history alone will often suggest that it is of a psychological origin.

The management is to determine and correct the underlying cause for the child's anxiety. When this is accomplished, the cough will disappear. During this period, do not ask the child why he is coughing, because often he really does not know. Asking him continually to stop coughing is like putting out the fire by adding wood. The cough usually intensifies.

Masses

Any mass in the neck may press on the windpipe, causing varying degrees of obstruction. These are very rare and are usually secondary to an abscess or tumor.

Investigations such as routine blood work, cultures, x-ray, ultrasound, CAT scan or MRI and perhaps a biopsy may be required to determine the origin of the mass; it is then treated accordingly.

Sudden Infant Death Syndrome (SIDS)

SIDS, also known as crib death, is the sudden, unexpected and unexplained death of an apparently healthy infant under one year of age. The peak incidence is between 1 and 6 months of age.

Investigations thus far have not found the cause of SIDS. It has been speculated that in SIDS, the infant's respiratory system center is not functioning properly. Normally, with decreasing amounts of oxygen (02) in the blood, the rate of respiration increases in order to increase O2 and lower carbon dioxide (CO2) levels. One thought is that in SIDS there is a lack of sensitivity of the respiratory centre to decreasing levels of O2. As a result, the level of CO2 may become high enough to depress the respiratory centre so that the infant stops breathing.

Some recent studies have shown that there may be a problem with the uptake of a hormone called serotonin in the respiratory centre that could be a causative factor. Further studies are required.

Predisposing factors:

Prenatal

- Maternal smoking during pregnancy
- Drug abuse during pregnancy
- Prematurity
- Multiple births
- Low birth weight for gestational age (less than 2.5 kg)
- Lack of prenatal care
- Teen mother

Postnatal

- Sleeping on tummy
- Exposure to secondhand smoke
- Overheating
- Bed sharing
- Sleeping on soft surfaces or the presence in the crib of any soft items (comforters, pillows, soft toys, etc.)
- Mild upper respiratory tract infections

Prevention

- It is **extremely important** that the air is able to circulate around the infant's mouth and nose.
- Maintain a clutter-free crib – no comforters or duvets, no side bumpers, no soft items that may result in the baby, becoming overheated, suffocated, strangled or entrapped.
- Have a tightly fitted bottom sheet.
- Swaddling is fine; however, if the infant can loosen the blanket then discontinue swaddling.
- Have no more than a 2-finger width between the mattress and the crib.

- Put baby down to sleep on his back.
- Share room (not bed) for up to 6 months.
- Breastfeeding, if possible, is optimal.
- Maintain a smoke-free environment.
- Use of a pacifier after one month of age or earlier is okay once breastfeeding has been well established. If expelled during sleep there is no need to reinsert.

After 6–8 months of age, when the baby is able to roll and has good head control, the likelihood of SIDS diminishes. Allow the baby to sleep on his stomach if he wishes to. At this age as well, it is probably safe to put some soft toys in the crib.

Sunscreen and Insect Repellent

The cold storms are over. Spring thus far has been cold and wet. Oh, for those sizzling summer days! They are just around the corner and we can hardly wait. Hold on! Summer is indeed great, but it does bring with it 2 major hazards: the sun and blood sucking bugs. I realize that you have been lectured time and time again about these 2 problems. Maybe if we read about them a few more times, the message will eventually sink in and we'll actually take action on the potential problems. So here follows my sermon on the subject.

Sunscreen

The sun, with its ultraviolet rays (UVA and UVB), does much more harm than good to our skin. The ultimate damage is cancer of the skin, This is the fourth most common cancer in the under- 39-years-of-age group.

Skin damage can result in early aging of the skin, wrinkling, discolouration of the skin with red or brown patches, broken blood vessels, leathery, dry skin, and loss of elasticity and "glow". The skin does not forgive or forget. One bad sunburn at a young age may have lifelong harmful effects.

Some children are at a higher risk than others. Fair-skinned children will burn more easily and tan less than those with darker-pigmented skin. They also are at a greater risk for developing skin cancer. Others at high risk are children with freckles or a large number of moles. Those who have blonde or red hair are also considered high risk.

Remember, sun damage occurs mainly between 11 a.m and 4 p.m. Clouds present little protection against UV rays, which easily penetrate them. Reflected light from the water, sand, stone, or metal surfaces further intensifies the sun's power. Although shade offers some protection, don't count on not getting burned. Even a dark tan will not protect you for long periods of time in the sun. An average tan will offer protection equivalent to an SPF of 2 in a sunscreen.

So what should we do? Stay inside? The answer is obviously no. But you must be sun smart. So here are some tips for you and your children to protect the family while enjoying the outdoors this summer:

Wear a broad-brimmed hat. Infant carriers, strollers, and carriages should be fitted with a sunscreen cover. Cover as much of the body as possible with light-coloured clothing. If you hold up a T-shirt and can see through it, the weave is not tight enough to protect from the sun.

Sunscreens should not be used on children less than 4 months of age. Keep babies less than 4 months of age out of the sunlight. Cover their whole body with loose-fitting, light-coloured clothes and a hat.

Try to avoid sun time from 11 a.m. to 4 p.m. Play as much as possible in the shade. Apply and reapply a sunscreen with a factor of at least 30 every few hours and more often if you are swimming or sweating. A higher sunscreen factor number does not actually mean that it is stronger. It only means that a person may remain in the sun for a longer period of time before the sunscreen requires reapplication. If it would take you or your child 15 minutes of sun exposure to develop a burn, for example, you multiply this number by the factor of the sunscreen. This, in theory, gives you the total time in minutes that protection will last.

Those with sensitive skin should use hypoallergenic sunscreens. If you are uncertain, rub some on a small area of the skin and wait a day. If there is no reaction, then it is safe for your skin. You may want to check with your pharmacist or doctor as to which product is best for your family.

Apply the sunscreen liberally 15–20 minutes prior to sun exposure and reapply frequently, especially if you are going into and out of the water and towel drying.

Always use a sunscreen with protection from both UVA and UVB rays. Avoid applying it to the area near the eyes (unfortunately, the eyelids are very thin and easily burned). Sunglasses with UV protection are advised even for young infants. Lip balm with a high SPF should be applied to the lips.

Insect Repellent

West Nile virus infection still poses a real health risk despite the massive effort to eliminate mosquito nesting areas and to raise public awareness about the use of insect repellents. Hopefully, this program will be instituted on a yearly basis.

Pesky bug bites may become a real "scratchy" problem. Remember, every time your child has discomfort from insect bites, you'll have the same discomfort too.

There are many products sold that decrease the insect population in our surrounding environment (patio and backyard). Unfortunately, bug zappers, ultrasonic gadgets and scented candles are not as effective as they have been advertised in keeping insects away. Botanical extracts applied to the skin, if anything, offer minimal protection and only for short periods of time (less than one hour).

They should not be used on children under 2 years of age.

At present, DEET is the best product being used to repel insects. A product with 5% concentration should offer approximately 2 hours of protection, 10% between 3 and 4 hours, and 30% protects for 6 hours. Increasing the concentration does not mean an increase in strength. It only increases the length of time that it gives protection.

Whether it is sunscreen or insect repellent, unscented products are best (attracts fewer bugs).

Insect repellent should be applied to the skin after the sunscreen.

Do not spray DEET on your child's skin directly; apply by hand only on exposed areas. Do not apply around the mouth and eyes. Do not apply where skin is broken. Spraying DEET on clothing (before worn) is an effective way to help prevent attracting insects.

Insect repellents should not be used on children less then 5 months of age. For those 6 months to 2 years of age a 5% solution of DEET should be used. For children 2–12 years of age use a 10% solution. For children over 12 years of age and adults, 30% is recommended. It may be reapplied 2 or 3 times a day. I do recommend that at night, one should bathe or shower well enough to remove any insect repellent that might still remain on the body.

The more you can cover up with light-coloured clothing the better. Tucking pants into your socks may not make you a style setter, but it does give the best protection against ankle bites.

A product that contains both DEET and sunscreen should be used solely as a repellent with regard to frequency of application.

Just a word about watching your child play at a playground, wading pool, or swimming pool. The operative word is *watching* – not reading, not socializing, not snoozing. Problems can occur in seconds, so always keep your full and complete attention on your child.

Teeth Grinding and Clenching (Bruxism)

It is unlikely that, for children, bruxism is as related to stress factors as it is for adults. For the child population the grinding of the teeth back and forth is more common than clenching.

It can begin as early as the child develops upper and lower teeth. The noise caused by the grinding may be more irritating than that of squeaking chalk on a blackboard.

Why infants do this is uncertain. It most likely is pleasurable and soothing for them.

Despite what your grandparents say, it is not caused by intestinal worms.

It is impossible to get the infant or child to stop on his own.

Although there is the possibility of later problems with the temporomandibular joint, this is very unusual in childhood.

The most common problem is wearing down of the teeth due to constant grinding. If this appears to be happening, a dental appliance should be worn during the times of grinding (usually sleep time).

Teething and Dental Care

The primary dentition consists of 10 upper and 10 lower teeth.

When does the first tooth erupt? This, as they would say in the old days, is the $64,000 question. The best and most truthful answer is – it will erupt when it erupts. Why do parents have the notion that if their infant does not "break" a tooth by a certain deadline then there is a concern? In normal, healthy infants I have seen the first tooth eruption as early as 3 months and as late as over 15 months of age. In fact, babies can be born with a tooth already erupted (oftentimes these have to be removed because they are loose and can possibly be aspirated into the lungs). In truth, breastfeeding mothers should feel blessed if their infant's tooth eruption is later rather than early (an infant latching onto mom's breast with sharp little teeth can be painful!). The order in which teeth erupt may vary. Most common is the arrival of a lower central incisor tooth. But, in fact, it is also quite normal for any of the upper or lower front 6 teeth to show themselves first. Thereafter, a new tooth usually arrives every 1–2 months. Please do not compare one infant with another. There is no race to be won or an award given for being the first baby on the block who has a tooth.

Teething can be a miserable experience for some infants (unfortunately, also for their parents) and not at all problematic for others. Why this is so is the second big question.

Symptoms of teething are numerous. Normally it begins with excessive drooling and chewing on the hands. Anything and everything goes into infants' mouths and is chewed upon, and I mean anything! **Tugging at ears** is a common symptom. The stools may become slightly loose. The gums may appear swollen and quite tender. A blood bubble may appear under the gum prior to the eruption of a tooth. This is usually without any symptoms. A mild red rash may appear around the mouth and around the anal opening. Varying degrees of irritability may be present.

Because of the wide range of symptoms, do not blame teething as the root cause for all that ails the child. If the child is excessively irritable, especially for a long period of time (several days), your doctor should be consulted to ensure there is no other problem.

Although some moms swear that their infant's temperature becomes elevated with teething, this is **very uncommon**. An elevated temperature should alert the parent that there is a possible medical cause that has to be dealt with, not teething.

There are a few things that can be done to help relieve the discomfort of teething. Rubbing his gums vigorously with a clean finger or washcloth, starting at 4 months of age, will help the teething process. Let the baby gnaw on his finger if he wishes. Use your knuckle as a substitute. Hard teething biscuits are quite useful. A teething ring that has been cooled in the refrigerator is an excellent tool to minimize discomfort. Do not freeze it. The occasional use of acetaminophen or ibuprofen may be required. I do not recommend over-the-counter medication that you apply to the gums to act as a local anesthetic.

Dental hygiene starts at birth. It is best to clean the gums and tongue after each feeding with a moist, warm piece of gauze. This will not only help prevent future gum disease, it will also get your infant used to having his gums cleaned. If done on a regular basis, there will be less resistance to the later use of a toothbrush.

If you want your child to have a million-dollar smile without spending a million dollars, dental care should be started when the first tooth erupts. It is a myth that you need not worry about caring for the primary teeth because the child will get a second set of teeth. Nothing could be further from the truth. Proper hygiene of your infant's gums and primary teeth is important to ensure the development of healthy secondary dentition and gums.

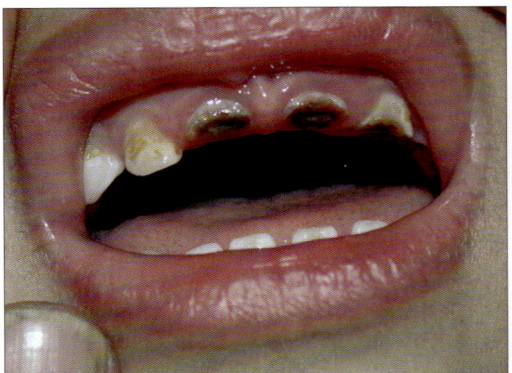 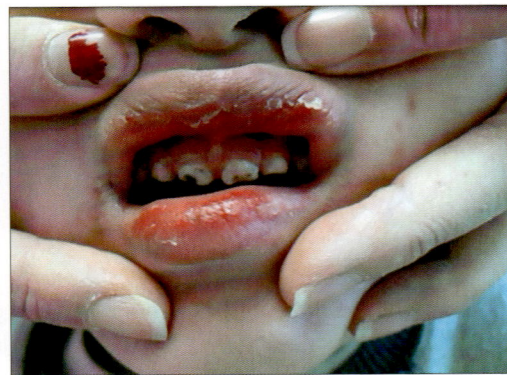

Night Bottle Dental Caries

To prevent dental caries, do not give the child a pacifier that is dipped in honey or any other sweetener. As well, do not leave any bottle of sweetened juice or milk in the crib for the baby to graze on periodically during the night. If a bottle must be left in the crib, use plain water only. During the day, again, do not allow him to walk around with a bottle or cup of milk or juice to continually sip upon.

At four months of age, even prior to the eruption of the first tooth, to ease the discomfort of teething start rubbing the gums vigorously twice a day with a clean finger or a wet, warm washcloth. After the first tooth has erupted, clean it daily the same way (clean the tongue as well). When there are four teeth, switch to a finger toothbrush. This is a rubberized device that fits over your finger like a thimble. This is an excellent way to keep the teeth clean and to massage the gums. Use water only. A small amount of toothpaste without fluoride is acceptable. When eight teeth have erupted, switch to a small toothbrush. Again, brush the teeth twice a day in an up-and-down motion. Allowing an infant to brush his own teeth will only result in his chewing the toothbrush – nothing else will be accomplished. However, you may allow him to hold the toothbrush while you hold his hand during brushing. Once his teeth are brushed, you may allow him to use the brush on his own. You will probably need a new brush every few months (or more frequently if he is a bristle chewer). At three years of age you should encourage your child, under your supervision, to brush his own teeth.

Some toddlers just will not open their mouth. It is clenched tight as a vise. They will more than happily put almost anything in their mouth except for a toothbrush (or food and medicine)! A massive struggle ensues each and every time during cleaning of the teeth. I fully understand your frustration. Here are a few tips that may help. Allow him to choose his toothbrush. Buy one that is his favourite colour or design. Let him watch you brush your teeth to demonstrate that it is harmless. There are a number of flavoured non-fluoridated toothpastes – try them. There are children who enjoy having their teeth brushed using a vibrating toothbrush. The noise and vibration may be enough to distract them during tooth cleaning. The bottom line is that dental care is important and a "battle" worth fighting and ultimately winning!

Fluoride toothpaste is not advised (if used, squeeze out no more toothpaste than the size of a matchhead). If excessive toothpaste is swallowed, over a period of time the excess amount of fluoride absorbed in the body may cause permanent pitting of the secondary teeth, even prior to their eruption. This condition is called fluorosis. When the child is four years of age and is capable of spitting out the toothpaste and rinsing his mouth, then toothpaste with fluoride can be safely used.

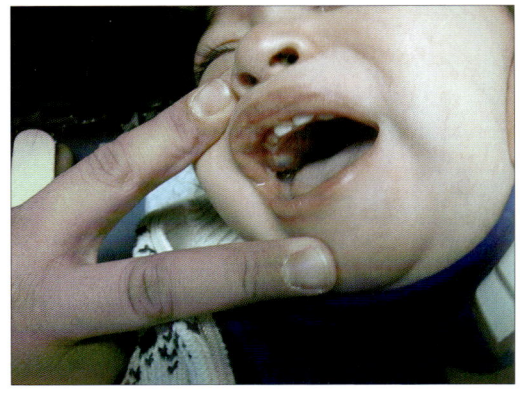

Blood Blister (Site of Tooth Eruption)

A visit to the dentist should take place within 6 months of the eruption of the first tooth. Certainly, it should take place before two years of age – the earlier the better.

As previously stated, one of the most difficult tasks a parent has is to brush their child's teeth. I am a firm believer that this "hassle" can be avoided if you start cleaning the gums early in life and the teeth (as they erupt) twice daily routinely. Starting early in establishing a normal day-to-day routine will result in a cooperative child.

P.S.: A big bravo to those who floss their children's teeth.

P.P.S.: Prior to the eruption of a premolar tooth, you may notice a bluish swelling in that area of the gum. It is non-tender. This is a hemorrhage under the skin and will disappear when the tooth erupts.

Temper Tantrums

Temper tantrums may begin as early as one year of age. Basically, they occur because a toddler wants to change a 'no' answer to a 'yes'.

Since infants are unable to communicate their displeasure verbally they will do so in the only way that they know – by crying, screaming, running uncontrollably, hitting, biting, kicking or banging their fists or head against the floor, wall or some other hard object.

It is bad enough when this occurs in private at home, when you are alone with your child, but it is more embarrassing when it occurs while you are visiting others, while you are at church, while at social events or any other public place, such as a mall. You feel that everyone's eyes are upon you. You imagine them thinking, "What is she doing to that poor child?" Their stares are penetrating and seem to imply that your parenting skills are questionable. You would like to crawl into a little hole. You never bargained for such "testing".

The fact is, however, most onlookers feel only sympathy for you. They may have gone through it themselves and know how it feels – just awful. They are thankful it is not them in that situation this time.

Tantrums often are directed, for the main part, toward one caregiver – usually the mother. Infants learn very early in life which caregiver is most likely to give in – again the mother.

So what do you do?

First of all, you must realize that temper tantrums of varying severity occur with most children. They are not a reflection of your particular parenting skills.

Don't give in only to prevent the child from embarrassing you. If the final word is "no" changing a "no" to a "yes" answer means that you are giving the power to your child. It will only encourage further tantrums. He will think, "This works for me; if I can get away with one tantrum, I probably am able to get away with many. If I scream loud and long enough, I will get what I want."

Often there are warning symptoms of an impending conflict of wills. This is the time when you have to take action to prevent it from escalating into a full-blown tantrum. One tactic you can try is to distract the child from what he wants. This may sound silly, but saying, "Look at the squirrel out the window" or "Look at the birdie on the sink!" The toddler most often can be distracted from his intentions. If you continue talking to him about what you saw he may forget what he is becoming angry about – a tantrum nipped in the bud. Believe it, this method works tremendously well if it is initiated while you can still get your child's attention, prior to the onset of the storm of a possible tantrum.

But what do you do in the presence of others, for example, in public at a grocery store? Of paramount importance, you do not give in to the child just to save face. If he is already in full-blown tantrum mode, excuse yourself, pick him up, screaming and kicking, and leave to go to a quiet" place. This place could be a washroom, your car or, in desperation, the nearest broom closet.

During a tantrum the child is not listening to you. This is not the time to reason with him. Never laugh at your child during a tantrum. Doing so will aggravate the situation and demonstrate to him that you do not care about his feelings. Instead say "I know you're feeling sad." Your main objective is to ensure that he does not harm himself. I should state that in 40 years of practice I have never witnessed any child harm himself no matter how hard he hits or bangs his head. I have seen, however, many a parent completely frazzled by their child's behaviour. Some parents are ready to cry, others are on the verge of violence themselves.

By at least 2-1/2 years of age and, hopefully, earlier, your child will be speaking and will be better able to express his feelings with words rather than physical actions – encourage this. When he cries, get down to his level, make good eye contact, speak quietly with as few words as possible, and listen to him. You can negotiate with him, but do not compromise your disciplinary principles. With negotiation no one loses and a lesson will be taught.

In the end, you are the teacher and your child the pupil – not the reverse. Stay in the driver's seat. Do not give the power to your child. If you do, no positive lesson will be learned.

Temper tantrums become less frequent by 2-1/2 to 3 years of age. If they continue beyond this time, the solution may be found in the manner in which you are handling your child during tantrums. However, other behavioural issues are often present in the family besides temper tantrums. These, along with the temper tantrums, should be addressed concurrently in order for compliance to take place. The power struggles that commonly exist are most often related to sleep issues, feeding issues or other behavioural issues.

If you find that you are unable to cope with your child's temper tantrums send out an S.O.S.!!! Consult with your doctor.

Testicles (Undescended)

Approximately 33% of premature boys and 3% of those born at term have one or both testicles undescended.

By 6 months of age, testes that will descend will, for the most part have descended. Certainly by one year of age a majority of those testicles will have descended into the scrotum.

If by 6-12 months of age, one or both testicles have not descended and cannot be felt at all, an ultrasound should be done to determine their location. If they are left undescended, there is an increased risk of testicular trauma, twisting of the testicle, cancer and a nonfunctioning testicle(s). When the child is older, there can also be a psychological effect from the absence of a testicle.

By 6–12 months of age, if one or both testicles, on ultrasound, are not present in the inguinal canal but higher up, then they should be surgically placed in the scrotum.

Retractile testes are ones that rest some of the time in the "penthouse" (i.e. in the inguinal canal above the scrotum), but often are found in the "boiler room" (i.e. the scrotum) during a warm bath. The vast majority of these will descend without any intervention before the time of puberty.

If retractile testes are not spending much time in the scrotum and are difficult to "milk down" into the scrotum, they should be considered as undescended testicles. Hormonal therapy may be considered between 4 and 6 years of age. The therapy consists of intramuscular injections given every 2 days for up to 6 doses. There are no side effects. If treatment is effective, the testes usually "thunder down" during therapy and remain in the scrotum. The success rate of hormonal therapy is low (approximately 30%) but is worth a try. If this therapy is unsuccessful, a urology consultation for a surgical opinion should be considered.

The management of undescended or retractile testes may vary depending on the training and experience of the doctors involved.

Throat Sore (Strep Carriers)

It is estimated that approximately 15%-30% of the population carry a strep bacteria in their throats. These carriers are asymptomatic and it is unlikely that they will transfer the bacteria to someone else and cause them to develop a strep infection.

So what does this mean? Every time a throat swab is done on such a child it will come back positive, because he is a strep carrier. It is also possible however, that the child may at some point develop an actual strep infection. In this case, it would be unclear whether the culture result is positive due to a true strep or because of the child's status as a strep carrier. It may also be difficult to determine whether the infection is viral or strep in origin. In fact though, the majority of throat infections are caused by viruses.

The following are the clinical criteria that I consider indicative of a possible strep carrier:

1. A child repeatedly has symptoms that are thought to be viral in nature and at the same time repeatedly has positive throat swabs for strep.

2. A child complains of recurrent sore throats; however, on examination of the tonsils, they do not appear infected, yet the throat swab is repeatedly positive for strep.

3. More than one member of a family are ill at the same time with sore throats and all are strep negative, except the child of concern.

4. A child has a positive strep culture but is not improving despite the use of an appropriate antibiotic, the appropriate dose, and proper compliance in taking the medication. The positive strep culture here is the "red herring", indicating a wrong diagnosis. Another cause for the symptoms should then be considered.

5. A child has a cold and/or eye infection and a sore throat, together with a throat swab which is positive for strep. Colds and eye infections, along with a sore throat, are most likely of a viral nature and are not due to a strep infection.

6. A child who has a positive throat culture for strep but does not complain of a sore throat.

If the child is suspected of being a strep carrier, then a throat swab should be done after a course of antibiotics has been completed. Alternatively, a throat swab may be done when the child is entirely well. In both these situations the culture should be negative. If it remains positive, the child is most likely a strep carrier. Further confirmation can be done by testing the blood to see if there has been a rise in the antibodies to strep 2–3 weeks after the infection. If there is no rise, then the infection was not due to strep bacteria. This further confirms that the child is a strep carrier.

If a child is identified as a strep carrier, every time he presented with a sore throat the doctor would most likely have to give him a course of antibiotics. The problem, therefore, is that the child would be receiving multiple doses of antibiotics that he might not require if the infection were viral.

The following are the options for managing a strep carrier:

• Do nothing. Each throat infection will be treated with antibiotics if the doctor feels it is caused by strep bacteria. Most strep carriers only carry the strep bacteria for varying lengths of time. I suggest a new toothbrush be used just before the end of treatment because the strep bacteria can remain for 4 days on the toothbrush and therefore perpetuate a strep-carrier state.

• A course of antibiotics normally used for a strep infection is prescribed for 10 days. For the last 4 days of treatment, an antibiotic called rifampin is added to the treatment regime. (Incidentally, rifampin may cause the urine and tears to have an orange tinge. This is expected and is not a concern. While taking rifampin, contact lenses should not be worn because they will become stained.) A few days after treatment has been completed, a repeat throat swab is done. If the strep has been eradicated, it will be negative; the patient is no longer a strep carrier.

• If the throat swab remains positive, then another course of antibiotic is indicated. Strep bacteria present very deep in the crypts of the tonsils and can be very difficult to eradicate. A 10–day course of clindamycin is the next step. Again, after antibiotic treatment, the throat swab should yield a negative result; the child is no longer a strep carrier.

• If the above protocols fail, then there are only 2 remaining choices. First is to recognize that the child is a strep carrier and treat only those infections that the doctor feels, on clinical grounds, are due to strep. The second option is removal of the tonsils.

To complicate matters further, those who have been successfully treated for being strep carriers may again become strep carriers. Similarly, as previously stated, strep carriers may revert to normal after a period of time without any treatment at all.

Management of the strep carrier may differ depending on the region in which you reside. Most physicians take a more conservative approach and treat each throat infection based on the clinical symptoms, inspection of the throat and the results of the throat swab, and do not try to eradicate the strep by the above measures.

Throat, Sore – Tonsillitis, Viral or Strep

The tonsils are located on either side of the posterior oral cavity. They vary from the size of very small peas to a size as large as walnuts. They, along with the adenoids, serve as a ring of tissue that prevents potential infective organisms from entering the lower respiratory tract. As a general rule, their size alone has little to do with the severity or frequency of infections. Small tonsils can have frequent infections with severe debilitating symptoms while large ones may become infrequently infected with only mild symptoms.

The tonsils may have many crypts (creases) on their surface. Within these crypts there may be soft to hard white secretions. These are found in normal tonsils and are not to be mistaken for infections.

Bacterial (strep) tonsillitis is very uncommon in children under one year of age and is infrequent until 3 years of age.

The vast majority of throat infections are viral in origin and therefore do not require antibiotics. Antibiotics are indicated only in patients with a proven beta hemolytic group A strep infection, that is, strep throat. A throat swab, therefore, is mandatory in all cases when a diagnosis of tonsillitis has been made on clinical grounds, to isolate a possible strep organism.

A child less than two years of age with symptoms suggestive of tonsillitis and white spots on the tonsils usually has a viral infection until proven otherwise – to reiterate, strep throat infections under 3 years of age may occur but are uncommon.

No child should be put on an antibiotic until a throat swab is done, and preferably not until that throat swab has proven positive for strep. Most culture results are available within 24 hours. Some clinics will do a rapid strep screen test. The results should be available within five minutes and are about 85% reliable for the diagnosis of strep infections. If the child is very ill, antibiotics may be started after the throat swab is done. If the throat swab returns negative, then the antibiotic should be discontinued. A similar approach may be used on long weekends when the results of the throat swab may not be available for a few days.

Caregivers should not pressure a doctor into prescribing antibiotics unnecessarily. Acetaminophen or ibuprofen may be given to relieve both fever and pain until the results of the throat swab are available and conclusive of a strep infection.

A typical strep throat more often presents in the child over 2–3 years of age. The child feels unwell, with fever and sore throat, and has difficulty swallowing. Swollen, tender neck glands are often present. Abdominal pain and headache are frequent. The child appears ill. On examination of the throat, the tonsils appear inflamed and swollen, with a grayish exudate. The soft palate and uvula also may be swollen and inflamed, with small hemorrhages on them. These are the typical clinical findings suggestive of a strep throat, but they are not diagnostic – a throat swab is still mandatory.

In a child who has a cold (with or without a cough) and is complaining of a sore throat – the sore throat is usually viral in origin. This is true as well with the child who is complaining of a sore throat and also has infection (conjunctivitis) in his eyes.

If two or more members of the family complain of a sore throat, the cause is usually viral.

The child who has all the symptoms and signs of strep throat and is also extremely tired, may have infectious mononucleosis (especially if the neck glands are very enlarged and tender). An enlarged spleen may be present. The diagnosis is confirmed by a blood test for mononucleosis ("mono"). There are other viruses that can give a similar picture. Children who have mono and are put on amoxicillin often develop a red rash on the body a few days after the medication is started. This is not an allergic reaction to Amoxil but it does characteristically occur in children with mono. No treatment for this is required. It will fade within a few days.

Supportive treatment for tonsillitis includes the use of acetaminophen or ibuprofen for pain and/or fever. The child should be encouraged to drink. Throat lozenges and gargling may help diminish the symptoms. The drug of choice is penicillin. Amoxicillin also works well. If there is an allergy to penicillin, there are other acceptable substitutions that will adequately treat the infection. These include clindamycin, azithromycin and clarithromycin. Once the child is well, he may return to his normal activity. This usually takes two days.

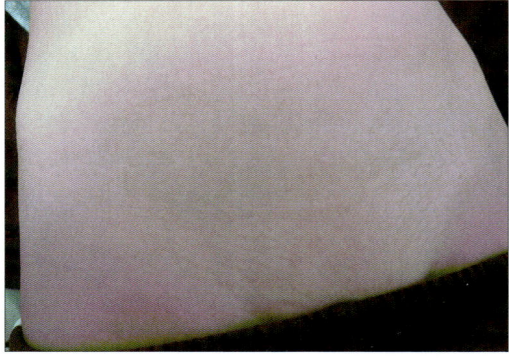
Scarlet Fever Rash

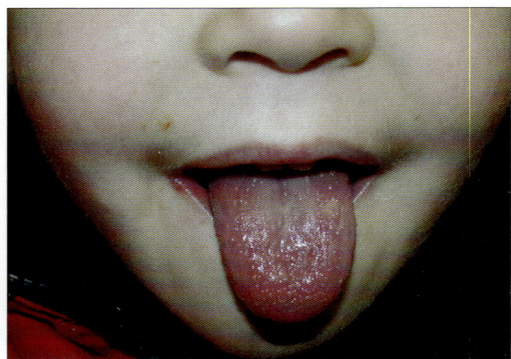
Strawberry Tongue

Scarlet fever is caused by only a few of the many different strains of beta hemolytic group A strep bacteria. The symptoms are the same as for other strep infections. However, within a day or two after the onset of the illness a faint rash may be present on the trunk of the child. The rash is heavier in the axillary (armpit) and suprapubic area (above the genitalia). It has a sand-paper feel to it. The area around the mouth may be pale. The tongue may have a strawberry-like appearance. The child may look and act ill. Peeling of the skin at the tips of the fingers may occur approximately 1 week later. It is extremely important that scarlet fever be recognized, because the strep strains that cause it are the very same strains that may result in rheumatic fever (heart damage) or acute glomerular nephritis (kidney damage). This is the one occasion when antibiotics should be started before the results of the throat swab are available. Early treatment of scarlet fever will prevent the complications mentioned above. With a strep infection there may be swelling and pain of one, or less often, more than one of the large joints. This is uncommon but does occur. Although joint swelling may also be a symptom of poststreptococcal rheumatic fever, more often it is just concurrent with strep strains that are not associated with rheumatic fever. Other diagnostic criteria must be present for the diagnosis of rheumatic fever. Diminishing of swelling in the joints usually occurs within 7–10 days.

The indications for removal of the tonsils are as follows:

1. Three or four proven strep infections occurring within a period of 8 to 10 months.

2. Several viral throat infections over a period of the year, during which the child was ill enough to miss a lot of school or daycare. I am excluding those children who just say "I have a sore throat" and are not really ill. Children, as well as adults, have varying pain thresholds – the "softies" versus the "toughies". Often it can be difficult for the physician to assess how ill the patient actually is. As a general finding, the younger the child, the more exaggerated are the symptoms described by the caregiver.

3. Peritonsillar abscess. Here the infection goes deep into the tonsils and underlying tissue. The child is usually very ill. Clinically, the diagnosis is confirmed by the examination of the oral cavity and noting a marked enlargement on one side of the tonsillar area. Hospitalization for IV antibiotics is required. Incision and drainage of the abscess may also be required. Once the infection is treated, the tonsils are usually removed a few weeks later.

4. In young children, the tonsils are often removed along with the adenoids if there is the additional presence of sleep apnea.

5. Very rarely there may be persistent or recurrent tonsillar bleeding or cancer of the tonsil. I have not yet seen either of these in 40 years of practice.

6. Tonsils are removed, if possible, to eradicate the status of "strep carrier" in a person who has persistent throat infections (see Throat, Sore – Strep Carriers).

7. Removal of tonsils will not increase a child's appetite. If, however, the child's tonsils are so enlarged that they are "kissing" each other and the child has great difficulty swallowing, then a tonsillectomy may be considered.

8. If there is a speech problem which is considered to be due to enlarged tonsils and/or adenoids then the tonsils/adenoids may have to be removed.

To be cautious, any child who has not had his primary immunizations and is complaining of a sore throat, as well as exhibiting other symptoms of tonsillitis, should receive medical attention early to rule out the possibility of diphtheria. With diphtheria a child is very ill with fever and has a marked difficulty in swallowing. As mentioned, it only occurs in those individuals who are not yet immunized.

Thrush-mouth – Monilia (Yeast) Infection & Monilia Diaper Rash

Monilia is a yeast infection. In infants, monilial infections occur most commonly in the mouth or the diaper area.

Thrush (Oral Monilial Infection)

Oral thrush is more prevalent in infants who are breastfeeding. It presents as whitish curds on the gums or lips that cannot be wiped off with the finger, whereas milk residue is easily removed with the finger. Frequently, the breastfeeding mother will notice a feeling of burning of her nipples (no rash will be present).

Thrush, in an infant, is not accompanied with any other symptoms (pain, feeding problems, digestive problems, fever, etc.).

Oral thrush should not be mistaken for a "milk tongue" in which the tongue is partially coated with a milk residue that is difficult to remove. The rest of the mouth (gums and lips) remain clean.

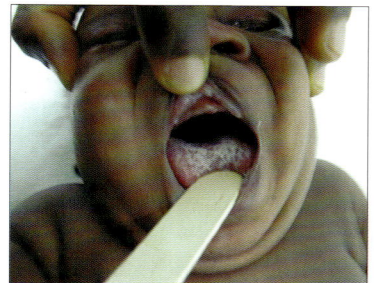
Coated tongue

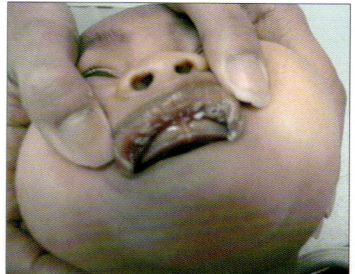
Thrush

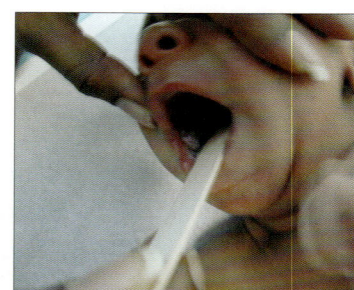
Thrush

Treatment

If the infant is bottle fed, then thoroughly sterilize the nipples before each feeding. The following medications can be used:

- Mycostatin suspension – this must be prescribed by the physician – 1 cc 4 times a day for one week – if no response, repeat for one more week.

- Gentian violet 1% – applied to all areas where the thrush is present, with a cotton stick, 4–6 times a day. This will turn the mouth purple. It stains, so wear old clothing (the stains do not come out). Use for 10 days.
- For mother's nipples – apply nystatin cream 4 times a day. It does not matter if the baby nurses when the cream is on the nipples, *or*
- Apply gentian violet 1% to nipples 4–6 times a day for 10 days (remember, it stains your clothing permanently).
- For persistent oral thrush the doctor may prescribe a course of fluconazole – this is given by mouth to the infant.
- If the thrush is on the lips as well as the mouth, the administration of oral medication will bypass the lips and thus be ineffective for this area. I suggest that mother uses a nystatin vaginal suppository (those used for women with monilia vaginitis) for the baby to suck on 4 times a day for 3 or 4 minutes. Clean the suppository after each use.

There are 2 conditions that may present with recurrent oral thrush that is resistant to the above therapies. These conditions are diabetes and an immune deficiency disorder. In 40 years of practice I have seen many cases of resistant thrush; however none of them was associated with either of these illnesses.

One side effect of inhaled steroids for asthma is the potential for developing oral thrush. It is recommended, if possible, to rinse out the mouth after each time inhaled steroids are administered. However, I cannot remember seeing a single case of oral thrush with the use of inhaled steroids, even in those who do not rinse their mouths (most of my patients do not rinse).

Monilia Diaper Rash

Unlike other diaper rashes, a monilia diaper rash has a distinctive characteristic appearance. It is a fiery red rash. The margins are quite defined. There may be several small satellite lesions on the skin around the rash. It spreads out, beginning at the base of the penis or around the vagina.

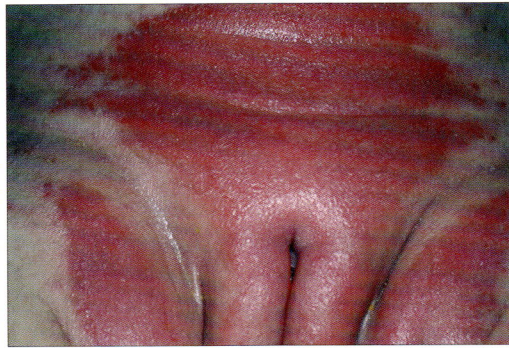

Yeast (Monilia) Diaper Rash

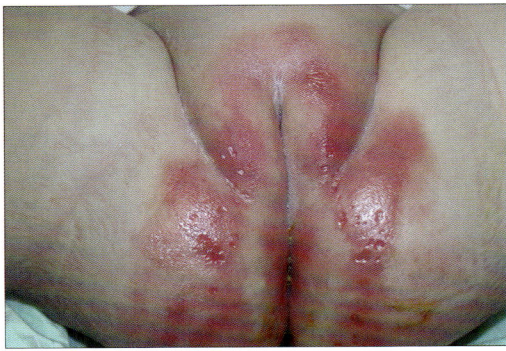

Ammoniacal Diaper Rash

Treatment

Exposing the rash to the air is very important.

Your doctor will order nystatin cream with or without hydrocortisone. Apply sparingly 3 times daily. It usually takes 7–10 days for the rash to disappear. A faint pinkish discolouration may persist for a few weeks. As with all other diaper rashes, exposing the area to the air as much as possible will help the healing process (this is more easily done with infant girls than with boys because of the distance the urine can flow).

Thumb Sucking and Pacifiers

The sucking reflex is one of the baby's natural instincts. It is functionally present for feeding. The sucking reflex, however, is also a powerful source of self comfort. Nothing is sacred – the knuckle, nose, arm or cheek. Anything, and I mean anything, that comes close to the mouth will be clamped onto.

The thumb has never received the recognition it deserves. When was the last time you heard "that's a fine-looking thumb"? It is essential for grasping, communicating (thumbs up is good; thumbs down is bad) and it can also be used for hitchhiking. Most important, it is a reliable, easily accessible object for sucking. It gives pleasure and security and has a very calming effect. Up to 60%–80% of infants suck their thumb. The vast majority of children stop by the age of 4; however, some will use it longer, usually exhibiting this behaviour when they are tired.

Generally, a pacifier is preferable to the thumb for sucking from the caregiver's point of view because with pacifiers it is easier to break the habit later on. However, the early introduction of a pacifier has some drawbacks. It is a time-consuming endeavour on the part of the caregiver to play the "pop in-pop out" game. As well, the early introduction of a pacifier before the infant is well established on the breast may, in some instances, not only shorten the duration of time a mother wishes to breastfeed but may lead to problems with breastfeeding itself (shorter and less frequent feeding). The use of a pacifier may also play a role in recurrent otitis media (middle-ear infections). One very positive factor is that it is thought that pacifiers may be helpful in the reduction of SIDS (sudden infant death syndrome). It is best to try to limit the use of the pacifier to times when the baby is fussy. A toddler who constantly has the pacifier in place will still develop language normally. However, speech may not be understandable when the pacifier is in place, and oral communication may be diminished. There may also be a delay in an infant or toddler's willingness to find other means for self-settling.

One thing that I find interesting is the different reactions of parents when a pacifier falls to the ground. Some will do nothing, some will wipe it off, others will use a spare pacifier or rinse it with water. Still others, for whatever reason, will, strangely, clean it off with their own mouths.

There are likely more germs in the caregiver's mouth than on the ground. It is most unlikely that any adverse reaction or infection will occur if you just wipe the pacifier clean and put it back into the infant's mouth.

A few words of caution if a pacifier is used. Make sure that:

- It meets the required standards for construction.
- It is the proper size for the child's age.
- It is orthodontically correct.
- It is checked periodically for dryness of the nipple or for a cracked nipple – if these are present discard the pacifier.
- Never hang a pacifier around the baby's neck by a string or chain – we do not want any accidental strangling.
- Never dip the pacifier in honey or other sweeteners – gum and dental disease will surely follow.
- Never threaten to take the pacifier away to obtain compliance – this is a cruel and unnecessary demonstration of your power. The result will have a negative impact on your parenting success.

How long should you allow the use of a pacifier or allow thumb sucking? By 4 to 4-1/2 years of age you should begin to discourage this habit. If sucking occurs only in the evening to help the child fall sleep, I would not be overly concerned.

Extensive sucking on either a pacifier or the thumb may lead to dental malocclusion (pushing the front secondary teeth forward) even before they have erupted. It may also push the hard palate up. This could lead to speech articulation problems. Both problems are directly related to the duration of time spent sucking, but more importantly, it is the degree of pressure (force) exerted by the sucking action that accentuates these problems.

How do you get the child to stop?

First, think about it from the child's point of view. He has had a readily available device for most of his life that is giving him much pleasure. Why in the world would he want to give it up without a titanic struggle?

It is easier to dissuade a child from using a pacifier than from using the thumb, which is conveniently and permanently attached. A carefully thought-out plan, along with very diplomatic negotiations, is required.

Negotiate for short periods of "time-out" (no sucking). Provide lots of praise and stickers as rewards. Slowly lengthen these time periods. Withdrawal should be gradual. Eventually, eliminate the evening need for a pacifier.

If the child is old enough, you may explain to him that the "pacifier fairy" will be coming to take it away while he is sleeping and leave something special in its place, for example, a small toy, book or puzzle. For the reluctant child who still wants to suck his thumb, try one or more of the following:

- A bandage or glove – this usually does not work because where there is a will there is a way, and the child will take it off soon after it is put on. A bandage could present a choking hazard. Do not use one when the thumb is being used to help settle for sleep.
- Dabbing non-toxic, bitter-tasting nail polish may be tried on the thumb and can be purchased at the local pharmacy.
- Rubbing garlic or onion on the thumb.
- Have the child hold on to a small toy during bedtime storytelling.

If none of the above suggestions is successful, orthodontic appliances from a dentist are easily available. These render thumb or pacifier sucking difficult to nearly impossible.

Maybe these babies are on to something! The sucking impulse is so strong that it continues in many adults for anxiety and stress control. The pacifier or thumb sucking is replaced by the cigarette, and a multi-billion-dollar industry is based on this compulsion. Oddly, there would be fewer health risks for adults if they were to follow the baby's lead for self-comforting – that is, suck their thumb or a pacifier.

Toilet (Potty) Training – Tricky, Very Tricky

You feel that you are ready to potty train your child. You have heard lots of conflicting advice as to when and how to accomplish this. You are somewhat confused but ready to give it a go.

For some, potty training is a breeze. For others it can be a very stressful time, especially in view of suggestions given to you by your "advisory staff".

Most children achieve bladder and bowel control between 2 and 4 years of age. Girls generally achieve control before boys. The average length of time from initiation of toilet training until it is fully accomplished is 3 to 8 months (and sometimes a much longer period). The sequence in which bowel and bladder training occurs is usually (but not necessarily) as follows – bowel control first, then bladder control during the day and, lastly, nighttime bladder control. Night control of the bladder may not occur until after 6 years of age or older. Bladder control is a neurophysiological (developmental) process. Although you may be able to help initiate and maintain urination dryness during the day using behaviour modification, nighttime training will take its own time.

On the parent's part, toilet training of a child requires a positive mental attitude, much patience and the investment of a lot of time. Never overtly demonstrate your disappointment about progress if it is not to your liking.

Potty training should never be attempted during a stressful time, for example, just before or after a move, or just after the arrival of a new infant.

Here are some signs that the child's toilet learning process may be initiated and that he is ready, willing and able to start:

- He understands the term(s) that you wish to use for the function that is being taught.
- He is able to remain dry for 4–6 hours.
- He is able to understand and follow simple commands.
- He has a desire to please, based on a positive relationship with his caregivers.
- He has the desire for independence in control of bladder and bowel functions.
- He seems uncomfortable when the diaper is wet or it contains a stool.

Now the adventure begins. Recognize that it is going to be harder and more frustrating for you than the child. After all, although you may think you have control over him, the real control over his bowel and bladder is purely his own.

Whether to start his training on a regular toilet with an infant toilet seat securely attached, or on a potty chair that sits on the floor, is your choice. It is important that the child feels secure and is not afraid. He should also be able to have his feet firmly planted either on the floor or on some other support so that he is able to use all muscles required.

Having him watch you use the toilet will help him to understand and be somewhat reassured that the toilet will not "swallow him up". Allow him to flush the toilet.

If there is any apprehension, go very slowly. If there is any reluctance, stop; he is not ready.

Place the child on the potty for a minute or so with the seat down while he is still fully dressed. A potty chair may be used as a regular chair so that he will become accustomed to it. Once he is comfortable with this, repeat the same with the seat up. Repeat both of these procedures with, and then without, a diaper. Place the contents of a soiled diaper into the potty to demonstrate its function.

Once this is completed, repeat the same process at specific times, for example, after waking in the morning, before and after naps, at mealtime, and at bedtime. This should be done approximately 6 times daily. Remember, do it just for 2–3 minutes – no longer.

The child needs to be praised whenever there is an expression of interest on his part in sitting on the potty. Begin watching for signals of the child's need to pee; for example, holding himself or herself; then encourage the use of the potty.

Remember the toilet is used for specific functions. Potty training is not the time for play, looking at books or colouring, for example. Certainly, talking with your child when he is on a potty is perfectly fine. Running water may promote the urge to urinate. Boys frequently like to sit on the potty to urinate before learning to stand. If nothing is accomplished within 2 minutes take the toddler off the toilet and try again later.

Once the child has used the potty successfully for 1 to 2 weeks, try switching him to training pants, and then, if he is doing well, to underwear. Remember, accidents are inevitable. Caregivers must be both patient and supportive. If there is a series of accidents, quietly return to the diapers. Try the process again after 2 or 3 weeks. At times there may be reluctance by the child to have a bowel movement. If this occurs, it is imperative that he or she be allowed to continue having bowel movements in a diaper. This will prevent a tendency toward having constipation and an experience of discomfort with the passage of the stool. If you allow constipation to develop, it is certain you will encounter a delay in the toilet training process. Toilet refusal means the child is not yet ready; therefore, back off and wait 1 to 2 months and then try again. Avoid negative reinforcement or punishment if accidents occur – in fact, expect them.

One little incentive to encourage compliance is to place a sticker or Cheerios at the bottom of the potty or in the toilet water. "Bombing" the sticker makes going to the bathroom fun and thus encourages the child to use the toilet. With boys, have dad compete with his son to see who does the best job at "bombing" (you lose one point if you splash on the seat and 2 points if you miss the toilet completely).

Some children are fascinated by the movement of water being flushed down the toilet. You can use this (allowing him to flush) as a reward for successful use of the toilet. Squirting coloured water into the toilet as if urinating may also enhance the child's interest in toilet use.

Remember, your child will progress on his or her own time schedule toward readiness to shed the diaper. Do not compare one child to another.

Night wetting may persist despite your expectations and your time schedule. Night wetting happens when the child is in a deep sleep and does not awaken with the signal of a full bladder. Restricting fluid intake after supper usually is ineffective. If you're able to wake the child up to go to the washroom before you retire, it can work occasionally and is worth a try. Remember there is a progressive maturation process that is physiologically necessary before complete night control is established. It may be well beyond 6 years of age before this occurs in some children.

All in all, there are no gold medals for being the first on the block to have a child potty trained.

If he were left on his own he would probably be self-trained at the same age regardless of all your efforts.

Tongue Tie (Poor Latch and Speech)

Underneath the tongue there is a web of tissue that connects the bottom of the tongue to the base of the mouth. This piece of tissue varies in size. It is called the frenulum. Tongue tie occurs when the frenulum is attached far forward, almost at the tip of the tongue.

On the bright side, he will have difficulty sticking out his tongue at people he dislikes when he gets older. On the dark side, he may have difficulty "blowing a raspberry" as an infant.

Tongue tie may interfere with an infant's ability to latch on to the mother's breast – the result being feeding difficulties.

If severe, it may also interfere with the child's speech articulation. Difficulty pronouncing sounds that require the tongue to touch the roof of the mouth may occur. Some examples are the /d/; /t/; /n/ and /l/ sounds.

Tongue tie is often overdiagnosed. If your infant's tongue can thrust forward enough to touch his lower lip there should be no problem with latching or articulating.

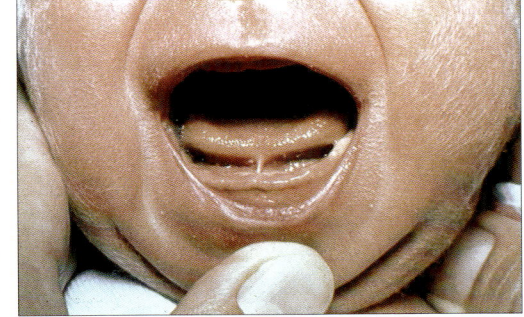

Tongue Tie

If the child is unable to touch his lower lip with his tongue and has difficulty in latching, the tongue tie should be released by snipping it with surgical scissors.

This procedure is most commonly done in an ear, nose and throat specialist's office. It is a minor procedure that takes only a few minutes. There may be slight discomfort and minimal bleeding. Infection is uncommon after a tongue-tie release.

If feeding problems were indeed due to tongue tie, then once released, there should be an immediate improvement in latching.

Torticollis (Wry Neck)

Congenital Torticollis

At 2–4 weeks of age, you or your doctor may feel a firm grape- to walnut-sized, nontender lump on one side of the infant's neck below the jawline. It is more common in infants born vaginally with a breech presentation.

The lump is a fibrous piece of tissue that has formed in the sternomastoid muscle of the baby's neck. It is not an enlarged lymph gland, tumor or cyst.

Its exact cause is uncertain. For some reason, during the birthing period there was a small hemorrhage in the sternomastoid muscle. The hemorrhage was replaced by firm, fibrous tissue – the lump. The baby's head may appear to tilt to the involved side and the chin appears to rotate to the opposite side.

Once diagnosed, treatment consists of physiotherapy. Physiotherapy involves gentle stretching of the sternomastoid muscle over a period of 1 to 2 months in order to stretch out the lesion. The physiotherapist will teach the parent how to do the exercises.

With early therapy, the resolution will be quicker. Best results are obtained when physiotherapy is started in the first 6 weeks of life.

If left untreated, by approximately 8 months of age the child's centre of vision will shift and no longer be where it normally would be. If the torticollis is surgically corrected after that time, the centre of vision will still be off, resulting in a visual problem.

Acquired Torticollis

Acquired torticollis is an inflammation of the sternomastoid muscle on one side of the neck. The inflammation is most likely viral in origin.

It occurs in a previously healthy child. There is no history of recent trauma. The usual story is that he wakes up in the morning complaining of a sore neck on one side. Because of muscle spasm, the head is tilted to the same side as the involved muscle and the chin is turned to the opposite side from the muscle involved. Commonly, it is tender to touch and painful if the child is asked to hold his head straight.

The treatment is the use of acetaminophen or ibuprofen for discomfort and ice on the affected muscle. It resolves within a few days.

Travel (Surf's Up) – Swimming

Not to brag, but I am somewhat of an authority on swimming. I still hold the Lake Simcoe record for the 10-metre dog paddle. My time was just under one minute. I was nosed out by a a 4-year-old; however, he was disqualified for using fins. It really does not matter that I was 18 years old at the time. A record is a record.

There are certain "nevers" that I have learned over the years. Never try to figure out your teenage daughter. Never teach your teen how to drive. Finally, never teach your own child how to swim.

There are two areas in which a child can learn to swim. One is in open water and the second is in an enclosed pool. The latter is a safer environment.

Starting to "waterproof" your child can begin as early as 4–6 months of age. A word of caution to parents of children who have already started to swim – no matter how well you think your child can swim, he or she should always be supervised, and supervision should continue until the child is at least 8 years of age. Less vigilance may be acceptable thereafter if you have additional support, such as certified lifeguards.

For the very best results, a certified instructor should be teaching your child. I personally prefer group lessons. Misery always enjoys company. A small class of 3 or 4 other children, hopefully of the same age and ability level, will help your child cope with the stress of learning how to swim in a much more casual and less intense atmosphere.

Some of you have home swimming pools. You are very fortunate. But this carries with it a tremendous responsibility: you are the sole person responsible for the safety of those swimming in the pool. This includes your own children, as well as guests. You are also responsible for pool safety 24 hours a day. Access to your pool may be easier than you think. Every year a few neighbourhood children may enter a pool when it is unattended and, unfortunately, a drowning may occur – a tragic and preventable accident. You are still responsible. You must ensure that all pool safety rules are known not only by your children but as well by any other parents and children who make use of your pool.

Whether the pool is chemically treated with chlorine or bromine is your choice. The latter is less irritating to the skin and eyes. Saltwater pools are an excellent choice – chemical reactions to the skin or eyes can be thus minimized.

If your child is not toilet trained, please have him wear the appropriate swim diaper. Nothing is more infuriating to your host than cleaning the bottom of the pool if your child has an "accident".

If the child is not able to swim in the deep water, be extremely cautious of flotation devices. Make sure that they are certified to be used for non-swimmers who may venture into deeper waters, and that they are the proper size for the child's weight – this is a must.

Wearing soft swim shoes at the beach will prevent foot trauma from stepping on stones or sharp objects that may not have been placed in the trash can.

Sunscreens are a must. A factor of at least 30 or more should be used. Reapply every 45 to 60 minutes – even those sunscreens that are specifically waterproof and meant for swimming.

Pain in the ear may occur shortly after swimming. If you pull on the outer ear and this elicits pain, the child has otitis externa (swimmer's ear). You can try to treat this with Buro-sol eardrops (these may be purchased over the counter). Two or 3 drops in the ear 4 times a day for 5 days should do the trick. If there is no improvement within 24 hours, an antibiotic/cortisone eardrop may be required (with a doctor's prescription). Swimming may be resumed when the child feels well enough. If swimmer's ear is a recurrent problem, preventative measures include using Buro-sol eardrops after each swim or using a hair dryer on low heat and pressure directed into the ear to ensure drying. Do not use cotton swabs to dry out the ear (impacting of wax may result).

Those children with tubes in their middle ear should not be excluded from swimming. Many can get by without any problems whatsoever. Drainage from the ear is a sign that contaminated water has entered the middle ear and has caused inflammation. A 5-day treatment with an antibiotic eardrop is required. Ear plugs are necessary to totally prevent water from entering the middle ear. I would start with those purchased from a drugstore that can be easily molded for your child's ear. If they continually fall out, an aqua band can be purchased from the drugstore and worn as a headband over the ears to prevent the plugs from falling out. These come in a variety of colours and are quite acceptable to the "style-conscious" child. Molded ear plugs for your child can be purchased but are more expensive – discuss this with your ear, nose and throat specialist.

Just another word of caution – an infant can drown in as little water as will fill a soup bowl. Never, ever leave a young child unattended in a bath, at a swimming pool or at the beach. Anyone who is responsible for a child while swimming should always take a CPR course and be recertified every 2–3 years.

Despite all of these cautions, water activities should be enjoyed. Swimming is a wonderful physical activity for your child. It also enhances both confidence and self-esteem. What could be better while having fun?

Travel Blues

It was 1947. Our family was about to take a "very long" car trip – an hour and a half to Hamilton, Ontario. We were in a 1945 two-door Dodge. I was squashed between both my brothers; we were squeezed together like sardines. It was a very hot summer day. Within two minutes of leaving I asked my dad, "How long is it going to be?" Five minutes later, I asked, "Are we there yet?" My older brothers took no mercy on me. They pinched me, pushed against me and said mean things, which I cannot repeat. I don't remember how many times my father said, "If you kids don't stop it, I'm going to pull over and you'll be in real trouble." We finally arrived and I heard my father mumble to my mother, "Never again." I still don't know what he was complaining about. After all, he was in the front seat and I was the one at the mercy of my brothers.

Travelling today is supposed to be a lot easier – especially for the parents. There are bigger and more comfortable cars. Everyone has his own seat. There is air conditioning and numerous entertainment tools – music CDs, storybook CDs, handheld games and individual or group videos. Mother is not just another passenger but an event coordinator. After all, if the kids are occupied and happy, so are Mom and Dad.

Is that the best scenario? Well, the answer is yes and no. Certainly, you can arrive at your destination a lot less hassled – that's the good. But I am a firm believer that when the opportunity arrives for children to learn, you should take hold of it. Children can benefit from having to make their own fun to pass the time. It develops creativity. The child is required to use his "inner resources" rather than just being entertained – to be active rather than passive. There may be fewer fights when watching a video but there are also fewer opportunities for "conflict resolution". However, having said that, kids are just kids and may fight like vipers over the channel or remote.

If you are driving in more remote areas with less intense traffic requirements, the following activities may be fun to try. Counting posts or license plate colours, playing word games, storytelling or singing songs may be old-fashioned but are also "mind builders". They can help to teach self-discipline, delayed gratification, digging deep to find a sense of fulfillment and the feeling of accomplishment that results. Now that is a learning experience – children who are spending the time using their minds rather than being involved in passive entertainment activities. Unfortunately, many of us have lost the patience and are unwilling to put in the effort to do these activities, especially with all our daily stressors. It must also be said that one must pay absolute, close attention to the road in most urban settings, with little distraction and utmost concentration.

You want to make the trip easy? Here are a few ideas. Rent a bus – a big one. Use earplugs. Rent a U-Haul and pile the kids in it (just don't forget to install air holes). Put sound-proofing Plexiglas between you and the children. Have someone else take the children to your destination. Seat them in a different section of the plane. You may get lucky and they'll be seated beside a pediatrician or child psychologist. If you really want to have a good time on your vacation, why don't you just leave them at home? I am quite sure you could think of many other ways to make your trip easier on you. Joking aside, I know that each and every one of you enjoys the company of your children and wants to spend quality time with them. What better way is there than on a family vacation? It is the getting there and back that is a major hassle.

In the end, will you have to compromise? Combine some of the old-fashioned techniques to keep your children occupied along with the newer media types of entertainment. Doing this is a win-win situation. Everyone is happy and your children learn something of value.

If your child has motion sickness in a car, place him in the middle of the back-seat (see Motion Car Sickness). On the plane, choose seats behind the wing, if possible. Take extra air sickness bags just in case. On the plane's departure and arrival, to prevent ear pain, have your infant drink and your older child chew gum or suck on a hard candy. Ear plugs, even for infants, are available to help prevent ear pain. Anti-vomiting medicine can be used if really necessary. I would certainly try giving it to the child prior to the trip to ensure that there are no adverse side effects. This also applies to any medication to help induce drowsiness and/or sleep – antihistamines or anti-vomiting medications share this common "sometimes beneficial" side effect. Consult your doctor. Patches worn to prevent vomiting are safe. Again, check with your pharmacist or doctor.

Just think of it – no matter how bad things seem they could always be worse – for example, having to contend with a frisky dog as well. At least you'll have plenty of stories to tell your grandchildren about how naughty their parents were as passengers when they were children.

Enjoy your trip – these opportunities for togetherness are priceless!!!

Travel Tips

Here are a few practical tips on how to make your vacation more enjoyable. Start with some basic guidelines – use common sense and "if in doubt – don't." If these tips are followed, read no further – have a great time! But just in case….

A vacation is a journey. It has a beginning and an end. It should be a memorable occasion. Involving your children with the planning of the entire journey will not only enhance the enjoyment of it but also yield an excellent learning experience for you all. The trip becomes an adventure. There isn't a child (or for that matter an adult) who doesn't love an adventure.

Before the trip you should discuss with the children in an age-appropriate manner your expectations of them – the "do's and don'ts" while away. Listen as well to their expectations. If you are visiting a foreign country that converses in a different language, it is always nice to learn a few words beforehand, such as "hello", "goodbye", "please" and "thank you". Teach the children about the politics, religion and culture of the area that you are visiting, keeping in mind their age and understanding level.

When travelling to a foreign country, the culture, behavioural expectations and laws may be different from those of your country and must be respected. It is very important that you acquaint yourselves as well, as your children with these differences to avoid potential problems. Examples would be dress codes in holy places, acceptable noise levels in public places, spitting on sidewalks and littering.

Waiting (waiting, waiting and more waiting) at airports can be a trying time for everybody. Children will accept the wait more readily if they are properly prepared beforehand. When walking inside the airport, it is a good idea to undo or take off their overcoats. You do not want anybody to have heat exhaustion before the trip has even begun. (The same goes for when the car is being warmed up for a long trip.)

The worst part of any vacation is the going and coming back. This is especially true when travelling with children. The younger they are and the more their number, the greater is the difficulty and strain on all, especially the caregiver(s). How many times have I heard a parent say, "Never again"? Yet we do it over and over again because the travel suffering is, hopefully, soon forgotten, but the memories (and photos) of the trip last a lifetime.

You as a parent must come up with the solution for travelling that best suits your children's needs. Whether it is a pillow and blanket, a cuddly bear, small books, magnifying glass, telescope or kaleidoscope, it is up to you (with the child's input).

There is nothing more exasperating than going on a long plane trip with an irritable infant or child. Although you may want them to sleep, all too often they are too excited to do so. You naturally are embarrassed that your children are disturbing the other passengers (crying, yelling, pushing on the seat in front of them or wanting to run up and down the aisle).

I am not generally partial to recommending sedation. However, there are cases when a mild sedative would be welcomed. Products such as Benadryl and Gravol are safe to use. I would suggest that they be tried before the trip to see their effect. Give it to the child at the same time you think that he would need it while on the plane. You can start with a double dose and repeat a single dose a few hours later if required. If it does the job you are set; if it does not, just keep your fingers crossed that all will be well. I am sure that you are well-prepared to entertain your child for the duration of the trip.

A miserable child makes everyone else within hearing range miserable as well. You can, however, only do what you can do. Most parents have been in the same situation. Try not to let this spoil your adventure.

A long car trip can be a pleasure (even if you take the children with you – a joke). Please do not rely solely on video games and DVD movies. It is a wonderful opportunity to play word games, read, have a singsong, colour, play "I spy", talk, share family stories, etc. – an excellent opportunity for "family time".

While vacationing in a cold climate, besides accidents that cannot be avoided, there are problems that can be averted. These include taking precautions against sunburn, windburn and frostbite. Ensure that all exposed body parts are well protected (use sunscreen or zinc oxide). If possible, do the activity with a "buddy". Depending on how cold it is, frostbite is a real possibility. Each member of the pair should check the other frequently for signs of frostbite. The early signs are, excessive redness followed by areas of pale skin which are numb to the touch. Exposed ears, the tip of the nose, the cheeks and the chin are the most common areas affected. One area that is often forgotten is the wrists. If the toes start aching they are probably frostbitten. If any of the above symptoms occur, go immediately to a warm area. Place your hands over the mouth, nose and chin and breathe in and out – the hot air will help the warming process. If the ears are involved, cover them. Place your toes in front of a warm fireplace. Never rub the affected area!

Travelling to a warm climate away from the frosty cold north also has health-risk factors. Most prevalent problems are posed by poor water safety. Children using a pool or playing by the ocean's edge must always be supervised – this is a given.

Sunburn, windburn, insect bites and stepping on jellyfish can be avoided if you take the proper precautions. You cannot overdose with suntan lotion. I would use no less than a 30 SPF or, better still, a 60 SPF. Apply liberally before going out and repeat often. A sun hat and sunglasses should be used by all. Remember that sun rays can be reflected from the water, sand and cement. Thick clouds offer only minimal protection from the sun.

If insects are going to be a problem, cover up the best you can. For children over 5 months of age DEET may be used (see Sunscreen and Insect Repellent). Check with your pharmacist or doctor as to the strength recommended for the age. Avoid using lotions near the eyes or on any open skin lesions.

If you are going to a foreign country, check with your doctor as to which vaccinations may be required. Do not wait until the last day to do this. Some vaccinations have to be started 2 or 3 months prior to departing on your journey. Preventative medication for malaria may be required.

A small first-aid kit is always a wise thing to take on your vacation. Hopefully, it will never have to be opened. It should include at a minimum the following: a lip balm, petroleum jelly, moisturizers, acetaminophen or ibuprofen of appropriate dosages and Gastrolyte or Cera powder (for diarrhea). Pepto-Bismol, in large doses, is a good remedy for diarrhea. Gravol may be used for vomiting. Also in your kit should be varying sizes of bandages, scissors, Polysporin ointment, 4 x 4 in. gauzes, disposable gloves and a hot/cold pack.

Some good news – infants under 4–6 months of age, and often older, have few problems with time change. They adapt quite nicely no matter where they are. Have a great adventure.

P.S.: Do not try to break in new shoes while you are on vacation.

Urinary Tract Infections

The urinary tract, from the lower extremity up, consists of the urethra, bladder, 2 ureters and 2 kidneys. An infection may occur in one or any combination of these parts.

Urinary tract infections are more common in females than males. The reason for this is that the urethra of a female is more exposed to a "hostile" environment. It is also shorter than the male urethra, allowing infections to climb into the bladder with greater ease. Proper hygiene also plays a role. The area around the female urethra is much more difficult to keep clean than the male counterpart.

Uncircumcised males under the age of one have an increased incidence of urinary tract infections compared to circumcised males.

Urethritis

Infection in the urethra presents as a burning sensation during urination. Blood may be visible in the urine (in males, if the urine stream can be observed, the blood often is apparent only at completion of urination). There are no other symptoms. Fever does not occur. Females whose labia are fused are more at risk for a urinary tract infection. In addition, bubble baths can be irritating to the urethra and lead to inflammation with subsequent infection. Overzealous cleansing – the so-called "hyper wiper" may also be the cause of irritation to the vulvar region.

Wearing tights, which can ride up between the labia, may be irritating. For females, wiping themselves from back to front, rather than in the reverse direction, can bring bacteria into the vulvar area. Lastly, pinworms may carry organisms from the rectum to the vaginal area, resulting in a possible urethritis, which in turn could result in an upper urinary tract infection.

Urethritis for males is more common if not circumcised. Patients will complain of a burning feeling at the tip of the penis. Usually, very little inflammation is evident on inspection. Warm water baths and drinking lots of cranberry juice will help during the next few days to resolve this condition.

Sexually transmitted diseases have occurred even in young infants. Depending on the circumstances, these must also be considered as a causative factor.

On urinalysis, there is usually some blood and protein in the urine and an increase in white blood cells. The urine culture is usually negative, meaning that the symptoms are either due to inflammation alone or, if infection is present, it is viral in origin. Only if the culture comes back as showing a significant single bacterial growth will treatment with antibiotics be required.

Urethritis symptoms usually last only a few days and then disappear. They may be intermittent in nature, with periods without symptoms. This depends on the underlying cause.

The treatment consists of acetaminophen or ibuprofen for discomfort, drinking lots of fluids including cranberry juice, along with frequent tepid baths.

Remember, antibiotics are only required if a significant number of bacteria are present in the urine culture. It is important that a urine culture be done before treatment commences. Otherwise, antibiotics which are unnecessary will be used for nonbacterial infections and may even be harmful (for example, an allergic reaction to the antibiotic, secondary diarrhea, or a yeast infection could occur).

With young girls who have repeated vaginitis I recommend treatment for pinworms, even without testing for them.

Upper Urinary Tract Infections – Bladder and Kidney

Depending on the age of the child, a urinary tract infection may present in a number of ways. In the infant who is unable to verbalize, the symptoms may also be common to many other illnesses. The symptoms may include irritability, a change in sleep pattern, loose stools, difficulty being pacified, abdominal discomfort and a decrease in appetite. The toddler who is not yet verbal may hold his/her hands over his/her "private" area while voiding. Foul-smelling urine may be present and the only clue to a possible urinary tract infection. Crying may occur on urination due to pain (because of the wearing of diapers, urination may not be seen by the caregiver and the connection not made). Older children who are toilet trained also may have accidents, both day and night; they may refuse to void and because of this have increased frequency of urination, passing only small amounts of urine at a time. Dysuria (pain on urination) is present.

A more specific indicator is the presence of an elevated temperature, especially when there is no other source of infection. Any infant under 1–1/2 to 2 years of age who has a fever lasting longer than 3 days without any other source of infection should be considered to have a urinary tract infection until proven otherwise. The younger the infant, the earlier the concern alert – especially for an infant less than 3–4 months of age. Any infant or toddler who has recurrent fevers lasting a short period of time (2 days or less) with no other symptoms should have a urinary tract infection ruled out.

Suspicion of a urinary tract infection arises from the history and the physical examination which shows no other source for the symptoms. Confirmation is made by urinalysis or the use of a urine dipstick. Both may show the presence of increased white cells, blood, protein, and bacteria in the urine. For the infant or toddler who is not toilet trained, the urine is obtained by placing a bag over the penis or vulva. For the child who is toilet trained, a urine specimen is obtained in a sterile specimen container. A midstream urine sample is preferable. No cleansing preparation has to be done prior to obtaining the specimen.

The urine specimen sent for culture and sensitivity testing, for a child who is toilet trained, should be a fresh specimen (less than one half-hour old), mid-stream if possible, and voided into a sterile container. It should be in the laboratory in less than a half hour after being obtained. The longer it sits, the greater the chance that bacterial growth will occur, which in turn may lead to a false positive result. Refrigerating the specimen will help delay the growth of bacteria until the specimen can be brought to the laboratory.

Any infant or toddler not toilet trained must have an in/out catheter specimen obtained for culture. This is done as an outpatient procedure at the hospital. A catheter is placed in the urethra and advanced to the bladder. The specimen obtained this way will have no contamination and therefore, hopefully, no false positive results. It is very important that the results of urine cultures obtained from bag specimens never be used to diagnose a urinary tract infection. Bag specimens are frequently contaminated, leading to misdiagnosis of a urinary tract infection. It is mandatory that the ultimate decision for determining the presence of a urinary tract infection be made by an in/out catheterization. I cannot overemphasize this. Although it is inconvenient, time-consuming and a somewhat uncomfortable procedure, an in/out catheter urine specimen must be done on all children who are not toilet trained.

Specimens obtained initially in non-sterile containers should never be used to diagnose a urinary tract infection, even if they are transferred immediately to a sterile container.

Treatment

Infants under 3 months of age are most often admitted to the hospital for IV treatment with antibiotics for up to 3 to 5 days and then are discharged on the appropriate antibiotic to be administered by mouth for a total of 10 days.

General measures consist of the use of ibuprofen or acetaminophen for fever/pain. Lots of fluids should be encouraged.

Treatment in the infant (over 3 months of age), toddler or child who is not ill may be delayed until the results of the urine culture and sensitivity tests are obtained. If the culture is positive, then the appropriate antibiotic will be prescribed orally to be administered according to the sensitivities.

If, however, the child is ill, once the culture has been obtained, an antibiotic may be initiated. If the culture shows that the bacteria present are resistant to the prescribed antibiotic it will be changed to the appropriate antibiotic. If the culture is negative, the antibiotic will be discontinued. With proper treatment the child should be markedly improved within 24 hours.

Follow-up and Investigations

I would certainly recommend that follow-up urinalysis and cultures be done after the child has been on antibiotics for 3 or 4 days to ensure that he is responding, and again a week to 2 weeks after the antibiotics have been discontinued to ensure that clearance has been maintained. However, in the real world, to put an infant who is not toilet trained through subsequent in/out urine catheterization is completely unrealistic. For these infants a bag specimen is fine. Depending on the results, a further catheterization specimen may be required. With those children who are toilet trained I would recommend similar follow-up as above. This would apply especially for a child who has had recurrent urinary tract infections.

All children under 2 years of age who have had an upper urinary tract infection should have an ultrasound of the kidneys to ensure that they are anatomically normal, and a catheter voiding cystogram to rule out any reflux going from the bladder up the ureters to the kidneys. All boys over 2 years of age who have an upper urinary tract infection should have similar investigations. There is still some controversy as to what follow-up investigations are required for girls with upper urinary tract infections. My view, ultimately, is that this decision should be made on an individual basis. Normally, when voiding there should be no reflux. With urination the bladder contracts to push urine out the urethra. There are no actual valves in the bladder to stop reflux of urine back up the ureters during the bladder contraction. However, because of the way the ureters are implanted in the bladder wall, with contraction of the bladder the ureteral openings are closed. With a single urinary tract infection the ability for this closure to function may be hampered. As a result, with each bladder contraction there may be a "backwash" of urine up the ureters. If the urine is infected with bacteria, the backwash may carry bacteria-laden urine upward, causing a kidney infection and possible kidney damage. The goal for management of a urinary tract infection is to prevent this from happening.

A voiding cystourethrogram (VCUG) involves a catheterization and injection of dye into the bladder. When the bladder contracts, the dye (if one or both ureter-bladder junctions are incompetent) will travel upward in the ureter(s) to varying degrees. The degree of reflux is graded. With increased reflux the grading is higher. Estimating the grade of reflux is important. With a bladder infection, if there is reflux up to the level of the kidneys, bacteria in the urine may cause an infection in the kidney – known as pyelonephritis.

If no reflux is present no further monitoring is required. If, however, there is reflux to the level of the kidneys, then monitoring the child for potential future urinary tract infections is important. Any fever lasting for more than 48 hours without an ostensible cause should be considered a urinary tract infection until proven otherwise.

After one year, the VCUG should be repeated if reflux was initially present. If the reflux has resolved, nothing further needs to be done. If, however, the reflux persists, a referral to a urologist should be made. The urologist most often will do a cystoscopy to examine the entrance of the ureters into the bladder to determine the degree of residual damage. Yearly VCUGs will be done. With continued reflux an anti-reflux surgical procedure will be carried out. This procedure, done in hospital, will prevent further reflux.

Prophylactic (preventative) use of antibiotics in a child who has recurrent urinary tract infections is no longer considered the standard of treatment. It has been found that with the routine use of prophylactic antibiotics, future urinary tract infections that occur may result from bacteria that have become resistant to standard antibiotics.

The above comments on the management of urinary tract infections are not cut in stone. Each child is considered on an individual basis. Management depends on the training of your individual doctor and what is considered to be the standard of care in the community in which he practices.

Vaginal Irritation and Discharge

The lining of the external genitalia before puberty is very thin and prone to irritation.

A clear, milky white discharge, which is often noted in a newborn's vaginal area, is normal. It will disappear within 1–2 weeks. No treatment is required.

There are a number of factors that may lead to irritation of the external genitalia. These include poor hygiene (wiping from back to front), soaking in bubble baths, and the overuse of scented soaps and wipes. Over-vigorous wiping during cleaning of the vaginal area may lead to irritation. Do not be a "hyper wiper". Tight-fitting synthetic tights may irritate the outer vaginal area. Irritation of the labia from stool or urine can also be causative factors.

Resulting symptoms typically include itchiness of the external genitalia, redness, and just generalized discomfort.

The combined symptoms above are diagnosed as vulvitis. There is little to no discharge.

Treatment

- Give frequent oatmeal or oilated baths.
- Discontinue bubble baths.
- Properly wipe from front to back.
- Use non-scented soap.
- Avoid tight undergarments (non-synthetic material is preferred).
- Expose the area to air as much as possible.
- Use loose-fitting diapers (do frequent changes).

- Apply a very thick coating of diaper ointment when the infant is wearing diapers or underwear (the thicker the better).

When the above symptoms occur in the presence of a large amount of discharge, especially if there is a foul odor, there is usually an additional yeast or bacterial infection known as vaginitis.

Yeast infections are most common in children under a year of age. The discharge, if present, is usually minimal. The skin around the vaginal area appears fiery-red with a well-demarcated margin between the rash and the normal skin. Small satellite (peripheral) lesions may be present.

Unlike for adult women, vaginal yeast infections from the use of antibiotics (which kill off the friendly bacteria as well as the nasty) are uncommon in younger children.

Treatment consists of the same measures as for treating vulvitis. A cream or ointment for the treatment of a yeast infection will be prescribed and cortisone may be mixed with the yeast medication to help decrease the inflammation. Treatment usually takes 7–10 days. Once healed, the skin may appear less pigmented. The pigment will return within a few months.

In children over a year of age, the presence of vaginal irritation along with a yellow to green discharge will necessitate the taking of a culture to rule out a bacterial infection. The most common bacteria checked for may be streptococcus (others may be present). Topical, as well as oral, antibiotics will be required.

Occasionally pinworms may enter the vagina, causing irritation and possible secondary infection. I feel it is prudent to treat any child who has recurrent vaginitis with treatment for pinworms, as well.

If there is no improvement within a few days it may be suspected that a foreign body is present in the vagina. As well, repeated intrusion of a foreign object into the vagina can result in persistent vaginitis. The repeated insertion of a foreign object may be the doing of the child. However, child abuse must be a consideration for any child who has recurrent vaginal infections.

Visiting Your Doctor

Like going shopping or going on an adventure trip, going to the doctor with your child (children) can turn out to be quite a trying experience. Details and arrangements must be made with military precision, and timing must be right to move the troops en masse. The visit may include mom, dad, baby and older siblings, and don't forget grandmother. Only Fido and the goldfish are reluctantly left behind. The journey, however, can be made more pleasant if the plan is put in place as long as possible prior to the visit.

Believe me, although it does not always seem that way, the doctor and his staff are there to help you. A successful doctor–patient relationship depends on the confidence you have in the doctor and his staff. This confidence usually is a result of good communication between both parties.

Remember, doctors are human too. They have their good days and, unfortunately, some bad ones. They have headaches and disagreements with their spouses (very occasionally), and are not infrequently tortured by their own children. As such days wears on, there is not a doctor who does not become a little more grumpy – for this we apologize! Most doctors truly understand and respect how long it takes you to prepare to get to their office, wait in their waiting room and do the reverse after your visit. Most also understand that when they are in the examining room with you, as far as you are concerned, you are their first and only patient of the day. You (the caregiver) want 100% of the doctor's attention. Speaking personally, I wish this were the case. I wish there would be no interruptions during the visit. I wish I could spend more time than I do with my patients. I can only hope that when the visit ends all of your needs will have been met and all of your questions answered to your satisfaction. Unfortunately, for many reasons, in the real world this does not always happen.

If you feel in any way upset or short-changed by your visit, always talk it over with the doctor to clear the air. Do not let it eat away at you. A doctor has only one personality to deal with hundreds of different personalities. Understanding works both ways. If you are upset, do not take your frustrations out on the staff. Similarly, if a problem arises with one of the staff, discuss this with the doctor.

If you do not quite understand the instructions given to you, do not be embarrassed to say so. If you feel further information or explanations are required – ask. If you feel the doctor does not understand you or underestimates your concern, then it is your responsibility to speak up. Most doctors these days are feeling rushed but are willing to spend the time to answer all your questions – either at your appointment or later with a phone call.

Here are some ways to get the "biggest bang for your buck" during your doctor's visit:

- Write down all questions before the visit.
- Have a pen and paper handy to jot down any notes.
- Keep the visit about the child you're bringing in (if you wish a second child to be seen, phone first to see if it is possible or let the secretary know when you check in, so that this child's chart can be pulled).
- If medications have been prescribed by another doctor, then bring them with you. Saying that your child is on the "pink medicine" is not helpful.
- If laboratory tests have been performed elsewhere, try to bring the results with you. If you're unable to do so, jot down the name of the lab or x-ray facility so that the results can be obtained. Saying that your child had blood tests and you think they were normal, again, is not helpful.
- If your child is particularly apprehensive, then inform the nurse. There are special techniques that can be used to handle the visit in the least upsetting way possible for the child.

• If your child is ill, then write down the symptoms in an organized way – day by day if possible. The doctor wants to know what the symptoms are and not whether the child was wearing red or blue socks when they occurred (an exaggerated example for sure, but all too often unnecessary information is given).

• If you feel your child is very ill, let the staff know immediately. Very ill children will always be seen first.

• If you feel your child has an infectious disease (chicken pox, for example) let the staff know so he will not wait in the common waiting room.

• If there has been an address, phone number or insurance number change, please inform staff upon arrival.

What to Bring to the Visit

• Insurance information.
• Extra diapers and wipes.
• A plastic bag to dispose of any soiled diapers. The odor of a soiled diaper thrown into the wastebasket will linger for hours. Have some consideration for the people who follow you.
• Remember to bring in your child's immunization booklet so it may be kept up to date.
• If grandparents or someone else is bringing the child in for the visit, provide them with a list of questions to be answered, and include a phone number where you can be reached if necessary (also the name to be used if a call is required to your place of work).
• Did not give the child anything to eat or gum to chew during the visit. We certainly do not want the child to aspirate from crying or choke on anything during examination of his mouth.
• If the child is to receive a reward for behaving well and the visit ends up being a disaster, then the child should not be rewarded – a lesson will be taught.
• If a form(s) is to be filled out, fill in as much as you can yourself. Do not wait until the very last minute for the form to be filled out. You cannot expect the doctor to fill it out on the spot. Other forms from other patients have to be filled out on a daily basis. They may need to be left to be picked up at a later date.
• Respect the doctor's equipment. These are not toys and are easily broken and quite expensive to replace.
• Please turn off your cell phone during the vist to the doctor.

Most doctors are fully booked 3, 4 or more weeks in advance for routine health examinations. So if you know that you require such an appointment, for example, an annual health examination, a well-baby visit, a presurgical checkup, or a pre-camp or school physical, please phone well in advance so that the date and time of your choice will be available. Waiting until the last minute, and then becoming upset with the doctor's staff because the time is not available, is not productive.

If you feel that you will require more time from the doctor than normally spent during a routine visit, please let the staff know. That way you may be given a longer appointment, for which the appropriate time required may be set aside to properly handle your concerns.

Ill children will always be seen the same day as a call. Restrict the discussion to this illness only. Any other concerns should wait for subsequent appointments.

Personally, I hate to wait a long time before seeing the doctor. I am sure you feel the same way, especially when you have young children with you. Long waits and inability to get through to the doctor because of the phone being continually busy are the 2 most common complaints patients have with their doctor's office. I completely understand and sympathize with you. All I can say is that we try to meet your needs as quickly as possible – unfortunately, the busier the doctor, the busier the phones.

Ultimately, no one wants a negative visit. It is not a pleasant experience for the child, for you, or for the doctor. As doctors, we do our best, but we need your help. You and your doctor are, after all, on the same team, with a common goal – to support your family and to meet its health needs in the best way possible.

Vitamin D

Vitamin D has been the subject of recent debate. At present the recommended dosages are:

- Breastfeeding mothers should take 800–1000 international units (IU) daily by diet and or supplement.
- Breastfed infants – 400 IU daily.
- Toddlers more than one year of age who drink less than one litre of vitamin D-fortified milk a day – 600 IU daily.
- All children and adolescents should receive 800 IU daily by diet and/or supplement.
- Pregnant women should have at least 800–1000 IU by diet or supplement daily.
- Adults over 50 would probably benefit from up to 2000 IU daily.

There is not enough exposure of the skin to the sun's rays during the winter to ensure that an adequate supply of vitamin D is produced by the body.

Vitamin D is not only important for normal bone development but is probably important in its association with the prevention of various diseases, such as multiple sclerosis, type 2 diabetes and some cancers. As more research is being done, vitamin D is seen to be an important link in the prevention, delay of onset or treatment of many other illnesses, especially those with an autoimmune origin.

I myself take 1400 IU of vitamin D as a daily supplement. I probably receive another 400–600 IU in my diet. The bottom line – if unsure of the vitamin D present in the diet, a supplement will do no harm.

Vitamins and Supplements

There is something I have wanted to reinforce to parents, and now I have the opportunity to do so – toddlers (one year of age), young children and teenagers who are healthy and are eating a well-balanced diet should not have to supplement their diet to maintain or improve health. Parents frequently ask me whether their children require any type of supplementation. "My child always looks tired." "What about the dark circles under his eyes?" "Certainly there must be something to help prevent him from getting so many colds!" "Will vitamins help him do better in school?" "Surely there must be something that I can give my child so that he will grow taller!" I could go on and on. Still, the question remains; what constitutes a well-balanced diet? Alas, I have the feeling that the majority of today's children, as well as adults, are not following a well-balanced diet. To be assured of complete nutrition, my recommendations at this time are to supplement your diet with any multivitamin and 400–2000 international units of vitamin D, depending on you and your child's age. Omega-3 fatty acid (DHA) would also be of benefit.

We all know from past experience that that which is "in" today is "out" tomorrow. The reverse is also true – that which is "out" today is "in" tomorrow. Our knowledge of what our bodies need in the way of optimal nutrition and nutritional supplementation is a rapidly advancing and ever-changing field.

Be aware though that everything comes at a price – not only to your wallet but there is the chance of doing harm as well to your child's body. An overdose of some supplements can be harmful (for example, excessive fluoride causes pitting of the teeth; kidney stones may result from overloading with vitamins). There are some supplements which can interfere with prescribed medications – always discuss this possibility with your pharmacist or doctor to ensure your child's safety.

To keep this as simple as possible, the following are well researched and generally recommended supplements for normal growth and development. I am not including those needed for the child with special nutritional needs.

Iron – All premature infants who were born before 34 weeks gestation require supplemental iron on a daily basis until one year of age.

All infants who are formula fed should have an iron-fortified formula. By the way, there is not enough iron in iron-fortified formulas to constipate a minnow, or to cause colic or any other digestive problem.

All infants, children, and adolescents who are on a low-iron diet (little meat, eggs, iron-fortified cereals and vegetables such as spinach) should be monitored for iron-deficiency anemia and supplemented accordingly. Women who have heavy menstrual cycles are also prone to iron-deficiency anemia.

Toddlers who drink large quantities of milk (cow's milk has a low iron content) to the exclusion of solids will surely develop a nutritional anemia within a few months due to low iron intake. Infants over one year of age should be restricted to no more than 20 ounces of milk a day in total. When their fluid intake is limited they will then still have an appetite for solids. Iron is found in meat (especially liver), eggs and spinach.

Vitamin D – All infants who are breastfed require supplementation with vitamin D from the first week or two after birth until they are weaned to formula. All formulas are enriched with vitamin D. When cow's milk is introduced, all infants should remain on vitamin D, 400 international units daily. It has been recently shown that vitamin D is not only important for bone growth but may be helpful in preventing other conditions, such as multiple sclerosis and type 2 diabetes. The recommendations, therefore, at present are that all infants, children and adolescents receive a minimum of 600-800 international units of vitamin D daily either by diet or vitamin supplementation. By the way, in Canada there is not enough exposure to sunlight for the body to stimulate the production of adequate quantities of vitamin D, even during the summer months.

Fluoride – If an infant's or child's water source is primarily bottled water or home-filtered water, fluoride may not be present. Check with the manufacturer of the bottled water or home filtration system used to see if fluoride is present in the water. If manufacturers cannot provide a satisfactory response, have your water analyzed for fluoride. Fluoride is important for proper tooth development. If a supplement is necessary, the dose will depend on the age and size of your child.

Fluoride treatment which is applied to the teeth is important to help prevent dental disease. This should be done on a regular basis as arranged by your dentist. The first visit to the dentist should be no later than 2 years of age and preferably by one year.

Folic acid – some milks, especially rice and goat's milk, are low in folic acid. Depending on the child's diet, supplementation may be required to prevent a folic acid deficiency.

Omega-3 (DHA) and Omega-6 (ARA) fatty acids – Breast milk contains these essential fatty acids. They have been shown to be important in retinal and neural development. This is most significant for premature infants. Studies have demonstrated that when comparing breast-fed children, regular formula-fed children and those fed with formulas fortified with these fatty acids, cognitive function of those who were breastfed and on formulas supplemented with fatty acids was higher than those fed routine formulas at 18 months of age. The data is just emerging concerning the beneficial effects of DHA and ARA on older children. Until this is sorted out, I feel it is prudent for formula-fed infants to be on an enriched fatty acid formula until one year of age. In the diet thereafter, 3 helpings of fish per week should supply all the fatty acids required.

There are a few myths concerning supplements that should be cleared up. Vitamins do not stimulate appetite. Vitamins will not increase growth. Vitamins will not prevent or alter the course of the normal cold.

You, as a caregiver may be under a lot of pressure to "vitaminize" or use naturopathic products to maintain the health of your children. This advice comes, not infrequently, from your non-elected "advisory staff" (your mother, mother-in-law, Aunt Minnie, neighbours and friends). As well, you are constantly being bombarded by advertisements, especially infomercials – the 21st-century counterpart to the old snake oil medicine man. Again, the best way to meet your child's nutritional needs is through natural food sources.

If you have any doubts concerning the dietary needs of your child, please consult a professional (the child's doctor or qualified nutritionist) before throwing away your hard-earned cash on unsuitable and/or potentially harmful supplementation.

Those caregivers who wish to keep their children on a vegetarian diet should have their child's diet reviewed by a nutritionist to ensure there are no deficiencies. Remember, ultimately you are the one who should be choosing what is going into your child's mouth. and not your child; it is not about a battle between you and your child, it is about being well-informed and making wise choices.

My advice to the parents who are concerned about supplementation is that if you model good lifestyle and eating habits, your child will follow your example.

P.S.: Keep all household medicinals out of reach of your children!!!

Vomiting and/or Diarrhea (Gastroenteritis)

"Itis" when placed after a word in medical terms means "inflammation". The medical term for vomiting is "gastritis". The term for diarrhea is "enteritis". If both vomiting and diarrhea are present at the same time, it is called "gastroenteritis".

All 3 of these conditions – vomiting, diarrhea or combination of both – are very common throughout infancy and childhood. Besides respiratory tract infections, they are perhaps the most common reason that the caregiver seeks medical advice.

For young infants under a few months of age, it is often difficult for a caregiver to determine if they are just spitting up or vomiting. Moreover, when do the stools, which normally appear loose and seedy, become diarrhea? If your infant has a change in pattern, then there probably is something that needs to be dealt with.

A problem is indicated if the spitting up becomes more frequent and the quantity increases. Similarly, if the stools become more frequent and more watery, then diarrhea is most likely the reason.

The majority of illnesses in infants who vomit or have diarrhea, or a combination of both, are the result of viral infections. Bacteria and parasites can also be the cause of gastroenteritis (usually enteritis alone). Medications (usually antibiotics) may cause loose stools of varying degrees.

Note: Infants under two months of age can become dehydrated quite quickly. The passing of one large watery stool may be enough to cause dehydration. As a general rule, infants under two months of age who are either vomiting or have diarrhea, or both, should receive medical attention.

Symptoms of dehydration – The earliest symptom of dehydration is a decrease in urine output (an infant who is having at least 4 good wet diapers is probably not dehydrated). The decrease in urine output is caused when the baby's body is trying to conserve water. Other symptoms indicating dehydration are a lack of tearing and extreme dryness of the tongue and mouth. Other reasons for concern include:

- An infant who is less than two months of age.
- Sunken fontanels and/or eyes.
- Refusal to drink.
- Skin pallor (pale), the skin feels cool or a bluish tinge underneath the nails is noticeable.
- Baby displays lethargy (increased weakness) or seems very irritable.
- Weak crying.
- Rapid breathing.
- Difficulty in arousing (awakening).
- Bile (dark green) or blood in the vomit.
- Presence of blood in the stools.
- Crampy abdominal pain.
- Projectile vomiting (shoots out like a firehose).
- If there is no improvement within 48 hours of onset of symptoms or worsening of the symptoms during this period of time.
- Elevated temperature (rectal – greater than 102.5°F or 39°C).
- Returning from travel outside of Canada and the USA.

If any of the above symptoms or concerns are present, the child should be seen by a doctor.

Viral causes are much more common than bacterial ones. This is usually the case if more than one person in the family has similar symptoms. Daycare settings are a haven for viral infections, including gastroenteritis.

Children with bacterial infections are usually more ill than those with viral infections. They often have a higher fever. The abdominal pain is crampy and more severe. Blood may be present in the stool.

Infants and children with gastroenteritis which starts before or within a few days after their return from travel outside of Canada and the United States should have a stool sent to be checked for bacteria or parasite infection. This is especially true if they are returning from the Middle East, India and its surrounding neighbours, the Philippines, China or Vietnam, Africa, Mexico or any other country where a specific "bug" is endemic (common).

Note: There are other conditions that may present with symptoms of acute onset of vomiting and/or diarrhea. These may not be infections.

Pyloric stenosis – This is more common in boys and presents as increasing episodes of projectile vomiting during or after feeding. It is usually painless, and the regurgitation does not contain blood or bile. It usually begins after the first week of life but seldom presents after 4 weeks of life. The diagnosis is made by history, physical examination and an ultrasound of the abdomen. The pylorus is a muscle found at the junction between the stomach and the small bowel. bowel. If the pyloric muscle goes into spasm after feeding this junction becomes blocked . Then when the stomach contracts to push milk into the small bowel, the force of the stomach contraction causes the milk to shoot out of the mouth in a projectile manner. Pyloric stenosis is a surgical emergency.

Bowel obstruction – This presents with the sudden onset of very severe abdominal pain. It is as if the child has been hit in the stomach with a cannonball. Dark green bile may be present if the child is vomiting. Bloody diarrhea (like currant jelly in appearance) may also be present. This is a surgical emergency.

With any gastroenteritis, the vomiting usually begins before the diarrhea, seldom the reverse.

Treatment – The purpose of treatment is to maintain hydration, prevent further dehydration and to rehydrate if necessary.

Over-the-counter medications (such as Gravol, Kaopectate or Imodium) should not be used in the treatment of vomiting and/or diarrhea in infants and toddlers. As well, any "homemade" remedies should not be used. Acetaminophen (Tylenol, Tempra and Panadol) as well as ibuprofen (Advil) may be given if fever is present. A prescription medication called ondansetron (1 dose) may be helpful for the child who has persistent vomiting and is unable to retain any fluids.

Breastfeeding of the infant is to be maintained during his illness. If the diarrhea is mild (2 to 3 small watery bowel movements daily) and the child does not appear ill, no dietary changes (including the elimination of milk) are required.

For moderate vomiting continue breast-feeding. Discontinue the formula and any solid foods until the vomiting has ceased. Offer the child oral rehydrating fluids – Pedialyte or Gastrolyte. These may be given as liquids or frozen as Popsicles. If you cannot find a flavour that the child likes, you may add unsweetened Jell-O or Kool-Aid powder (a 1/4 to 1/2-teaspoon) for taste. Carbonated or uncarbonated beverages such as pop, juice, Kool-Aid, fruit juices and the so-called sports drinks, such as Gatorade, should be avoided. None of these beverages contains the appropriate balance of water, salt, and sugar required, and may, as a result, worsen the child's illness.

The following is a guideline for the approximate required amounts of oral rehydrating fluids to prevent dehydration:

- Up to 6 months of age – 30 to 90 mL (1–3 ounces) every hour.
- 6 months to two years of age – 90 to 120 mL (3–4 ounces) every hour.
- Over two years of age – 120 to 240 mL (4–8 ounces) every hour.

Once the vomiting is under control, the child may go back onto a completely normal diet without any restrictions (this includes milk).

Stool samples may be required to determine the cause of the illness – bacterial, viral or parasitic. Not every case of gastroenteritis requires stool analysis. It is only recommended if the following descriptions fit:

- If the child is in daycare and others there have similar symptoms.
- Child has severe cramps.
- There is blood in the stool.
- He has recently returned from foreign travel other than to the USA and Europe.
- The child is immunocompromised or on medication that could affect his immune system.
- Child is experiencing repeated bouts of gastroenteritis over a short period of time.

There is no specific medication to prevent or cure gastroenteritis caused by a virus. Anti-diarrheal agents should be avoided. They may only mask symptoms, leading a caregiver to falsely believe that their child is improving when, in fact, this is not the case.

Antibiotics may be used for specific bacterial or parasitic infections only.

The mainstays for preventing the spread of gastroenteritis are the following:

- Frequent handwashing by the patient and the caregivers.
- The frequent use of antiviral and bacterial hand rubs.
- No sharing of food or anything else that goes in the mouth.
- Frequent cleaning of surfaces the infected child is in contact with (for example, the change table).

If the diarrhea persists for more than one week with only minimal improvement, I suggest the following: Continue breastfeeding. Place the child on a lactose-free milk and a dairy-free diet (no cheese or yogurt, which contain lactose) for 10 to 14 days and then return to the normal routine. Lactose-free cow's milk and formula are readily available. Soymilk or soy formula are helpful only because they are lactose-free and not because of the presence of soy per se. All other lactose-free dairy products may be used (cheese, yogurt, etc.).

The reasoning behind this is as follows: The small intestinal lining is covered with a very fine film that contains the enzymes necessary to digest food. One of these enzymes is called lactase. It is responsible for breaking down lactose sugar, present in milk and dairy products. Without the presence of lactase the lactose will not be broken down and, subsequently, will not be absorbed into the body. The presence of too much lactose may cause persistent diarrhea. Placing the child on a lactose-free diet gives the intestinal lining time to "heal" and regain the ability to produce needed digestive enzymes such as lactase. If this is allowed to occur the diarrhea ceases.

The use of a probiotic for 5 days will help to restore the normal beneficial flora and friendly bacteria of the bowel. This will in turn lessen the severity and duration of the illness.

With diarrhea, the skin around the child's buttocks area may become quite raw and irritated. To prevent this or to treat it if it occurs, apply a very thick layer of diaper paste and also make sure to change his diaper more frequently than usual.

The above suggestions are some guidelines only. It is impossible to cover every situation. What is most important is that if you feel your child is ill with gastritis, enteritis or gastroenteritis, you need to seek medical attention at once.

Warts

Warts are a result of a viral infection in the skin. They normally do not occur in children under 3–4 years of age and are often found on the bottom of the feet (plantar warts) or on the hands and fingers

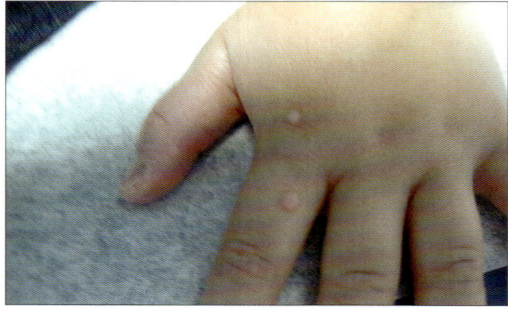

Hand Wart

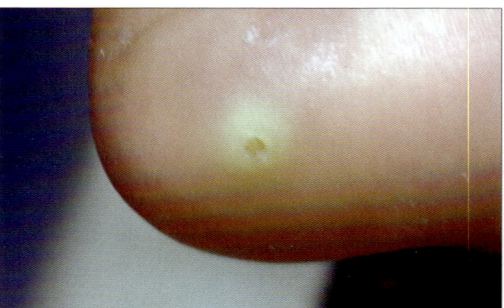

Plantar Foot Wart

where they appear as a small raised area on the skin. Plantar warts have little black specks in the centre. Plantar warts are often mistaken for calluses. Calluses are usually found on the edges of the large toes or on the ball of the foot below the large toe.

Warts are not related to poor hygiene. My grandfather told me they are caused by stepping on a frog. However, science has not backed this up as yet.

They are not very contagious from person to person, but may spread from one area to another on the child who has the wart.

Most often there are no symptoms. If the warts are large and found on the bottom of the foot, some discomfort may be felt due to pressure.

Treatment varies depending on the presence of symptoms and the wart's location. If no symptoms are present and they are left entirely alone, they will disappear. Unfortunately, it may take up to several years for this to occur. If they are symptomatic or cosmetically unacceptable, there are varying treatments:

• Any over-the-counter medication may be used as directed. Use an emery board to file the wart down twice weekly.

• Duct tape – this works well for warts on the finger. Wash the wart area well and with an emery board file the wart down as much as possible. Wrap the wart in black duct tape. Do not remove for one week. After one week remove the tape, wash the wart and file down as before. Reapply the duct tape for one further week. Continue the treatment weekly until the wart is gone. It may take up to 2 months.

• Cantharidin may be applied to the wart by the doctor and covered with tape for one day. The treatment may have to be repeated monthly for 3–4 treatments. If the wart is not gone at that time this method is discontinued.

• For very large warts, numerous warts covering a small area, or those that are resistant to the above treatments, alternative therapies, which are usually carried out by a dermatologist, may be necessary. These include:

• Liquid nitrogen

• Removal by laser

• Surgical removal

Index

Note: A page reference in bold type indicates the location of the main article for that topic.

abdomen
    acute pain, **13–16**, 318, 366
    chronic pain, **16–18**
abscess, 31
accidents. *See* falls; toilet training
acetaminophen (Tylenol/Tempra), 109, 191–92
adenoids, 120, 306–7
adhesions, 14
    labial, 232–33
adrenal glands, 45
Advil (ibuprofen), 109, 191–92
"advisory staff", **37–38**, 97, 108, 364
    as anxiety cause, 35, 108, 178
Alimentum. *See* formula, hydrolyzed
allergies, **18–27**. *See also* hives
    to animals, 41, 43
    to antibiotics, 185, 289
    as asthma triggers, 39, 41–42
    breastfeeding and, 19, 21, 22–23, 41, 151
    and conjunctivitis, 160
    desensitization treatments, 26, 46
    and eczema, 151
    to foods, 19–20, **21–24**, 42, 175, 177, 215
    formula and, 19–20, 21, 23–24, 151, 170
    medications for, 26–27, 156
    seasonal, **24–27**
    severe, **18–21**
    testing for, 26, 175
alternative medicine, **27–29**, 364. *See also* herbal remedies
    for abdominal pain, 18
    for asthma, 46
    for conjunctivitis, 160
    for ear infections, 146
    for head lice, 202
    for hives, 213
    and immunization, 219

aluminum (in vaccines), 221
anaphylaxis, **18–21**
anatomy
    of newborns, 265
    orthopedic problems, **269–73**
anemia
    hemolytic, 230
    iron deficiency, 362–63
    nutritional, 279, 363
    sickle cell, 14
animals, 41, 43, 215
ankles, 271
antacids, 128
antibiotics, **29–32**
    allergies to, 185, 289
    for colds, 30, 109
    for ear infections, 31, 142–44, 145
    for fevers, 30, 185
    necessary, 30–31
    prophylactic, 357
    for strep throat, 334
antihistamines, 156
anti-inflammatories
    for asthma, 43–46, 48–49
    for eczema, 154–56
anxiety, **32–38**, 312
    in children, **32–34**, 135
    as pain cause, 17
    in parents, 35, 108, 130, 178, 216
    postpartum, **34–37**
    about school, **33–34**, 131–33, 135
    separation, 33
    about vaccinations, 222–24
apnea, 306
appendicitis, 13
appetite. *See* eating habits
ARA. *See* omega-3 and -6 fatty acids
articulation, 308
asthma, **38–52**
    antibiotics and, 30
    bronchiolitis and, 79
    bronchodilators for, 43, 44, 48–49
    colds and, 41, 50
    diagnosing, 39, 40–41, 47–48

environment and, 24, 42, 49
exercise-induced, 41, 44, 52
inhalers for, 43–46, 50–51
managing, 40, 42–46
medications for, 40, 43–46, 48–49, 51
peak flow meter monitoring, 50
preventing attacks, 50–51
Singulair and, 44, 51, 52
treatment problems, 46–50
triggers, 39, 41–42, 49–50, 52
viral-induced, 41, 50
attention deficit disorder (ADD), 244
audiograms, 205
autism, **52–55**, 194, 221
testing for, **255–56**

babies. *See* infants; newborns
baby blues, **34–37**
back, 266
bad breath, **58–60**, 218
balanitis, 275
barrier creams, 285, 286, 368
baths, 56–57, 235, 285, 290–91
beach, 294, 297, 348. *See also* swimming
bed bugs, **60–61**
bed sharing, **61–62**, 70, 302–3, 304, 305
bedwetting, 344
behavior, 90, 95, 331. *See also* discipline; misbehavior
belly button, 56–57, 262
bilingualism, 311–12
Bio Gaia, 112
birthmarks, **62–64**, 259, 316
bladder, 342, **354–57**
bleeding
in mouth, 295
from nose, **268–69**, 295
under skull, 199–200
from vagina, 263
blessed thistle, 73–74, 114
blood
Rh incompatibility, 230
spitting up, 72, 318
from umbilical cord, **117–18**
body mass index (BMI), **64–65**, 239

body odor, 218
booster seats, 85
booster shots. *See* vaccinations
bottle feeding, **166–67**. *See also* formula
of breastfed babies, 69, 76–77
intake amount, 127, 166
at night, 77–78, 167, 178, 235, 304
sterilization needs, 164–65, 177
with sweetened liquids, 167, 304, 329
weaning from, 77–78, 171
bowels
control of, 342
obstructed, 15–16, 210, 318, 366
parasite infections, 194–95, **280–81**
twisted, 14–15, 211
brain
calcification in, 63
development of, 166, 180
injury to, 198–200
breastfeeding, **65–78**. *See also* breast milk; breasts
advantages, 66–67, 177
and allergies, 19, 21, 22–23, 41, 151
and jaundice, 72–73, 231
medications during, 73
mother's diet and, 70, 75, 113, 128, 151, 165–66, 180, 318
problems with, 36, 71–74, 345
of sick babies, 366
and sleep issues, 301, 302
supplementing, 66, 68–69, 74, 165
support for, 68
weaning from, 69–70, **75–78**
breast milk, 67, 177
colostrum, 67, 68
expressed, 68, 74, 76–77, 167
storing, 167
supply, 70, 71, 73–74, 114, 126–27
breasts
of mothers, 71–73, 339
of newborns, 265, 266
breathing. *See also* bad breath
breath-holding, **78–79**
through mouth, 59, 306

noisy, 108, 264, **320–22**
snoring, **305–7**
bronchiolitis, **79–81**
bronchitis, 30, **81–82**
bronchodilators, 43, 44, 48–49
bruxism, 326–27
burns, 292–93, 297

café au lait spots, 64
calcineurin inhibitors, 154–55, 156
calluses, 369
candy, 214
canker sores, **82–83**
carotenemia, **85**
car seats, **84–85**
car sickness, **83–84**, 350
celiac disease, **85–86**
cellulitis, 31
cephalohematoma, 264
cereals, 171, 172–73
chalazion, **162–63**
cheese, 174
chicken pox, **86–89**, 136, 227, 228
vaccination for, 89, 225, 227
childproofing, **290–91**
children. See also parenting
communicating with, 97, 99–100, 311, 331
empowering, 132–33
need for structure, 95, 300
negotiating with, 99, 331
overindulged, 215–16
overprotected, 96, 216, 237, 319
power struggles with, 92, 100, 300, 303, 331–32
sedentary, 237, 241
chin, 287
chiropractic, 146
chlamydia. See yeast infections
choking, 174
chordee, 276
chromosome abnormalities, 194
cigarette smoke, 42
circulatory system, 264. See also blood
circumcision, **101–5**

cleanliness. See hygiene
clindamycin, 334
clothing
for cold weather, 107
eczema and, 153–54
for sun protection, 325, 326, 352
cochlear implants, 207
colds, **105–11**
antibiotics for, 30, 109
and asthma, 41, 50
dairy products and, 109
and flu, 109–11
red flags, 107–8
treatment, 106–7, 109–10
cold sores, 82, 229
cold weather, 107, 110, 352
colic, **111–13**, 127–28
colostrum, 67, 68
communication, 307
with children, 97, 99–100, 311, 331
with doctor, 130, 359–60
complementary medicine. See alternative medicine
concussion, **198–200**
conjunctivitis, 135, **159–60**
constipation, 16, 17, **113–17**, 344
as diarrhea cause, 116
diet and, 114–15, 168, 173
cord blood, **117–18**
cornea (scratched), 128
corticosteroids. See steroids
co-sleeping, **61–62**, 70, 302–3, 304, 305
cough, **118–21**. See also croup
asthma as cause, 47–48
during feeding, 318
as habit tic, 120, 322
medications for, 30–31, 48
persistent, 48–49, 59, 81–82, 119–20
whooping, 31, 48, 120, 136, 225
CPR, 291
cradle cap, **121–22**
CRAP (chronic recurring abdominal pain), **16–18**
croup, **122–25**
crying, **125–30**, 303. See also colic; sleep
cup feeding, 77–78, 168–69

cysts, **162–63**

dairy products. *See also* milk
    allergies to, **22–24**, 128, 170, 318
    cheese, 174
    and colds, 109
    and constipation, 114–15, 168
    and gastroenteritis, 368

daycare, **130–37**. *See also* school
    anxiety about, 33, 34, 131–33
    choosing, 130–31
    as illness source, 133–34, 136–37
    sick children and, 134–37

decongestants, 48, 146

DEET, 297, 326

dehydration, 289, 365, 367

dental care, 59–60, **328–30**
    early, 167, 178, 235, 328, 329
    fluoride and, 170–71, 177, 179, 363
    night bottles and, 167, 178, 235, 329
    sippy cups and, 169

dentists, 330

deodorant, 218

dermatitis
    atopic (eczema), **150–57**
    seborrheic, 122

dermoid cyst, **162–63**

development. *See also* autism
    brain, 166, 180
    language, 138, 139, **310–15**
    milestones, **137–40**, 204, 313–15
    motor, 138–40
    neurological, **255–56**
    physical, 64–65, 178, 180, **196–97**, 241
    social, 314–15
    speech, **307–10**, 345

DHA. *See* omega-3 and -6 fatty acids

diaper creams, 285, 286, 368

diaper rash, **284–87**
    common, 284–86
    and crying, 127
    monilial, 339–40
    staphylococcal, 286–87
    streptococcal, 281, 286
    treatment, 285

diapers, 285, 347

diarrhea, **364–68**. *See also* gastroenteritis
    constipation as cause, 116
    and dehydration, 289, 365
    formula type and, 169, 170
    probiotics and, 234, 368
    and school attendance, 135–36

diet. *See also* eating habits; food
    of breastfeeding mother, 70, 75, 113, 128, 151, 165–66, 180, 318
    and constipation, 114–15, 168, 173
    gastroenteritis and, 366–67, 368
    healthy, 242–43
    and obesity, 239–40
    during pregnancy, 151, 180
    salt in, 240
    and school success, 243–44
    supplements for, **361–64**
    vegetarian, **179–81**, 364

diphtheria, 338

discipline, **89–92**, 93, 97–98. *See also* misbehavior; parenting
    methods, 89–91, 98
    punishment as, 87, 89, 92, 98
    threats as, 92, 98

dislocation, 294

doctors, 129–30, 359–60
    visits to, **358–61**

domperidone, 74, 114

ear infections, **140–47**, 295–96. *See also* ears; ear tubes
    antibiotics for, 31, 142–44, 145
    as crying cause, 128
    and hearing loss, 205
    preventing, 145, 147
    swimming and, 146–47

ears, **140–50**. *See also* ear infections; hearing
    air travel and, 350
    cleaning, 57–58, 147, 149, 150, 235, 261
    drops for, 251
    plugs for, 148, 350
    thermometers for, 182
    wax in, 57–58, **149–50**, 235, 261

ear tubes, 144–45, 146, **147–49**

eating habits. *See also* obesity
    picky, 179, **277–80**
    refusing food, 176
    self-feeding, 278
    struggles over, 278
echinacea, 106
eczema, 24, **150–57**, 165, 228
    preventing, 151–54
    treatment, 152–56
eggs, 175
Elidel, 154–55
enemas, 115, 116
English as a second language (ESL), 311–12
enterovirus, 197–98
environment
    and asthma, 24, 42, 49
    and seasonal allergies, **24–27**
    stimulating, 310
epiglottitis, **157–58**, 321–22
epinephrine, 20–21
erythema toxicum neonatorum (ETN), 259
esophageal reflux, 59, 128, **317–19**. *See also* spitting up
exercise. *See* physical activity
eyes
    cleaning, 58
    cornea (scratched), 128
    cysts, **162–63**
    drops for, **160–61**
    foreign bodies in, 292
    infections, 135, **159–60**
    insect bites around, 293–94
    of newborns, 58, 261–62
    squint, **161–62**
    styes, **162**
    tear ducts, **158–59**, 262

falls, 198–200, 291, 294
family, 130, 240. *See also* "advisory staff"; grandparents
fathers, 36, 56, 74
feeding, **163–81**. *See also* bottle feeding; breast-feeding; food
    cough during, 318
    by cup, 77–78, 168–69
    of infants, 67–68, 126–27, **163–78**
    problems with, 176–77, 317
    schedule for, 67–68
    by tube, 69
feet, 270, 272
    cold, 264
    flat, 271
    hypermobile, 271
    in-toed, 265, 270–71
    protecting, 294, 348
    skin problems on, 154, 287–88
fenugreek, 73–74, 114
ferberization, 302–3. *See also* sleep
fever, **181–92**. *See also* temperature; *specific illnesses*
    antibiotics and, 30, 185
    controlling, 186–87, 191–92
    medical advice on, 184–86
    medications for, 186–87, 191–92
    prolonged, 186
    and school attendance, 136
    as seizure cause, **187–89**
    teething and, 127, 181, 328
fifth disease, 189–90
first aid, 291, 297, 352
fish, 175, 177
fitness. *See* physical activity
flu, 109–11. *See also* colds
    vaccination for, 43, 110–11, 157
fluids. *See also* milk; water
    intake, 114, 178, 279
    rehydrating, 367
fluoride, 170–71, 177, 179, 363
Fluticasone, 45
folic acid, 363
food. *See also* diet; eating habits; *specific foods*
    allergies to, 19–20, **21–24**, 42, 175, 177, 215
    finger foods, 174–75, 280
    homemade, 171
    insufficient, 126–27
    intolerances, 17, 18, **85–86**, 112–13, 169, 170, **233–34**
    introducing, 20, 21, 23, 171–76, 277–78
    as reward, 174, 178, 239, 242, 278

safe handling of, 296
foreign bodies, 125, 291, 292, 321, 358
foreskin, 57, **273–75**, 277
    circumcision of, **101–5**
    problems with, 274–75
formula, **166–67**
    and allergies, 19–20, 21, 23–24, 151, 170
    as breastfeeding supplement, 66, 68–69, 74
    and colic, 112–13, 128
    and constipation, 114
    and diarrhea, 169, 170
    hydrolyzed, 20, 21, 23–24, 128, 151, 170
    iron supplementation, 165, 177, 362
    lactose-free, 112–13, 169–70, 368
    soy, 19–20, 23, 112–13, 169–70
    storing, 168
    thickening, 128
    for vegetarians, 180
    vitamin content, 165
fractures, 128, 294
fragile X syndrome, 194
frenulum, 74, 260–61, 345
friends. *See* "advisory staff"
frostbite, 352
fruits, 173–74

gait, **269–73**
gallstones, 13–14
gastroenteritis, **364–68**. *See also* diarrhea
    diet in, 366–67, 368
    and lactose intolerance, 169, 170
    preventing spread, 367
    rotavirus as cause, **289–90**
    and school attendance, 135–36
    treatment, 31, 366
gastrointestinal system, 194–95, 262, **280–81**
Gastrolyte, 367
genitals, 247, 263. *See also* genitals, female; genitals, male; masturbation
genitals, female. *See also* specific parts
    cleaning, 57, 218, 235, 353
    irritation of, 129, 280–81, 353, **357–58**
genitals, male. *See also* circumcision; specific parts
    cleaning, 218, 277

    irritation of, 129
    structural problems, **275–77**
German measles, **247–48**
germs, **234–36**
giardiasis, 194–95
gingivitis, 82
glands. *See also* lymph nodes
    adrenal, 45
    parotid, 254–55
gluten intolerance, **85–86**
glycerine suppositories, 115, 116
goat's milk, 170
grandparents, 241, 279
granuloma, umbilical, 211
gripe water, 112
growth, 64–65, 178, 180, **196–97**
    "growing pains", 195–96

habits
    bad, 299–300
    as tics, 120, 322
hair, 57, 218, 260
hairy nevus, 64
halitosis. *See* bad breath
Halloween, **213–15**
hay fever, **24–27**
head. *See also* scalp
    flattened, 193, 304
    injury to, **198–200**, 294
    swelling of, 264
headaches, 200, **202–4**
head lice, 136, **200–202**
hearing, **204–7**. *See also* ears
    devices for, 206, 207
    impaired, 205–7, 313
height, 195–96. *See also* growth
hemangioma, 63–64
hepatitis A, **207**
hepatitis B, 136, **207–9**
herbal remedies, 28, 73–74, 106, 112. *See also* alternative medicine
hernia, **209–11**
    hiatus, 318
    incarcerated, 13

inguinal, 210–11
umbilical, 210, 262
herpes simplex, 82, 160, **229**
herpes zoster, 86, 88, 225–26
Hirschsprung's disease, 114
HIV, 136
hives, 20, 44, **211–13**. *See also* allergies
holidays, **213–16**
home
environment, 42–46, 49, **290–91**
safety concerns, 200, 213, **290–91**
homeopathic medicine. *See* alternative medicine
honey, 175
hordeolum, **162**
hydrocele, 209–10
hydrocortisone, 154–55. *See also* steroids
hygiene, **216–19**, 234–36
genital, 277, 353
for pacifiers, 340–41
hypospadias, 275–76

Iberogast, 112
ibuprofen (Advil), 109, 191–92
illness, **234–36**. *See also* infections; *specific illnesses and causes*
viral, 110, 119, 133–34, 136–37
imagination, 96
immune system, 165, 217, 235–36. *See also* immunization; lymph nodes
immunization, **219–27**. *See also* vaccinations
advisability, **219–22**
pain prevention, **222–24**
routine, **224–26**
immunotherapy, 26, 46
impetigo, 31, 135, **227–28**
Infantcol, 112
infants. See also newborns; spitting up
feeding, 67–68, 126–27, **163–78**
needs, 299–301
overweight, 240, 242
premature, 362, 363
vaccinations for, 223
infections. *See also* infections, bacterial; *specific conditions*
fungal, 155–56, **287–88**

parasite, 136, 194–95, 366
preventing, 234–36
and school attendance, 135–36
viral, 30, **197–98**, **253–54**
infections, bacterial
antibiotics for, 31
diaper rash caused by, 281, 286–87
and eczema, 155–56
scarlet fever, 30, 336–37
strep throat, 30, 31, 135, **332–34**, 335
symptoms, 365–66
influenza. *See* flu
inguinal hernia, 210–11
inhalers (asthma), 43–46, 50–51
injuries. *See* falls
insects
bites from, 61, 292, 293–94, 325–26
repellents for, 297, **325–26**
in-toeing, 270–71
intussusceptions, 15–16
iron. *See also* anemia
as dietary supplement, 181, 362–63
as formula supplement, 165, 177, 362

jaundice. *See also* carotenemia
in breastfed babies, 72–73, 231
in newborns, 56–57, 72–73, **229–32**, 261
treatment, 232
juices, 114, 115, 173

Kawasaki disease, 190–91
kidneys, 13–14, **282–84**, **354–57**

labia, 218, **232–33**
lactose intolerance, **233–34**
and colic, 112–13
gastroenteritis and, 169, 170
language development, 138, 139, **310–15**
laryngomalacia, 320
laxatives, 115, 117
legs, 195–96, 265, 270–71
lice, 136, **200–202**
lungs. *See* respiratory system
lymph nodes, 190–91, **245–46**

March break, **215–16**
mastitis, 72
masturbation, 246–47
M-CHAT (Modified Checklist for Autism in Toddlers), 255–56
mealtimes. *See* eating habits; food
measles
    German (rubella), **247–48**
    red (rubeola), **248–49**
    vaccination for, 221, 225, 227, 248, 249
meatitis, 129
meats, 173, 174
meconium, 68, 262
medications. *See also* antibiotics
    administering, 160–61, **249–51**
    for allergies, 26–27, 156
    for asthma, 40, 43–46, 48–49, 51
    during breastfeeding, 73
    for colds, 106–7, 109–10
    for colic, 112
    ear drops, 251
    eye drops, **160–61**
    for fever, 186–87, 191–92
    for flu, 110
    for gastroenteritis, 31, 366
    measuring, 186
    for motion sickness, 84, 350
    oral, **249–51**
    for pneumonia, 282
    at school, 136
    suppositories, 115, 116, 186, 192
    before vaccinations, 223
meningococcal illness, **251–53**
milk
    as allergy cause, **22–24**, 128, 170, 318
    and colds, 109
    and constipation, 114–15, 168
    cow's, 168, 170
    goat's, 170
    intake, 168, 178
    introducing, 168, 177
    rice, 170
    soy, 177
mineral oil, 115, 122
misbehavior, 90–91, 92, 97–100. *See also* discipline; parenting
    consequences for, 90, 91, 97–100
molluscum contagiosum, 253–54
Mongolian spots, 62–63, 259
monilia, **338–40**
mononucleosis (infectious), 336
mosquitoes, 325
mothers. *See also* breastfeeding; pregnancy
    as hepatitis B carriers, 208, 209
    support for, 36, 56
motion sickness, **83–84,** 350
motor development, 138–40
mouth. *See also* teeth
    breathing through, 59, 306
    injuries to, 295
    lips, 287, 325
    of newborns, 260–61
    tongue, 58, 74, 260–61, **345**
    ulcers in, **82–83**
    yeast infection in (thrush), 45, 72, **338–39**
mucus
    in upper airway, 108, 264
    vaginal, 57, 263
mumps, **254–55**
    vaccination for, 221, 225, 227, 248, 249
mutism, 33, 312
myringotomy, 144, 146, **147–49**

nails, 58, 235, 265–66
naturopathic medicine. *See* alternative medicine
navel, 56–57, 262
neck
    mass in, 322
    twisted, **345–46**
neurofibromatosis, 64
neurological (nervous) system, 264
    development of, **255–56**
    problems with, **52–55**, 129
newborns, 56–58, **258–67**. *See also* infants
    anatomy, 265, 269–73
    bathing, 56–57
    breasts of, 265, 266
    feeding, 67–68, 126–27
    fluid intake, 114
    hair, 260

hearing, 204
hepatitis in, 208
infections in, 230
jaundice in, 56–57, 72–73, **229–32**, 261
kidney obstruction in, **282–84**
siblings and, **257–58**
skin, **56–58**, 259–60
vaccinations for, 208–9
weight loss/gain, 68, 71, 114
night bottles, 304
    and tooth decay, 167, 178, 235, 329
    weaning from, 77–78
night sweats, **267**
night terrors, **267–68**
nipples (baby's), 265, 266. *See also* breasts
nose
    cleaning, 58
    congested, 108, 261, 306
    foreign bodies in, 291, 292
    runny (postnasal drip), 60, 120
nosebleeds, **268–69**, 295
Nutramigen. *See* formula, hydrolyzed
nutrition. *See* diet; food
nuts, 175, 176

obesity, **238–41**, 242, 306. *See also* overweight
obsessive compulsive disorder (OCD), 33
omega-3 and -6 fatty acids, 41, 70, 75, 151, 165–66, 363–64
1, 2, 3 method, 91, 98
orchitis, 254
orthopedic problems, **269–73**
otitis externa, **146–47**
otitis media, 31, 128, **140–46**
    diagnosing, 141–42, 149–50
Oval drops, 112
overweight, 64–65, 163–64, 240, 242, 306. *See also* obesity
oxytocin, 67

pacifiers, 302, 304, 329, **340–42**
pain
    abdominal, **13–18**, 318, 366
    controlling, 191
    "growing", 195–96
    from vaccinations, **222–24**
panic disorder, 33
paraphimosis, 275
parenting, **89–101**. *See also* children; discipline
    and consistency, 91, 94–95, 177, 279, 300
parents, 56. *See also* fathers; mothers
    anxiety in, 35, 108, 130, 178, 216
    as role models, 89, 94, 179, 235, 238, 241–42, 280
    and sleep problems, 301
    stress and, 46, 130
parties, 214
parvovirus B19, 189–90
peanut butter, 175, 176, 177
Pedialyte, 367
penis, **273–77**. *See also* foreskin
pets, 41, 43, 215
phimosis, 274–75
phobias, 33, 135, 222
physical activity, **236–38**, 241, 243, 244–45, 297
    and asthma, 41, 44, 52
    lack of, 237, 241
picky eaters, 179, **277–80**
pilonidal sinus, 266
pink eye, 135, **159–60**
pinworms, 58, **280–81**
plagiocephaly, 193, 304
plantar warts, 368–69
play, 96, 139, 215–16
playgrounds, 297
pneumonia, 31, **281–82**
poison ivy/oak, 296
pollen. *See allergies*, seasonal
port wine stain, 63
postnasal drip, 60, 120
post-traumatic stress syndrome (PTSD), 33
potty training, 115, **342–45**
prednisone. *See* steroids, oral
Pregestimil. *See* formula, hydrolyzed
pregnancy
    and asthma, 42
    blood incompatibilities, 230
    diet during, 151, 180
    disease exposure during, 88, 190, 208, 247–48

Premarin cream, 232–33
probiotics, 112, 115, 165
    and diarrhea, 234, 368
Protopic, 154–55
prune juice, 114, 115
punishment, 89, 92, 97, 98. *See also* discipline
pyelectasis, **282–84**
pyloric stenosis, 317–18, 366

rash, **284–89**. *See also* diaper rash
    allergic, 20, 288–89
    causes, 227, **287–88**, 296
    in mononucleosis, 336
    of newborns, 259
recess, 244–45
reflux. *See also* spitting up
    esophageal, 59, 128, **317–19**
    silent, 318
Relenza, 110
respiratory syncytial virus (RSV), 79
respiratory system. *See also* breathing
    illnesses of, **79–81**, 135, **281–82**
    of newborns, 264
retropharyngeal pouch, 59
rheumatic fever, 336–37
ribcage, 265
rice milk, 170
rifampin, 334
ringworm, **287–88**
roseola, 185, **288–89**
rotavirus, **289–90**
routine, 95, 300
rubella, **247–48**
rubeola, **248–49**

safety
    away from home, 133, 297, **319–20**
    at the beach, 294, 297, 348
    fall protection, 200
    with food, 296
    at Halloween, 213–14
    at home, 200, 213, **290–91**
    in summer, **291–97**, 324–26
    swimming, 297, 347, 352
    tips, **296–97**

    in winter, 352
Salbutamol. *See* bronchodilators
salt, 240
scabies, 136
scalp, **121–22**, 136, 200–202. *See also* hair
scarlet fever, 30, 336–37
school, **243–45**, 307. *See also* daycare; teachers
    anxiety about, **32–34**, 131–33, 135
    nutrition and, 243–44
seborrhea, **121–22**
seizures (febrile), **187–89**
self-esteem, 33, 92, 95–96, 99, 100
self-feeding, 278
separation anxiety, 33
shampoos, 122
shellfish, 175, 177
shingles, 86, 88
shoes, 270, 272
shyness, 33
sibling rivalry, 91, **257–58**
SIDS (sudden infant death syndrome), 193, 300, 322–24
Singulair, 44, 51, 52
sinus, pilonidal, 266
sinusitis, 31, 60, **297–99**
sitting position, 272–73
skin. *See also* baths; dermatitis; rash
    birthmarks, **62–64**, 259, 316
    cleaning, 285
    discolored, 85
    infections, 227–29, 253–54
    moisturizing, 153, 156–57
    molluscum contagiosum, **253–54**
    of newborns, **56–58**, 259–60
skin tags, 262, 263
"slapped face fever", 189–90
sleep, **299–305**. *See also* co-sleeping
    amount needed, 244, 299
    bedwetting during, 344
    breastfeeding and, 301, 302
    encouraging, 301–5
    night terrors, 267–68
    position for, 300
    problems with, 300, 301, 306

smegma, 273–74, 277
smoking, 42
snacks, 278, 279. *See also* eating habits; food
snoring, **305–7**
soy milk, 177
soy protein allergy, 19–20, 22–23
speech development, **307–10**, 345
spider nevi, **316**
spitting up, 59, 113, 128, **316–19**
    of blood, 72, 318
    causes, 128, 364–65
splinters, 292
sports, 199, 200, 241
sprains, 294
squint, **161–62**
startle reflex, 264
STDs (sexually transmitted diseases), 353
stem cells, **117–18**
sterilization (bottle feeding), 164–65, 177
steroids
    for asthma, 43–46, 48–49, 50, 51, 339
    for eczema, 154–55, 156
    inhaled, 43–46, 50, 51, 339
    oral, 44, 45, 46, 48–49, 51, 154
    topical, 122, 154–55, 156, 286
stings, 292
stones, 13–14
stools, 127, 178. *See also* constipation; diarrhea
    blood in, 15
    of infants, 75, 113
    of newborns, 68, 262
    withholding, 115–16, 344
stool softeners, 115, 117
strabismus, **161–62**
strawberry birthmark, 63–64
streetproofing, 133, 297, **319–20**
strep carriers, 337
strep throat, 30, 31, 135, **332–34**, 335
stress, 46, 130. *See also* anxiety
stridor, **320–22**
Sturge-Weber syndrome, 63
stuttering, 309–10
styes, **162**
suffocation, 62
summer, **291–97**, 324–26, 346–48

sun protection, 297, **324–25**, 326, 352
supplements (dietary), 168, 170, **361–64**
    for breastfed babies, 70, 75, 165, 177, 363
    while breastfeeding, 66, 68–69, 74, 165
sweating, 218, **267**
sweets, 214, 278
swimmer's ear, **146–47**, 295–96
swimming, 148, **346–48**
    safety measures, 297, 347, 352

Tamiflu, 110
tantrums, 78, 91–92, **330–32**
teachers, 244–45. *See also* school
tear ducts, **158–59**, 262
teeth, 295, **326–30**, 341. *See also* dental care; teething
    grinding, 326–27
teething, 174, **327–28**, 341
    as fever cause, 127, 181, 328
telangiectasia, **316**
temper. *See* tantrums
temperature (body), 182–84, 192. *See also* fever
Tempra (acetaminophen), 109, 191–92
testicles, **332**
    hydrocele, 209–10, 263
    orchitis, 254
thermometers, 182
thimerosol, 221
throat (sore), 30, **332–38**. *See also* epiglottitis
thrush, 45, 72, **338–39**
thumb sucking, **340–42**
tics, 120, 322
time out, 90, 98
tinea corpus, **287–88**
tinnitus, 206
toe walking, 271–72
tofu, 173, 181
toilet training, 115, **342–45**
tongue
    cleaning, 58, 261
    tied, 74, 260–61, **345**
tonsils, 334, 337. *See also* adenoids
    tonsillitis, 334–35, 336
toothpaste, 167, 171, 329

torticollis, **345–46**
trachea, **320–22**
    tracheitis (croup), **122–25**
travel, **346–52**
    by air, 349, 351
    by car, **84–85**, **348–50**, 351
    to cold climates, 352
    to foreign countries, 350–51, 366
    games for, 349, 351
    motion sickness, **83–84**
    tips, **350–51**
    vaccinations for, 209, 225, 352
    to warm climates, **346–48**
tube feeding, 69
Twinject, 20–21
Tylenol (acetaminophen), 109, 191–92

ulcers (mouth), **82–83**
umbilical granuloma, 211
umbilical hernia, 210, 262
umbilical stump, 56–57, 262
underfeeding, 126–27
underweight, 64
urethra, 275–77, 353–54
urinary tract infection, 31, **353–57**
    causes, 280–81
    symptoms, 128–29, 185–86, 354
    treatment, 355
urination, 128–29, 263, 276–77, 354
urticaria, 20, 44, **211–13**

vaccinations, **224–26**
    for adults, 225–26
    booster shots, 225
    for chicken pox, 89, 225, 227
    fear of, **222–24**
    for flu, 43, 110–11, 157
    for hepatitis A, 207
    for hepatitis B, 208–9
    for infants, 208–9, 223
    for meningococcal illness, **251–52**
    MMR (measles, mumps, rubella), 221, 225, 227, 248, 249
    for rotavirus, 290
    routine, **224–26**
    side effects, 187, 226–27
    for travel, 209, 225, 352
    for whooping cough, 225
vagina
    bleeding from, 263
    discharge from, 57, 263, **357**
    vaginitis, 358
varicella, **86–89**, 136, 227, 228
    vaccination for, 89, 225, 227
vegetables, 173
vegetarian diets, **179–81**, 364
veins, spider, **316**
Ventolin. *See* bronchodilators
viruses. *See also* colds; coughs; illness, viral
    enterovirus, 197–98
    parvovirus B19, 189–90
    respiratory syncytial virus (RSV), 79
    West Nile virus, 325
vitamins, 165, 178, 180, **361–62**, 364. *See also* specific vitamins
vitamin C, 106
vitamin D, 361–62, 363
    as breastfeeding supplement, 70, 75, 165, 177, 363
    as dietary supplement, 168, 170
vocal cords, 320–21
voice, 309
voiding cystourethrogram (VCUG), 356–57
volvulus, 14–15
vomiting, 317–18, **364–68**
Von Recklinghausen disease, 64
vulvitis, 357–58

walking, **269–73**
warts, **368–69**
water (drinking), 170–71, 177, 179
water safety, 297, 347, 352
weaning, 69–70, 75–78, 171
weight, 163–64, 196, 318
    and body mass index, **64–65**, 239
    excessive, 64–65, 163–64, 240, 242, 306
    insufficient, 64
    loss of, 240, 279
    of newborns, 68, 71, 114
West Nile virus, 325

wheezing, 47
whooping cough, 31, 48, 120, 136, 225
windpipe. See trachea
winter, 107, 110, 352

yeast infections, 159, **338–40,** 358. *See also* thrush
yogurt, 174